Concise
Electrotherapy
Principles and Practice

Roshan Lal Meena, BPT, MPT (Orthopedics)

Lecturer, Department of Physiotherapy
Pandit Deendayal Upadhyaya
National Institute for Persons with Physical Disabilities
4- Vishnu Digmbar Marg, New Delhi 110002
(Affiliated to University of Delhi)

Concise **ELECTROTHERAPY** Principles and Practice

Published by
Roshan Lal Meena
@ Publishing rights with
Roshan Lal Meena
Pt. Deendayal Upadhyaya
National Institute for Persons with Physical Disabilities
4 – Vishnu Digmber Marg, New Delhi 110002

Correspondence Address
524A, Gaur Green Vista Nayay Khand – 1, Makhanpur Village, Indirapuram, Ghaziabad, UP 201010
Email roshan7leo@yahoo.com
Email roshanmanju00@gmail.com
91-9811368079, 91-9899777041

Disclaimer
Care has been taken to confirm the accuracy of the information present and to describe generally accepted practices, however, the author is not responsible for errors or omission or for any consequences from application of the information in this book and make no warranty expressed or implied which respect to the currency, completeness, or accuracy of the contents of the publication. Application of this information in particular situation remains the professional responsibility of the practitioners; the clinical treatment described and recommended may not be considered absolute and universal recommendations.
The author has made every effort to ensure that the selection of parameters and dosages set forth in this text are in accordance with the current research, recommendations and practice at the time of publication. However, any updates in the further research, and amendments in the government regulations to maintain the minimum standards in the practice, the reader is urged to keep himself or herself updated and recommend the parameters and doses as per the current practice and regulations. The author does not assure any liability for any injury and or damage to person or property arising from or related to use of material in this book.

Request for purchase of additional copies in bulk may be solicited at roshan7leo@yahoo.com or call at 9899777041, 9811368079

First Edition 2017
ISBN : 978-93-5279-241-2
Typeset by: Suman Teppala, 8447730242
Printed at: Deep Colours Scan (P) Ltd., M.: 9899058094

Dedicated to

Professor P K Prabhakar

Former Head of Physiotherapy Department
Pandit Deendayal Upadhyaya National Institute for Persons with Physical
Disabilities For his kindness and for his endless support when I joined
the Institute. His devotion to the profession will always be remembered.

Preface

The use of electrotherapy continues to have greater importance in patients with various musculoskeletal disorders and injuries. The practice of therapeutic modalities has been remarkably extended to the wide range of musculoskeletal, neurological, cardiovascular and obstetrician and gynecology ailments.

The concept for this book has evolved from a desire to generate and provide a comprehensive text for the students of physical therapy, physical therapists, and other rehabilitation practitioners. The text is arranged and organized systematically from basics to the advanced and evidenced based practice.

The readers may begin with the first chapter which describes the understanding of pain and functional limitations caused by pain. Each therapeutic modality is described with its various sources of production, physical characteristics, therapeutic uses, adverse effects and applications. The classification of modalities is based on the depth of penetration of heat, frequency of currents and source of energy. The book covers almost all the therapeutic modalities practiced world widely by the physical therapists.

It is written in simple and clear form with images and diagrams to give the reader a more realistic representation of the modalities. I hope the readers will find the text to be an adequate to formulate and design appropriate parameters of the therapeutic modalities for various musculoskeletal disorders, neurological disorders and sports injuries.

Acknowledgement

I must first recognize my friend C S Ram who had originally shared an idea of writing of book in 2002. My first book titled "Concise Exercise Therapy" published in 2006 was appreciated by many of physical therapists and students of physical therapy. This appreciation has inspired me to write a book on electrotherapy.

I would like to thank my wife, Manju, my son, Hardik and my daughter Mayara, who supported and encouraged me in spite of all the time it took me away from them. I thank my parents who have encouraged me to work hard to accomplish the task and objectives to achieve peace of mind.

I express my deep sense of gratitude towards my head of Physiotherapy department Mrs. Manda Chauhan, Associate Professor, Mrs Rajani Kalra, Assistant Professor and other seniors and colleagues. I would like to thank Samiya Sidiquee, Aasra Praveen, Ojas Bhateja and Sachin Gupta for their help in the process of editing the chapters. My special thank to Mr. Shagun Aggarwal, Dr. Suraj Kumar and Mr. Tarun Kumar for reviewing the chapters. I express my profound regard to Dr. Dharmendra Kumar, Former Director of the Institute for his kind appreciation and support in writing the book.

I thank Suman Tapplan, for designing the book and cover pages without that it would never find its way to the printing press and to the web. I also thank to Mr. Sandeep Malhotra Director, Deep Colour Scan Pvt. Ltd. for his valuable support and getting the book printed.

Last and not least: I beg forgiveness of all those who have been with me over the course of the years and whose names I have failed to mention."

Contents

immersion method, fluid fluid method, application parameters – coupling medium, frequency, intensity, continuous mode, pulsed mode, duty cycle, Beam non uniformity ratio, irridation time and surface area, half layer value, Phonophoresis, combination therapy, recent trends in ultrasound application, ultrasound in fracture healing, extensor carpi radialis tendinitis,

Section II Superficial Tissue Heating Modalities

5. Moist Heat, PWB, Contrast Bath and Fluidotherapy

Introduction, heat transfer methodsn – conduction, convection, radiation, physiological effects, Paraffin Wax Bath – physical characteristics, therapeutic effects, paraffin wax bath unit, contraindications, application, deep immersion technique, dip and immersion, direct pouring method, bruishing or painting method, toweling or bandaging method, Purification of wax, Moist Heat Therapy, Physiological effects, indications, contraindications, dangers, moist heat unit, moist hot packs, application, Contrast Bath, contrast bath unit, indications, contraindications, Fluidotherapy,

6. Electromagnetic Raditions-UVR and IRR

Introduction, production, Mercury Vapor, Kromayer lamp, Fluorescent lamp, Theraktin lamp, PUVA, physiological effects, determining minimal erythemal dose, doses calculation, treatment procedure, indications, contraindications, Infra red Radiation, production, physical characteristics – reflection, transmission, absorption, physiological effects, therapeutic uses, contraindications, dangers, application

Section III Therapeutic Currents

7. Faradic, Galvanic, Iontophoresis and Russian-Low Frequency Currents

Introduction, classification direct, alternating currents, low Frequency currents – faradic currents, surge faradic current, waveforms, interrupted direct currents, physiological effects, nerve depolarization, resting membrane potential, polarity, therapeutic uses, contraindications, motor point, faradism under pressure, strength duration curve, Rheobase, chronaxie, iontophoresis.

Chapter 01

PAIN, FUNCTIONAL LIMITATION AND ASSESSMENT

Pain has been viewed by physiologists as a distinct sensation from temperature and other cutaneous senses.[1,2] It is defined as an unpleasant sensation and emotional response associated with actual or potential tissue damage. It is a complex phenomenon encompassing sensory, emotional, motor, and cultural components.[3,4] Pain that leads to functional limitation and disability produces anxiety for the patient and can be a source of conflict with spouses, family members, friends, and coworkers.[5] Pain is the signal that is recognized by the brain which can be given due regard immediately by withdrawing the part of the body to protect it. Pain is sometimes neglected by individuals if its intensity is mild. The potential damage to the tissues sometimes does not produce pain till a significant disability or movement disorder is produced. Such pain arriving late in the course of a disease, or produced by dysfunction or rewiring of the nervous system, has no survival value and can even have adverse health effects and lead to disability.[6] Hence pain is a significant signal or indication which must be respected by withdrawing the body part from the stimuli to protect the body and seek medical attention for determination of its source, type and management

Source of Pain

Pain is a complex phenomenon hence; it is not always possible to determine its source reliably as it is originated from one or several structures or systems of the body. The subjective pain is not associated with the objective findings. It is, therefore, necessary, for the clinician to have a very clear concept of possible source of pain, diligently elicit an accurate and lucid history to determine the source of pain. Pain may either be localized, referred, or radicular. These three patterns of pain are mostly found in the spine. The localized and referred pain is also produced by the viscera. The localized pain is experienced by the patient directly over the lesion. The referred and radicular pain is experienced, distal to the lesion. The radicular pain which is originated from the nerve roots or nerves has distinct features such as parasthesia, numbness, tingling and weakness. These symptoms are provoked by the specific nerve root or nerve stretching.

Somatic Pain – The somatic pain may either be mediated through the faster conducting A-delta afferent neurons or the slower C fibers. The somatic pain may either be superficial or deep. The superficial pain originates from the skin and it is localized. A tender point can easily be elicited. The pain from the muscles, ligaments, tendons, joints fascia and periosteum is deeply situated and tends to be more diffuse. It may also be localized. The somatic pain is associated with the protective muscle guarding, and may be aggravated with the movements at end ranges. The deep pain is thought to be mediated through C fibers, although there is probably overlap between deep and superficial receptor systems.

Visceral Pain – Viscerogenic pain is originated from viscera such as kidneys, the pelvic viscera, lesions of the lesser sac, lungs, heart and retroperitoneal tumors. Pain originated from the viscera is often poorly localized and is characterized as an aching or gripping sensation associated with sympathetic effects, such as the pain associated with angina pectoris. The pelvic and abdominal viscera may refer the pain to the low back area, whereas pain from the heart may be perceived in the left shoulder and arm. The movements of the spine and extremities do not aggravate or relieve the viscerogenic pain. To get rid of pain, patients often walk around. The parietal pain associated with the peritoneum, pleura, and pericardium is innervated by the A-delta fibers are accompanied by superficial tenderness and reflex rigidity, as seen in the abdominal rigidity of acute appendicitis.

Vascular Pain – Pathological changes in the vessels and arteries may produce similar symptoms as of musculoskeletal tissues, however, they are differentiated for their distinct feature such as boring, throbbing and heaviness situated deeply. Pain from intermittent claudication is perceived in the calf, which is aggravated by walking and relived with standstill. Similarly pain from the superior gluteal artery insufficiency and abdominal aortic aneurysm is perceived in the lower extremity. The pain is aggravated by walking and is relieved with rest.

Psychogenic Pain – Although patients with pure psychogenic type of pain are rarely seen in clinical practice but failure to consider may lead to serious errors in diagnosis and management. The patients with psychogenic pain are very anxious, tend to overexpose their problem. They are usually demonstrative, use their hands to point out various painful areas. Fear, anxiety, and depression is capable of amplifying pain and environmental stress can give rise to or amplify pain.[7] Anxiety, depression, anger and aggressive behavior may provoke substantial autonomic, visceral and skeletal activity, which can enhance pain sensations.

Receptors

There are many pain carrying neurons which receive noxious stimuli from the skin, joints, and muscles and carry them to the higher centers for interpretation.

Skin – Several small free nerve ending receptors situated in the skin which are able to respond to the mechanical, thermal, and chemical stimuli. There are three types of receptors in skin which carry pain to the higher centers. High threshold mechanoreceptors –These receptors receive strong mechanical stimuli but do not respond in normal skin to heat, irritant chemicals, or extreme cold. *Polymodal Nociceptors* – these receptors receive strong mechanical stimuli, and also noxious heat and irritant chemical. *Cold Nociceptors* –Cold receptors receive extreme cold stimuli but do not respond to the strong mechanical, heat and chemical stimuli. The pain from skin is diameter myelinated A-delta neurons and small diameter, un-myelinated C fiber neurons.

Muscles – Similar to the skin, A-delta and C-fibers are situated in the muscles. In addition to the above pain receptors there are pain sensitive units in the muscles which receive information of muscle guarding and soreness and carry it to the higher centers.

Joints – The physical properties of the joints is maintained by various encapsulated receptive units situated in and around the joints. The subcutaneous receptors similar to the skin receptors are also present in the skin but they are slightly different from them in terms of functions.

Theories

Many authors have proposed pain perception and transmission theories. One of the oldest theories of pain was postulated by Aristotle, who believed that pain was a reaction to excessive stimulation.

Specificity Theory

In 1894 Von Frey proposed a doctrine of specific nerve energies- the specificity theory of pain. The doctrine implied that each sensory modality was sub-served by morphologically specific nerve endings. Von Frey includes four distinct types of sensation at the skin: warmth, cold, touch, and pain. He identified free nerve endings as pain receptors based on their widespread distribution in the skin. According to the theory the specific nerve endings always elicit an identical sensation no matter how it is stimulated. The specific stimulation is transmitted along specific pathways in the spinal cord to reach specific projection areas in the brain, where it is appreciated/recognized.

Pattern Theory

Pattern theory first formalized by Goldscheider in 1894 is based on empirical observation. The absence of specific pain receptors, pathways, or groups of neurons dedicated to the transmission of painful stimuli is its basic assumption.[8] According to the theory there is a group of nerve ending and associated nerve fibers which form a pain spot. The stimulation of pain spot with the sufficient intensity and frequency produces pain which results in initiation of train of impulses in the pathways.[9] Summation of neural impulses is relayed to the cerebral structures concerned with localizations and interpretation of intensity. In 1943 Livingston expanded on the pattern theory to explain how pain could occur long after an initial injury.[10] The drawback of the theory was that receptor specialization does not exist to a great extent.

Gate Theory

In 1965 Melzack and Wall proposed the gate theory of pain which they subsequently reviewed in 1978. They originally postulated that interneurons in the substantia gelatinosa in the dorsal horn of the spinal cord acted as a gate to modulate sensory input.[10] This theory has been credited with rekindling interest in electrical control of pain and inspiring research with important scientific and clinical ramification.[11] The essence of this theory is that small diameter myelinated A-delta neurons and small diameter, un-myelinated C fibers also known as pain carrying nociceptives project to the spinal cord where they synapse directly or via interneurons with the transmission cells (T cells) in the dorsal horn of the grey matter. The T cells relay the small diameter pain carrying sensation to the higher centers.

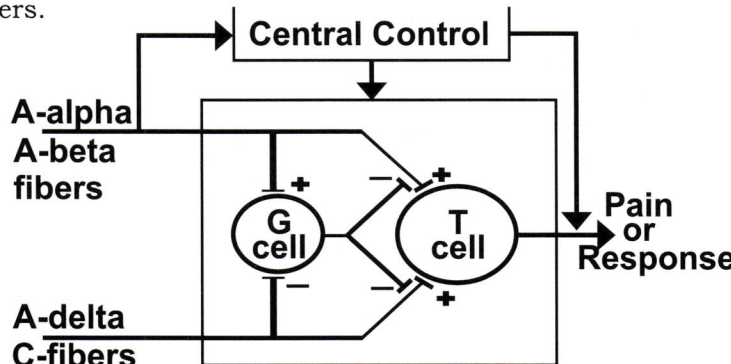

Fig.1.1 Schematic Diagram. Pain gate Control

Large diameter myelinated A beta and alpha fibers also known as pain inhibiting fibers arise from the peripheral part and terminate on   T cells through substantia gelatinosa of the spinal cord. The stimulation of the mechanoceptors large diameter fibers inhibit   the nociceptors at the T cells and prevent transmission to the higher centers. The inhibitory input caused by activation of the large diameter, mechanosensitive afferent is said to close the gate to nociceptor transmission. This is also known as "Pain Gate Control Theory"[19].

Pain, Functional Limitation and Assessment

Assessment of Pain

Pain is a very complex and subjective experience. A comprehensive assessment is required to determine the source of the pain. Many authors have designed tests and measures to quantify pain and attempts have been made to objectify the pain experience. However, no scale is made to assess the pain objectively as it is the experience of an individual which is explained to the examiner, hence, the assessment of pain remains subjective.

Examination

Examination is the process in which clinical data or findings are gathered by obtaining a lucid history, performing a relevant system review, selecting and administering special tests and measures. Examination has two parts subjective and objective. The subjective examination includes gathering clinical data from the patient by asking the question and observing the body part carefully. The examiner makes efforts in gathering accurate clinical data that may give clues in making a clinical diagnosis and determining an appropriate scheme of management. The objective examination consists of palpation, accessory movements, joint play movements, passive movements, and special tests performed on the patient to reproduce the symptoms and to determine the source of pain.

Evaluation

Evaluation is the dynamic process in which the therapist makes decisions on data gathered during the examination. Evaluation includes interpretation of the subjective and objective examination findings to understand the source or cause of the patient's impairments, disorder, functional limitation and disabilities. It is one of the critical stages in clinical decision making. The clinical data may also be analyzed to determine the progression and stage of the signs and symptoms, and stability of the condition.

Diagnosis

It is the process in which the examiner analyzes the clinical data gathered during the subjective, objective examination and evaluation; and organizing them into cluster, syndrome, or categories to help in determining the appropriate intervention and strategy for each patient.

Prognosis

Prognosis is the determination of minimal improvement to maximal improvement expected at various intervals during the course of physical therapy intervention. The prognosis depends upon the health, underlying conditions and age of the patient. A healthy patient shows faster improvement in the sign and symptoms than a patient who is having a history of underlying pathological condition such as diabetes of the same age.

Interventions

Intervention is the purposeful and skilled physiotherapeutic approach of various methods, and modalities administered towards the patient in order to improve pain, symptoms and functional limitations.

Clinical Decision Making

Clinical decision making is the dynamic process which involves vertical thinking and lateral thinking. Vertical thinking is characterized by logical sequential predictable thinking. It is also known as conventional thinking or process of gathering clinical data or information from the patient. It stays within a problem space. Lateral thinking is concerned with the generation of new idea, and with looking things in a different way. It tends to restructure the problem space, the lateral thinking focuses not only on the problem space but also on the proximal and distal parts of the problem space. The physical therapist's assessment is more inclined to the clinical decision making.

Numeral Rating Scale (NR)

The patient is given a scale marked from 0 to 10 or 0-100. Zero is no pain and ten or hundred is worst possible pain which is not tolerable. The patients are asked to tell the point that best describes their level of pain on the scale.

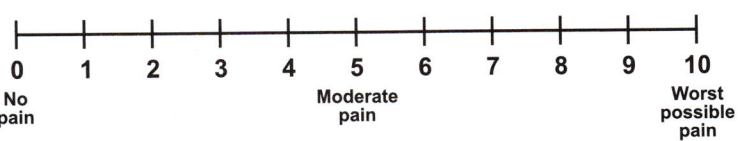

Fig.1.2 Numeral Rating Scale

Pain, Functional Limitation and Assessment

Verbal Rating Scale (VRS)

The verbal rating scale consists of a list of adjectives describing different levels of pain intensity. An adequate VRS of pain intensity should include adjectives that reflect the extremes of this dimension; from 'no pain' to 'extremely intense pain' and sufficient additional adjectives to capture gradations of pain intensity that may be experienced between these two extremes. Patients are asked to read over the list of adjectives and select the word or phrase that best describes their level of pain on the scale.

Visual Analogue Scale

A verbal analogue scale consists of a line, usually 10cms long whose ends are labelled as the extremes of pain - 'no pain' to 'worst pain'. Visual Analogue Scale may have specific points along the line that are labelled with intensity denoting adjectives or numbers. Those scales that use adjectives are called graphic rating scales. Patients are asked to rate their pain along the line that best represents the intensity of their pain. This distance between the number end and the mark provided by the patient is measured and this gives the pain intensity score.

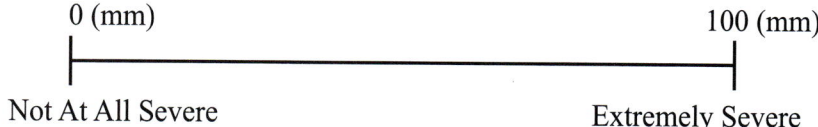

Fig.1.3 Visual Analogue Scale

In order to use pain-rating scales well clinicians need to appreciate the potential for error within the tools, and the potential they have to provide the required information. Interpretation of the data from a pain-rating scale is not as straightforward as it might first appear.[12] The most commonly used pain assessment instruments are pain scales.[13-14]

Williamson A and et al. reviewed three pain rating scales. This review aims to explore the research available relating to three commonly used pain rating scales, the Visual Analogue Scale, the Verbal Rating Scale and the Numerical Rating Scale. All three pain-rating scales are valid, reliable and appropriate for use in clinical practice, although the Visual Analogue

Scale has more practical difficulties than the Verbal Rating Scale or the Numerical Rating Scale[15] There is much evidence to support the validity of VAS for pain intensity. Such scales demonstrate positive relations to other self-report measures of pain intensity[16-17]

McGil Pain Questainer

The McGill pain questionnaire was developed at McGill University by Melzack and Torqerson in 1971. The scale is also known as McGill pain index. It is a self report questionnaire that helps the clinician in describing the quality and intensity of pain that the patient experiences. There is a list of words which describes the complaint of the patient. The patients carefully observes the list of words or the questionnaire and selects three words from groups 1-10 that best describe their pain, two words from groups 11-15, a single word from group 16, and then one word from groups 17-20. After completing the questionnaire, the patient will have selected seven words that best describe their pain. The patient can use some words more than once.

Questionnaire

Group	Words
1	Flickering, Pulsing, Quivering, Throbbing, Beating, Pounding
2.	Jumping, Flashing, Shooting
3	Jumping, Flashing, Shooting
4	Sharp, Cutting, Lacerating
5.	Pinching, Pressing, Gnawing, Cramping, Crushing
6	Tugging, Pulling, Wrenching
7	Hot, Burning, Scalding, Searing
8	Tingling, Itchy, Smarting, Stinging
9	Dull, Sore, Hurting, Aching, Heavy
10	Tender, Taut (tight), Rasping, Splitting
11	Tiring, Exhausting

Pain, Functional Limitation and Assessment

12	Sickening, Suffocating
13	Fearful, Frightful, Terrifying
14	Punishing, Grueling, Cruel, Vicious, Killing
15	Wretched, Blinding
16	Annoying, Troublesome, Miserable, Intense, Unbearable
17	Spreading, Radiating, Penetrating, Piercing
18	Tight, Numb, Squeezing, Drawing, Tearing
19	Cool, Cold, Freezing
20	Nagging, Nauseating, Agonizing, Dreadful, Torturing

Pain Quality Assessment Scale (PQAS)

There are different aspects and types of pain that patients experience and that the examiner measure. The patient can experience pain as sharp, hot, cold, dull, and achy. Some pains may feel like they are very superficial (at skin-level), or they may feel like they are from deep inside your body. The pain quality assessment scale helps in measuring the sharp, hot, cold, dull, achy, shooting, numb, tingling, cramping throbbing and radiating. PQAS has twenty rating scales of different types and quality of pain. Each rating scale has ten score.

1. Please use the scale below to tell us how intense your pain has been over the past week, on average. Zero is no pain, where ten is the most intense pain sensation imaginable

    No pain 0 | 1 | 2 | 3 | 4 | 5 | 6 | 7 | 8 | 9 | 10 The most intense pain sensation imaginable

2. Please use the scale below to tell us how sharp your pain has felt over the past week. Words used to describe sharp feelings include "like a knife," "like a spike," or "piercing."

    Not sharp 0 | 1 | 2 | 3 | 4 | 5 | 6 | 7 | 8 | 9 | 10 The most sharp sensation imaginable ("like a knife")

Pain, Functional Limitation and Assessment

3. Please use the scale below to tell us how hot your pain has felt over the past week. Words used to describe very hot pain include "burning" and "on fire

Not hot 0 | 1 | 2 | 3 | 4 | 5 | 6 | 7 | 8 | 9 | 10 The most sensation imaginable ("burning")

4. Please use the scale below to tell us how dull your pain has felt over the past week

Not dull 0 | 1 | 2 | 3 | 4 | 5 | 6 | 7 | 8 | 9 | 10 The most sensation imaginable

5. Please use the scale below to tell us how cold your pain has felt over the past week. Words used to describe very cold pain include "like ice" and "freezing."

Not cold 0 | 1 | 2 | 3 | 4 | 5 | 6 | 7 | 8 | 9 | 10 The most cold sensation imaginable ("freezing")

6. Please use the scale below to tell us how sensitive your skin has been to light touch or clothing rubbing against it over the past week. Words used to describe sensitive skin include "like sunburned skin" and "raw skin."

Not sensitive 0 | 1 | 2 | 3 | 4 | 5 | 6 | 7 | 8 | 9 | 10 The most sensitive sensation imaginable ("raw skin")

7. Please use the scale below to tell us how tender your pain is when something has pressed against it over the past week. Another word used to describe tender pain is "like a bruise."

Not tender 0 | 1 | 2 | 3 | 4 | 5 | 6 | 7 | 8 | 9 | 10 The most tender sensation imaginable ("like a bruise")

8. Please use the scale below to tell us how itchy your pain has felt over the past week. Words used to describe itchy pain include "like poison ivy" and "like a mosquito bite."

Not The most itchy itchy 0 | 1 | 2 | 3 | 4 | 5 | 6 | 7 | 8 | 9 | 10 sensation imaginable ("like poison ivy")

9.   Please use the scale below to tell us how much your pain has felt like it has been shooting over the past week. Another word used to describe shooting pain is "<u>zapping</u>."

Not shooting 0 | 1 | 2 | 3 | 4 | 5 | 6 | 7 | 8 | 9 | 10 The most shooting sensation imaginable ("zapping")

10.   Please use the scale below to tell us how numb your pain has flet over the past week. A phrase that can be used to describe numb pain is "like it is asleep"

Not numb 0 | 1 | 2 | 3 | 4 | 5 | 6 | 7 | 8 | 9 | 10 The most numb sensation imaginable ("asleep")

11.   Please use the scale below to tell us how much your pain sensations have felt electrical over the past week. Words used to describe electrical pain include "<u>shocks</u>," "<u>lightning</u>," and "<u>sparking</u>."

Not electrical 0 | 1 | 2 | 3 | 4 | 5 | 6 | 7 | 8 | 9 | 10 The most electrical sensation imaginable ("shocks")

12.   Please use the scale below to tell us how tingling your pain has felt over the past week. Words used to describe tingling pain include "<u>like pins and needles</u>" and "<u>prickling</u>."

Not tingling 0 | 1 | 2 | 3 | 4 | 5 | 6 | 7 | 8 | 9 | 10 The most tingling sensation imaginable ("pins and needles")

13.   Please use the scale below to tell us how cramping your pain has felt over the past week. Words used to describe cramping pain include "<u>squeezing</u>" and "<u>tight</u>."

Not cramping 0 | 1 | 2 | 3 | 4 | 5 | 6 | 7 | 8 | 9 | 10 The most cramping sensation imaginable ("squeezing")

14.   Please use the scale below to tell us how radiating your pain has felt over the past week. Another word used to describe radiating pain is "<u>spreading</u>."

Not radiating 0 | 1 | 2 | 3 | 4 | 5 | 6 | 7 | 8 | 9 | 10 The most radiating sensation imaginable ("spreading")

15. Please use the scale below to tell us how throbbing your pain has felt over the past week. Another word used to describe throbbing pain is "pounding."

Not throbbing 0 | 1 | 2 | 3 | 4 | 5 | 6 | 7 | 8 | 9 | 10 The most throbbing sensation imaginable ("pounding")

16. Please use the scale below to tell us how aching your pain has flet over the past week. Another word used to describe aching pain is "like a toothache".

Not aching 0 | 1 | 2 | 3 | 4 | 5 | 6 | 7 | 8 | 9 | 10 The most aching sensation imaginable ("like a toothache")

17. Please use the scale below to tell us how heavy your pain has felt over the past week. Other words used to describe heavy pain are "pressure" and "weighted down."

Not heavy 0 | 1 | 2 | 3 | 4 | 5 | 6 | 7 | 8 | 9 | 10 The most heavy sensation imaginable ("weighted down")

18. Now that you have told us the different types of pain sensations you have felt, we want you to tell us overall how unpleasant your pain has been to you over the past week. Words used to describe very unpleasant pain include "annoying," "bothersome," "miserable," and "intolerable." Remember, pain can have a low intensity but still feel extremely unpleasant, and some kinds of pain can have a high intensity but be very tolerable. With this scale, please tell us how unpleasant your pain feels.

Not unpleasant 0 | 1 | 2 | 3 | 4 | 5 | 6 | 7 | 8 | 9 | 10 The most unpleasant sensation imaginable ("intolerable")

19. We want you to give us an estimate of the severity of your deep versus surface pain over the past week. We want you to rate each location of pain separately. We realize that it can be difficult to make these estimates, and most likely it will be a "best guess," but please give us your best estimate.

How Intense Is Your Deep Pain?

No deep 0 | 1 | 2 | 3 | 4 | 5 | 6 | 7 | 8 | 9 | 10 The most intense deep pain sensation pain imaginable

How Intense Is Your Surface Pain?

No surface 0 | 1 | 2 | 3 | 4 | 5 | 6 | 7 | 8 | 9 | 10 The most intense surface pain sensation pain imaginable

20. Pain can also have different time qualities. For some people, the pain comes and goes and so they have some moments that are completely without pain; in other words the pain "comes and goes". This is called intermittent pain. Others are never pain free, but their pain types and pain severity can vary from one moment to the next. This is called variable pain. For these people, the increases can be severe, so that they feel they have moments of very intense pain ("breakthrough" pain), but at other times they can feel lower levels of pain ("background" pain). Still, they are never pain free. Other people have pain that really does not change that much from one moment to another. This is called stable pain. Which of these best describes the time pattern of your pain (please select only one):

Functional Limitation

Pain greatly affects the activities of daily living. Pain in the shoulder may limit the hand of the individual to reach to the back of spine to fasten bra, to the head to comb hair, to the back pocket (gluteal region) to place wallet. Pain in the knee joint can cause gait abnormalities, reduce tolerance to standing, difficulty in climbing and descending stairs. The limitation in the functional activities such as reduced tolerance to standing due to knee joint osteoarthritis and difficulty in walking due to prolapsed intervertebral disc result in difficulty in performing the task at the work place. No appropriate treatment for improving functional limitation can cause disability. The osteoarthritis and prolapse intervertebral disc is the primary impairment and reduce tolerance to standing and difficulty in walking is the secondary impairment. The physical therapist administers appropriate physical modality to prevent and improve the secondary impairment (functional limitation).

The physical therapist administers physical therapeutic modalities to eliminate functional limitations and disability in collaboration with the therapeutic exercises. American Physical Therapist Association (APTA) has defined functional Limitation as restriction of the ability to perform a physical action, activity, or task in an efficient, typically expected, or competent manner.[18] Nagi Model has referred functional limitation as restriction in performance of basic tasks that includes basic activities of daily living (BADL) such as personal hygiene, feeding, dressing and instrumental activities of daily living (IADL) such as preparing meals, house work, grocery, shopping.

Assessment of Functional Limitation

Many functional scales and questionnaires have been designed in the literature for the assessment of functional limitation and disability resulting from primary impairment or and pain. The scales not only help in assessing the pain subjectively but also provide significant feedback of the progression or improvement in the pain and symptoms. The periodical reevaluation of the functional limitation by using the functional scale enables therapist to determine appropriate scheme of therapeutic modality.

Oswestry Functional Scale

The Oswestry Disability Index (ODI) is an index derived from the Oswestry Low Back Pain Questionnaire used by clinicians and researchers to quantify disability for low back pain.

Oswestry Disability Index has been extensively tested, and shown a good psychometric properties, and applicable in a wide variety of settings. Hence, it is considered by many clinicians as a gold standard for measuring degree of disability and estimating quality of life in a person with low back pain. Oswestry Disability Index was published first by Jeremy Fairbank et al. in 1980 (Fairbank JC, Couper J, Davies JB. The Oswestry Low Back Pain Questionnaire. Physiotherapy 1980; 66: 271-273). The current version was published in 2000, (Fairbank JC, Pynsent PB. The Oswestry Disability Index. Spine 2000 Nov 15;25(22):2940-52.ODI) is a self completed questionnaire contains ten questions or items concerning activities of daily living. Each question or item is followed by six statements 0 to 5 describing different potentials scenarios in the patients day to activities. The first statement (0) carries no score. The each statement from 1-5 carries 1-5 scores. Statement 1 indicates least disability and last statement (5) indicates severe disability. The patient checks the statement which most closely resembles their disability. The scores of all statement are summed, then multiplied by two to obtain the index (range 0-100). The zero is equated with no disability and 100 is the maximum disability possible

Interpretation

1. 0%-20%: Minimal disability: This group can cope with most living activities. Usually no treatment is indicated, apart from advice on lifting, sitting posture, physical fitness, and diet. In this group some patients have particular difficulty with sitting, and this may be important if their occupation is sedentary, e.g., a typist or truck driver.

2. 20%-40% Moderate disability: This group experiences more pain and problems with sitting, lifting, and standing. Travel and social life are more difficult and they may well be off work. Personal care, sexual activity, and sleeping are not grossly affected, and the back condition can usually be managed by conservative means.

3. 40%-60%: Severe disability: Pain remains the main problem in this group of patients, but travel, personal care, social life, sexual activity, and sleep are also affected. These patients require detailed investigation.

4. 60%-80%: Crippled: Back pain impinges on all aspects of these patients' lives—both at home and at work—and positive intervention is required.

5. 80%-100%: These patients are either bed-bound or exaggerating their symptoms. This can be evaluated by careful observation of the patient during medical examination.

Neck Disability Index (NDI)

Neck disability index has been designed to determine as to how the neck pain has affected the ability of an individual to manage activities of daily living. There are total ten sections and each section has five score (0-5). The first statement of each section carries no score. The last score of each section carries five score. The patient needs to mark the statement which describes the problem most closely. It is not mandatory to attempt all the sections if the statements do not describe the problem.

Section 1: Pain Intensity
- I have no pain at the movement
- The pain is very mild at the moment
- The pain is moderate at the moment
- The pain is fairly severe at the moment
- The pain is the worst imaginable at the moment

Section 2: Personal Care (Washing, Dressing, etc)
- I can look after myself normally without causing extra pain
- I can look after myself normally but it causes extra pain
- It is painful to look myself and I am slow and careful
- I need some help but can manage most of my personal care
- I need help every day in most aspect of self care
- I do not get dressed, I wash with difficulty and stay in bed

Section 3: lifting
- I can lift heavy weight without extra pain
- I can lift heavy weight but it gives extra pain
- Pain prevents me lifting heavy weight off the floor, but I can manage if they are conveniently placed, for example on a table
- Pain prevents me fro lifting heavy weight but I can manage light to medium weight if they are conveniently positioned
- I can only lift very light weight
- I cannot lift or carry any thing

Section 4: Reading

- I can read as much as I want to with no pain in my neck
- I can read as much as I want to with slight pain in my neck
- I can read as much as I want with moderate pain in my neck
- In cannot read as much as I want because of moderate pain in my nexk
- I can hardly read at all because of severe pain in my neck
- I cannot read at all

Section 5: headaches

- I have no headaches at all
- I have slight headaches, which come infrequently
- I have moderate headaches, which come infrequently
- I have moderate headaches, which come frequently
- I have severe headaches, which come frequently
- I have headache almost all the time

Section 6: Concentration

- I can concentrate fully when I want to with no difficulty
- I can concentrate fully when I want to with slight difficulty
- I have a fair degree of difficulty in concentrating when I want to
- I have a lot of difficulty in concentrating when I want to
- I have a great deal of difficulty in concentrating when I want to
- I cannot concentrate at all

Section 7: Work

- I can do as much work as I want to
- I can only do my usual work, but no more
- I can do most of my usual work, but no more
- I cannot do my usual work
- I can hardly do any work at all
- I cannot do any work at all

Pain, Functional Limitation and Assessment

Section 8: Driving

- I can drive my car without any neck pain
- I can drive my car as long as I want with slight pain in my neck
- I can drive my car as long as I want with moderated pain in my neck
- I cannot drive my car as long as I want because of moderated pain in neck
- I can hardly drive at all because of severe of pain in my neck
- I cannot drive car at all

Section 9: sleeping

- I have no trouble sleeping
- My sleep is slightly disturbed (less than one hour sleepless)
- My sleep is mildly disturbed (1.2 hours sleepless)
- My sleep is moderately disturbed (2-3 hours sleepless)
- My sleep is greatly disturbed (3-5 hours sleepless)
- My sleep is completely disturbed (5-7 hours sleepless)

Section 10: Recreation

- I am able to engage in all my recreation activities with no neck pain at all
- I am able to engage in all my recreation activities, with some pain in my neck
- I am able to engage in most, but not all of my usual recreation activities because of pain in my neck
- I am able to engage in a few of my usual recreation activities because of pain in my neck
- I can hardly do any recreation activities because of pain in my neck
- I cannot do any recreation activities at all

Shoulder Pain and disability Index (SPADI)

The shoulder pain and disability index has been designed to determine the level of difficulty the patient has after pain in the shoulder joint. SPADI has two scales pain scale and disability scale.

The pain scale has five sections and each section has ten scores (0 -10). Zero is no pain at all and ten is the worst pain imaginable. The patient needs to circle the score (between 0-10) of relevant section which describes the problem most closely. All sections are not necessary to be attempted if the statements do not describe the problem.

Pain scale

How severe is your pain?

1. At its worst?
    0   1   2   3   4   5   6   7   8   9   10
2. When lying on the involved side?
    0   1   2   3   4   5   6   7   8   9   10
3. Reaching for something on a high shell?
    0   1   2   3   4   5   6   7   8   9   10
4. Touching the back of your neck?
    0   1   2   3   4   5   6   7   8   9   10
5. Pushing with the involved arm
    0   1   2   3   4   5   6   7   8   9   10

Disability Scale - The disability scale has total eight sections and each section has ten scores. Zero is no pain at all and ten is the most difficulty to perform activity. The patient needs to circle the score (between 0-10) of relevant section which describes the problem mot closely. All sections are not necessary to be attempted if the activity do not describe the problem

How much difficulty do you have?

1. Washing your hair?
    0   1   2   3   4   5   6   7   8   9   10
2. Washing your back?
    0   1   2   3   4   5   6   7   8   9   10
3. Putting on an undershirt or pullover sweater?

0   1   2   3   4   5   6   7   8   9   10

4.   Putting on a shirt that buttons down the front?

0   1   2   3   4   5   6   7   8   9   10

5.   Putting on your pants?

0   1   2   3   4   5   6   7   8   9   10

6.   Placing an object on a high shelf?

0   1   2   3   4   5   6   7   8   9   10

7.   Carrying a heavy object of 10 pounds?

0   1   2   3   4   5   6   7   8   9   10

8.   Removing something from your back pocket?

0   1   2   3   4   5   6   7   8   9   10

REFERENES

1. Mountcastle, VB: Pain and temperature sensibilities. In Mountcastle, VB (ed): Medical PhysiologyVol 1, ed1 3, CV Mosby, St Louis, p348.

2. Hardy, JD, Wolff, HG, and Goodell, Pricking pain threshold in different body areas. Proc Soc Exp Biol Med 80:425, 1952.

3. Craig AD. Pain mechanism: labeled lines versus convergence in central processing. Annu Rev Neurosci 26:1-30,2003.

4. Price, DD. Psychological and neural mechanism of the affective dimension of pain. Science 288 (5472):773-786, 2002.

5. Carrie M. Hall, Lori Thein Brody. Therapeutic Exercise Moving Toward Function. Lippincott Williams and Wilkins, Philadelphia.

6. DershJ, Polatin PB, Gathchel RJ. Chronic pain and psychopathology: research finding and theoretical considerations. Psychomat Med 64(5):773-786,2002.

7. Weisenber, M; Pain and Pain Control. Psychol Bull 84:108,1977. Selye, H: The stress of life. Mc Graw-Hill, New York, 1976.

8. Meryl Roth Gerish, Electrotherapy in Rehabilitation, contemporary Perspective in Rehabilitation, FA Davis Company, Philadelphia.

9. Luce JM, Thompson RL II, Getto CJ, et al: New concepts of chronic pain and their implication. Hosp Pract. April 1985:113.

10. Bernadette Hecox, Tsega Andemicael Mehreteab, and Joseph Weisberg, Physical Agents, Comprehensive textbook for Physical Therapist, Appleton and Lange, Norwalk, Connecticut.

11. Roger M. Nelson, Karen W. Hayes and Dean P. Currier, Clinical Electrotherapy, third edition, Appleton and Lange, Stamford, Connecticut.

12. Williamson A[1], Hoggart B. Pain: a review of three commonly used pain rating scales. J Clin Nurs. 2005 Aug;14(7):798-804.

13. Galer BS, Jensen MP. Development and preliminary validation of a pain measure specific to neuropathic pain: The Neurogenic Pain Scale. Neurology 48 (2):332-338,1997.

14. Price DD, McGrat PA, Rafii A, Buckingham B. The validation of visual anologue scales as ratio scale measures for chronic and experimental pain. Pain 17(1): 45-56, 1983.

Pain, Functional Limitation and Assessment

15. Williamson A[1], Hoggart B. Pain: a review of three commonly used pain rating scales. J Clin Nurs. 2005 Aug;14(7):798-804.

16. Jensen. M.P., Karoly, P., Braver, S., 1986. The measurement of clinical pain intensity: a comparison of six methods. Pain, Pain 27, 117-26.

17. Paice, J.A., Cohen, F.L., 1997. Validity of a verbally administered numeric rating scale to measure cancer pain intensity.. Cancer Nurs, Cancer Nurs 20, 88-93.

18. American Physical Therapy Association. A guide to physical therapist practice, I: A description of patient management. Phys Ther. 1995;75:709-764.

19. Roshan Lal Meena, Exercise Therapy Principles and Practice, Second Edition. Peepee Publishers and Distributors, New Delhi, pp 107.

Chapter 02

Shortwave Diathermy

The term diathermy is derived from two Greek words dia and thermy, dia means through and thermy means heat or through heating. It is an electromagnetic therapeutic modality most widely used by the clinicians for deep heating effects, increasing local blood flow, increasing nutrients, removing metabolites at large areas and increasing extensibility of tissues.

The first generation of diathermy devices, designed during the 1920s were termed longwave diathermy. It was designed to produce electromagnetic waves at frequencies ranging from 500KHz to 10MHz. The use of longwave diathermies diminished after arrival of the shortwave diathermy a second generation diathermy in the 1930-1940s. Later, the third generation diathermy, microwave was also introduced. Initially, microwave diathermy of 2450MHz was allowed to practice in physiotherapy. The advantage of third generation diathermy is that it is much easier to focus on the body, thus providing much more localized heating effect. However, its low depth of penetration into the tissues has been the main reason of lesser use in physiotherapy practice. The new microwave diathermy with the frequency of 915MHz which has a depth of penetration similar to the short wave diathermy and ultrasound have also been introduced to the physiotherapy practice.

Shortwave diathermy produces electromagnetic energy at 27.12 million cycles per second with wave length of eleven meters. Electromagnetic radiation at frequency of 27.12Mhz is not capable of depolarizing motor nerves or eliciting a contractile response from innervated or denervated skeletal muscles. This is an important reason why such a high frequency is used in diathermy application.[1] The short wave diathermy in the range of radiofrequency has non ionizing radiation in the tissues, which means that there is insufficient energy concentration to dislodge orbiting electron from atoms. Such energy may or may not be perceived cutaneously.

Diathermy with its longer wavelength and lower frequency, penetrates more deeply than infrared, which has shorter wavelength and higher frequencies.[2] The higher wavelength character of the shortwave diathermy allows more potent heating effects at deeper structure without affecting the skin and subcutaneous tissues significantly.[3]

The use of shortwave diathermy in physiotherapy practice has been declined for the last decade due to safety concerns in some western countries. Emission of unwanted stray radiation during therapy, which affects patients, operators, and other people in the vicinity of the device, is likely the main reason for the decline in shortwave diathermy.[15] There is also a misbelieve among the practitioners that shortwave radiation of the diathermy causes miscarriage in the physiotherapists who are concerned with the application of the diathermy.

Production

Short wave Diathermy has two circuits primary and secondary.

Primary circuit: - Primary circuit also known as the machine circuit consists of a power supply, a step up and step down transformer, a rectifier, oscillating and radiofrequency power amplifier designed to modify the output of the unit to levels required by the secondary coil. The primary circuit converts the house current (110V and 60Hz) into high voltage and high frequency (27.12Mhz) by the help of a rectifier and an oscillating circuit. The transformer contains a primary and oscillator coil which is physically in close proximity to the secondary or resonant coil of the secondary circuit. The modified high frequency current is transmitted through the cable to the secondary circuit.

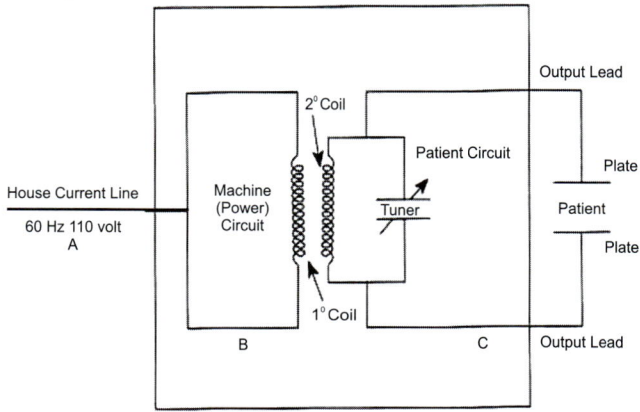

Fig: 2.1 Simplified diagram of a short wave diathermy unit with a patient positioned between the condenser plates. A. A representation of AC house current for the machine circuit. B. The machine circuit which includes the transformer, rectifier, power amplifiers and primary coil (1°coil) radio frequency oscillator of the machine circuit. C. The patient circuit, which includes the secondary (2°coil) transformer coil, the tuner, high frequency out put leads, and condenser plates.

Secondary Circuit: - The secondary circuit known as the patient circuit consists of secondary oscillating coil or electrodes and tissue of the patient. When both primary and secondary circuit are tuned to the same resonant frequency, the energy would be most efficiently transmitted from the high frequency generator circuit to the patient circuit. The movement of the patient or the electrodes during the treatment session can change the resonance between the patient and the device circuit. The tuning knob on the equipment is rotated to either direction to tune both the circuits. When both the circuits are tuned the output indicator will be at the maximum point. Some diathermy equipments are designed so that tuning is adjusted automatically. The outcome is similar to what occurs when a radio is tuned to receive a clear signal from a specific station.[3] The primary and secondary circuits are tuned manually or with the help of output indicator. The secondary circuit is of two types – condenser and induction.

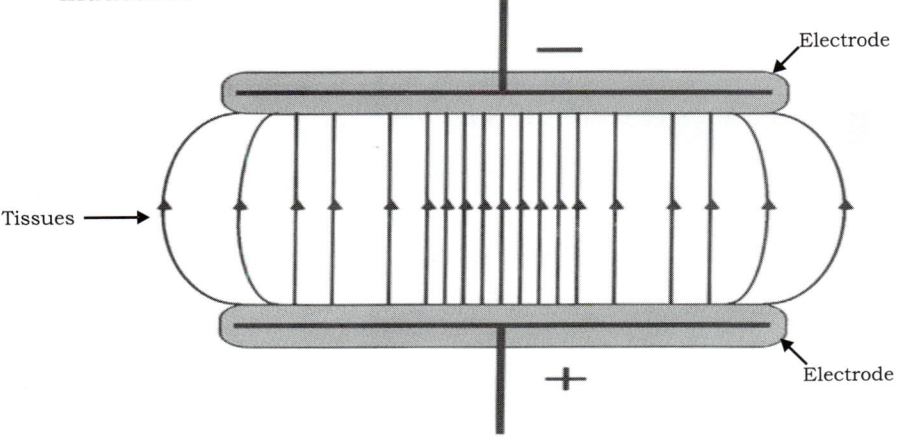

Figure: 2.2. A Secondary circuit or patient circuit.

Condenser Field

The high frequency current is imposed on the pair of opposite charged electrodes which in turn produce electromagnetic energy. A strong electrical field is generated between the plates, which is greater near the capacitance plates or electrodes and diverges further from the plates.

The electrical energy will cause ions and dipole molecules within the tissues to change the direction every time the charge on the plates and the direction of the electrical field changes. The faster the current changes the direction (i.e. the higher frequency), the smaller the actual movement of particles from their original position. The frequency of the back and forth oscillation of ions matches the output frequency of the generator[3]. The dipole molecules are randomly situated within the body tissues. When the pair of opposite charged condenser or capacitance plates generate electrical field in the tissues, the dipole molecules rotate in the direction dictated by their polar charge.

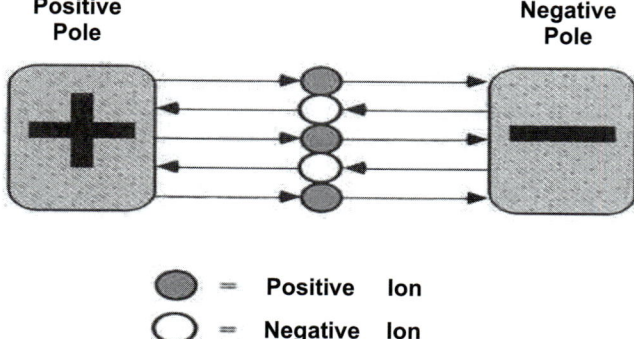

Figure 2.3 Dipole molecules Direction toward which dipole rotate according to the change in polarity of the plates. The positive end of the dipole is always toward the negatively charged plate.

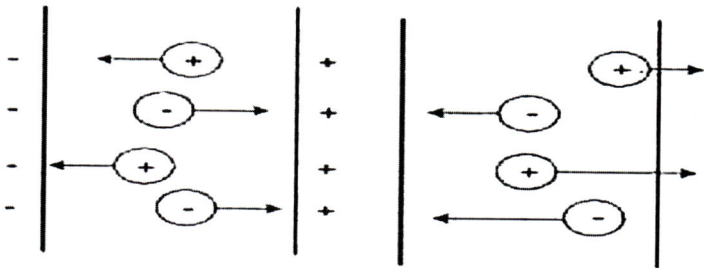

fig: 2.4 the dipoles change direction as the current changes direction.

Dipole molecules contain negative and positive ions, which rotates towards the opposite charged capacitive plate. As the capacitive plates change the charge the dipole molecules also change their direction, which results in rotation of the dipole molecules and that rotation of the dipole molecule produces heat in the tissues. The heat production in the tissues is proportional to the impedance of the tissues. The tissues with the greater impedance to the molecular activity would receive strong heating effects such as fat.

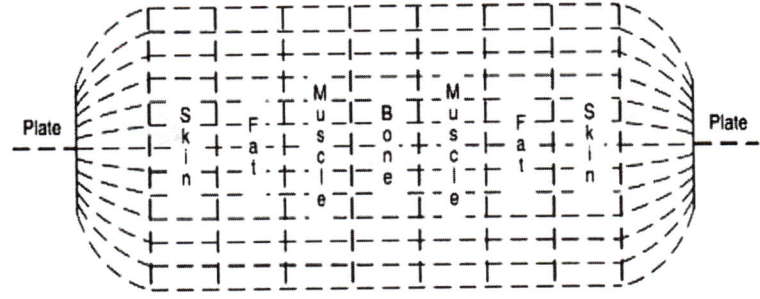

Figure: 2.5 Uniform distribution of the electric field, there is a gap between plates and skin. Reducing gap can produce strong electrical field in near the plates or electrode.

Induction Field Method

The high frequency current is imposed on the induction metal shaped coil, which has properties of high conductivity. The induction metal (plates) shaped into coil are mainly of monode (one flat plate) and the hinged dipode (positioned on one to three sides of a body part). Application of high frequency current on the coil produces strong magnetic field by the coil which in turn produce small, circular shaped electric currents known as eddy currents. The direction of the magnetic field changes as the direction of the current changes. The current is distributed evenly throughout the various tissues at any given distance from the induction. The strong eddy current activity occurs in the low impedance tissues.

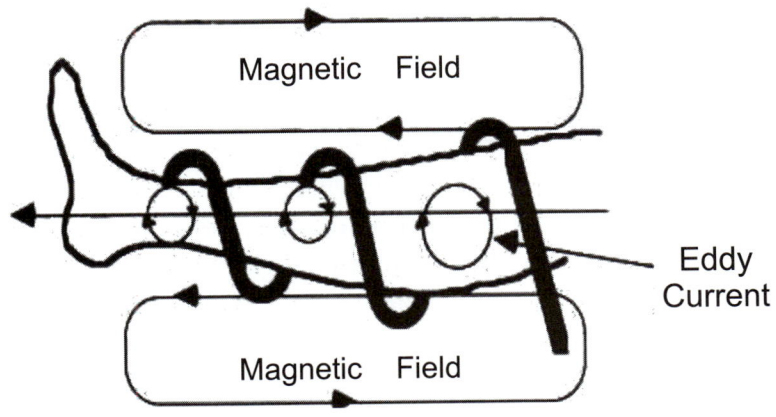

Fig: 2.6 Induction Field Method of application of short wave diathermy

The higher the electrolyte contents in the tissues the lower the impedance. Therefore, the muscle which has higher electrolytes (blood) can be heated more easily than fat, bone collagen tissues.[4]

The basic difference between condenser field diathermy and induction field diathermy is that, with induction field diathermy, a strong magnetic field is produced by the patient circuit which then induces an electrical current within the body part (treatment area). Whereas; the condenser field diathermy, produces electric field between the condenser plates. The body part (treatment area) is positioned in an electric field generated by two condenser plates. With the condenser field diathermy the heat production in the tissues is proportional to the impedance of the tissues. The tissues with greater impedance to the molecular activity would receive strong heating effects such as fat.

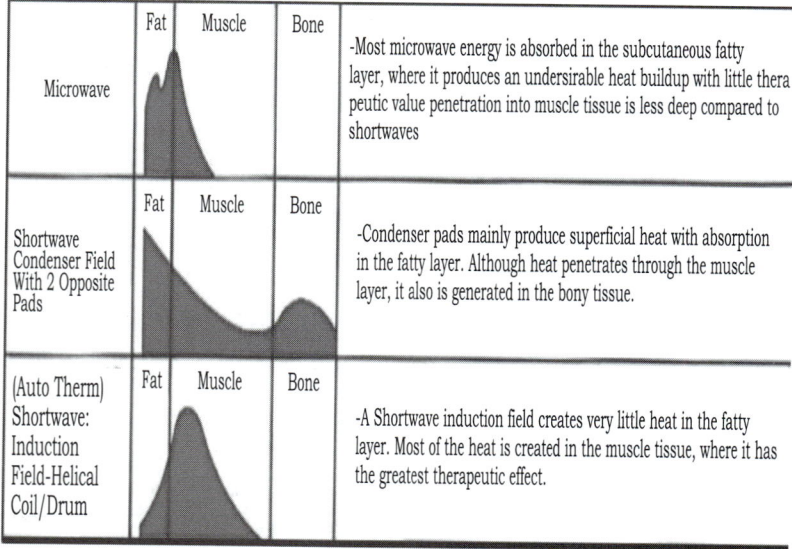

Figure: 2.7 The schematic diagram of condenser and induction field method. depth of distribution of electrical field (heat).

On the other hand the induction field diathermy produce strong eddy current activity in the low impedance tissues. The higher the electrolyte contents in the tissues, lower the impedance. Therefore, the muscle which has higher electrolytes (blood) can be heated more easily than fat, bone collagen tissues.

Pulsed Short Wave Diathermy

Pulsed Short Wave Diathermy is a cyclical interruption of the high frequency current that reduces the energy in the tissues in comparison to continuous short wave diathermy. The energy is transmitted in bursts of pulse trains which are separated from successive pulse train by an "off time". Therefore, each pulse train (on time) is followed by a brief period of 'off' time. The frequency of the pulse train may vary from one to 700 pulses per second[5]. The cyclical break in the transmission of electromagnetic waves does not allow thermal effects in the tissues. The PSWD is used for its stirring effects on the ions, molecules, cell membrane and metabolic activity of cells. This helps in increasing the overall rates of phagocytosis, transport across cell membrane and enzymatic activity. The physical characteristics of PSWD are similar to the SWD. The pulse length normally varies from 25- 400 microseconds.[6] The pulse period consists of on and 'off' time.

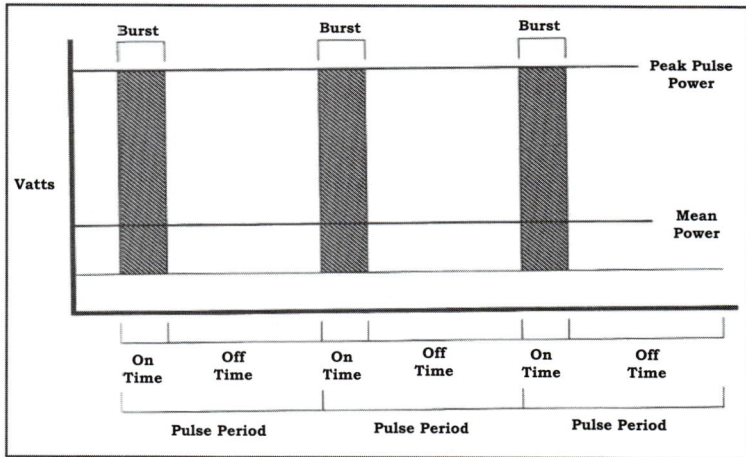

Figure: 2.8 Pulse Diathermy with Pulses/curapluse.

Physiological Effects

Short Wave Diathermy is most widely used for its uniform marked elevation of temperature in the deep situated tissues. Uniform distribution of the electrical field between the two electrodes has ability of producing heat in the tissues evenly situated between the two electrodes in case of capacitance and mono electrode in case of induction method, however, tissue temperature rise depends on the position of the electrodes, the type of tissues being exposed (as the body is composed of homogenous tissues) intensity, treatment time and the type of shortwave field (induction or capacitance).

Thermal Effects:- The most efficient mechanism involved in the conversion of the high frequency current to heat is the mechanism of increased ionic motion. The soft tissues contain billions of charged particles (molecules) or ions such as sodium (Na^+), Potassium (K^+) and chloride (Cl^-). A pair of opposite charged plate electrodes (capacitance) are placed on the body, which attract opposite charged molecules to oscillate about a mean position. The oscillation of the charged molecules at the mean produce kinetic energy which is converted into heat.[7]. Tissues containing high properties of charged molecules will in theory be heated most during the SWD exposure.

The dipole molecules are randomly situated in the body tissues. When a pair of opposite charged plate electrodes are placed on the body, a strong electrical field is generated between the electrodes. If the body part is placed between the electrodes, a strong electrical field is produced in the tissues. Dipole molecules contain negative and positive ions, which rotate towards opposite charged capacitative plates. As the capacitive plates change the charge the dipole molecules also change the direction, which results in rotation of the dipole molecules. Therefore dipole molecules which have opposite ions, rotate in the direction of the opposite charged electrodes. The rotation of the dipole molecules of tissues with the change of frequency of the current results in increase in molecular kinetic energy, which results in increased tissue temperature. The tissue with greater impedance to the molecular activity would receive strong heating effects in case of capacitance field method. The increase in tissue temperature produces following indirect effects in the tissues.

Increase Blood Circulation:- The rise of temperature in the superficial structures (skin) and muscles was studied by using the radioactive sodium. The study found that average increase of the tissue temperature in the skin and muscles was 5.3 and 5.2 respectively[8] The rise in tissue temperature above 40 degree Celsius causes vasodilatation which results in increase in blood circulation, increased supply of oxygen and nutrients to the local area.

Increase Metabolic Rate:- A rise of temperature of 1degree centigrade would increase the metabolic rate by 13 percent. The increase in metabolic rate increases the demand for the oxygen and food stuff and also increases the output of waste products, including metabolites.

Increase Motor Nerve Conduction:- There is significant increase in the motor nerve conductivity following application of diathermy. This relaxes the muscles and increases its efficiency of contraction. The increase in the motor nerve conductivity is not because of stimulation of the nerve but it is due to increase in tissue temperature. This is also to note that the short wave diathermy has no stimulating effects on the nerve, as it's a non ionizing radiation.

Fall in Blood Pressure:- The application of short wave diathermy at an appropriate intensity and duration elevates the temperature, causes vasodilatation and increases blood circulation in the local area where it is applied. However, if the application of SWD covers a large area for longer period of time, this can contribute to significant decrease in the viscosity of the blood and leads to fall in the blood pressure.

The magnetic field in the tissues by the induction method produce small circular shaped eddy currents in the tissues which tends to be more intense close to the treatment applicator and less intense as the field spreads into deeper tissues. However there is less heating effects in the subcutaneous tissues than the muscles. The amount of heating occurs in those tissues having the lowest impedance and the greatest eddy current density or activity. The magnetic field technique is particularly effective for heating tissues with higher conductivities and high electrolyte contents, particularly those well perfused with blood, such as muscles. Therefore, the induction method of application does not produce much heating effects in the fat, collagen fibers and bone as these structures contain low amount of electrolytes.

Indications

The short wave diathermy is most frequently used in the treatment of musculoskeletal disorders.

I.   The thermal effects of the short wave diathermy help in increasing blood flow, relieving pain and spasm, increasing extensibility of the collagenous tissues, increasing nutrients at the local area, removing metabolites, decreasing swelling or edema, and resolution of the inflammation.

ii. Pain especially over the large areas of body such as low back or upper back region.

iii. Secondary muscle spasm associated with pain and stiffness.

iv. Chronic inflammatory pelvic diseases.

v. Arthritic conditions such as osteoarthritis, rheumatoid arthritis (PSWD), Ankylosing spondylitis.

vi. Promoting acute healing including wound healing (Pulse short wave is most commonly used for).

vii Chronic musculoskeletal injuries to reduce pain and swelling or edema.

Clinical uses

Pain Modulation – The pain modulation effect of thermal short wave diathermy is similar to other heating modalities, such as decreasing muscle spasm, accelerating metabolic responses to acute injury, increasing the pain threshold to damaged tissue and influencing pain reception through sensory afferents. Mild heating with SWD in patients with knee osteoarthritis has been shown to reduce both pain and sac thickness.

Wound healing – Pulsed short wave diathermy has been shown to increase local microcirculation in both healthy subjects and around the wound margins in patients with diabetic ulcers[9-10] increasing microcirculation, but still being in the subthermal range, include increasing local tissue oxygenation, nutrient transportation and phagocytosis. PSWD has been shown to accelerate fibroblastic activity, collagen deposition, and tissue healing in animal[11-12]. The limited numbers of human studies that have been performed to date indicate it is likely that non-thermal PSWD enhances the rate of wound healing.

Contraindications

i. Any metal in the field, near the field including jewellery

ii. Cardiac Pace maker

iii. Over the Artificial joints

iv. Pregnant women

v. Direct by over the tissues with contents of high level fluid such as eyes and testes.

vi. Over the face of the patient wearing contact lenses

vii. Malignancy

viii. Over the area of sensory deficit

ix. Poor blood perfusion – such as in arterial insufficiency of the extremities, may not adequately allow for heat dissipation.

x. Hemophilia

xi. Over the active bleeding

xii. The therapist may be cautious in case of patient wearing moist clothes, accumulation of sweating and over the low back area in patient who is menstruating, over the area of growing epiphysis.

Application

Short wave diathermy is applied by two methods capacitance where two electrodes are used and inductance with mono or diplode electrodes.

Capacitance: - A pair of plate electrodes enclosed with an appropriate insulator is placed over the desired area to be treated. There are mainly two types of electrodes used for the therapeutic purposes. Flexible metal plates – These are also known as malleable electrodes, these are flat metal sheets covered with a thick layer of rubber. A felt like material is used to ensure that a sufficient spacing is retained between the electrodes and tissues. The flexible electrodes are connected with the cables. Rigid Metal Disks – These are the flat round shaped metal electrodes covered with the plastic covers. The rigid metal disks are attached with adjustable arms of the equipment. There are three major methods of placement of electrodes on the body tissues.

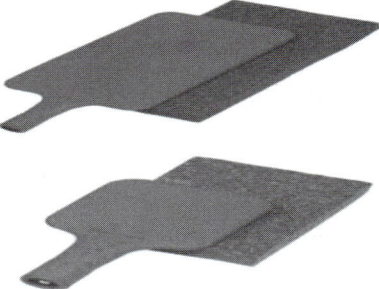

Figure: 2.9a flexible plate electrodes.

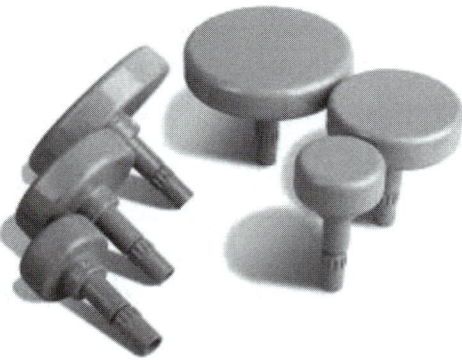

Figure: 2.9b Rigid metal Disc electrodes.

Contraplanar (Transverse) Method : - The electrodes are placed on each side of the body such that they face each other. For example, to treat the knee ailments each electrode is placed on medial and lateral aspect or anterior and posterior aspect of the joint. The distance between electrodes and skin should be 2cm to 4cm. To maintain the distance a layer of towel is placed between the skin and electrodes. The rigid metal disks electrodes do not require towel layer as the electrodes are enclosed with the plastic covers and attached with adjustable arms to positions them, therefore, distance can be maintained with the adjustable arms.

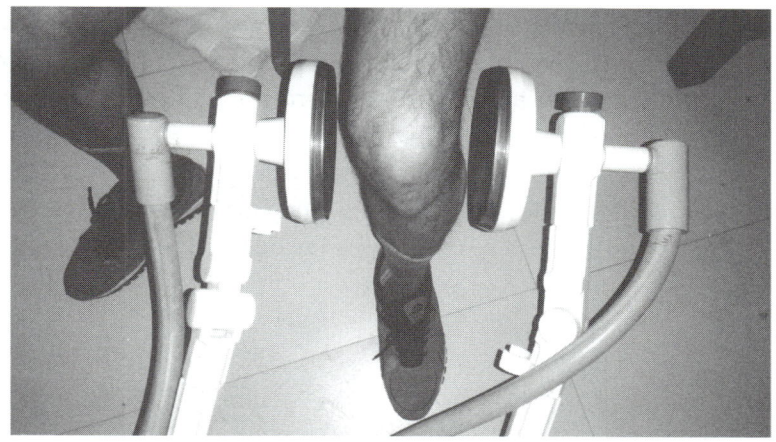

Figure: 2.9c. Contraplaner method, placement of disc plates on tissues

Coplanar Method:- Both the electrodes are placed on the same side of the area to be treated. For example, to treat the non specific low back pain, each electrode is placed on the left and right paravertebral region of the lumbar spine. There should be an appropriate space between the two electrodes as the electric field follows the route of least resistance or through the blood vessels, which contain high proportions of ions. If the distance between the electrodes is less, the electric field will pass directly between the electrodes or over the skin only. Therefore, to produce electric field in the deep tissues the space between the two electrodes and the space between the electrodes and tissues must be appropriate.

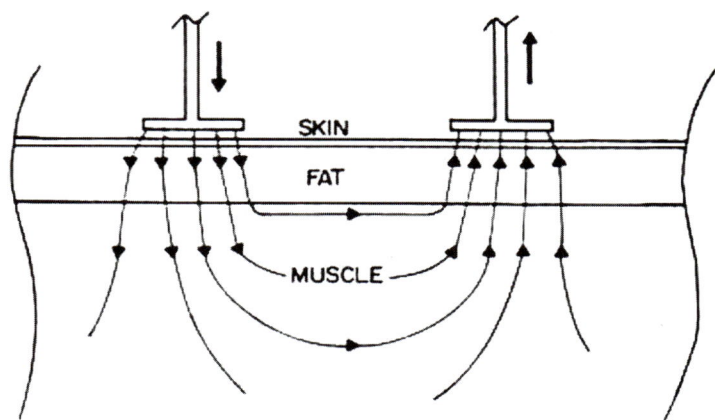

Fig: 2.9d. Coplanar Method, Electrodes are placed on same side of the treatment area

Longitudinal Method: - Each electrode is placed at each end of the extremity. For an example, to treat the lower leg one electrode is placed under the ankle (palmer surface) and other electrode is on the tibial condyles superiorly, while the knee joint is flexed at 90 degrees. The electric field in this method will be produced in the same direction of the tissues. The tissues lie parallel to the electric field and thus produce less resistance to the current flow

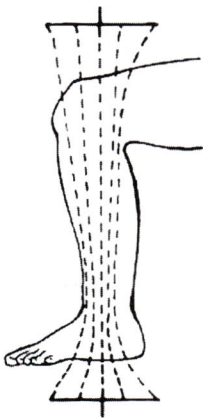

Fig. 2.9e. Longitudinal method.

Cross Fire Method:- The cross fire method involves treatment of four surfaces of the same joint or area in two equal treatment times. For an example, to treat the knee joint ailments first half of the treatment involves the medio-lateral aspect of the joint, which is followed by second half of the treatment on the anterioposterior aspect of the knee joint.

Bowmen's Method:- The method is advised for pelvic inflammatory disease (PID). PID is an inflammatory disease of the upper part of the female reproductive system namely uterus, fallopian tubes, and ovaries, and inside of the pelvis. The treatment is divided into the two parts. In the first part of the treatment the patient is positioned in crook lying. One electrode is placed over the sacrum and other electrode over the infra pubic area. In the next part of the treatment the patient is positioned in sitting, and the electrode over the infrapubic area is shifted to the ischial tuberosity.

The position of the electrodes over the tissues greatly affects the electromagnetic field. The following points should be taken into consideration while placing the electrodes in the capacitance field method:

I. **Space between the electrodes:** - There should be an optimal space between the electrodes to produce uniform electric field in the tissues. Direct placement of the electrodes on the body surface can produce high electric field near the electrodes that would produce excessive heat in the superficial area. This can lead to burn. If the distance between the electrodes and body surface is too large this may weaken the field strength. Therefore, an optimal distance between the electrodes and the body surface should be 2cm to 4cm. This can be achieved by placing a towel layer between the body surface and electrodes. However, plate electrodes do not require any spacing as it is already maintained with in the plastic covering.

ii. **Size of the electrodes:-** The electrodes should be of equal size. The unequal sized electrodes would produce non uniform electrical field in the tissues. The smaller size electrode would produce more heating in the tissues compared to its counterpart large electrode. The size of the electrodes should also be slightly larger than the treatment area, as the electric field is less uniform at the edge of planes, therefore; outer part would not receive electromagnetic waves. There are three different sizes of the electrodes provided by the distributors small, medium and large.

Induction Field Method- The induction method uses single plate electrode which is shaped into the coil. There are two arrangements of coils monode and diplode. A monode (drum) is an electrode which is basically arranged in one plane, whereas, the hinged diplode electrode is arranged into one to three planes. The diplode (drum) covers the treatment area from three parts, however it is a single hinged plate electrode shaped into the coil. A strong magnetic field is produced by the patient circuit, which then induces an electrical (eddy) current within the body part. The space between the coiled conductor and the surface of the drum is fixed so a single layer of towel laid on the body part provides adequate spacing.

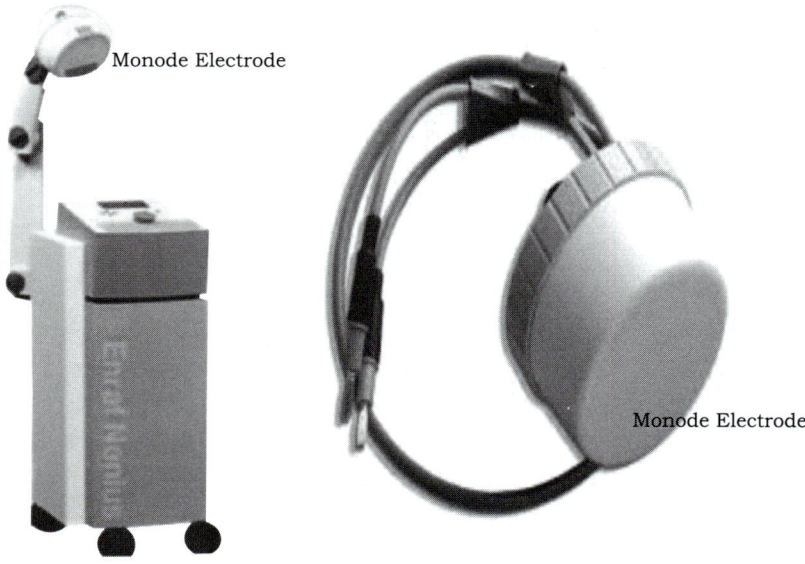

Monode Electrode

Monode Electrode

Fig: 2.10 shortwave diathermy with monode electrode.

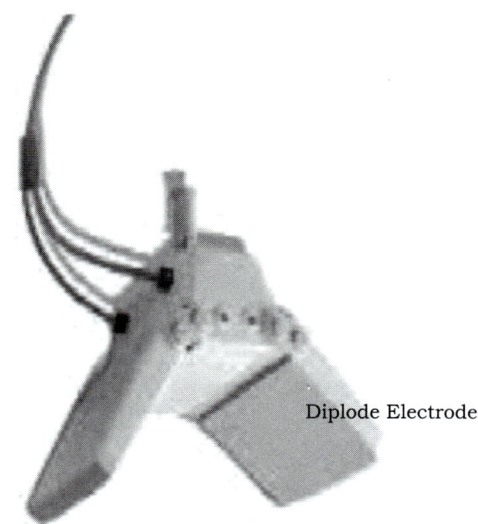

Diplode Electrode

Fig: 2.11 Diplode electrode

Shortwave Diathermy

Doses

It is not clinically possible to measure the amount of electromagnetic energy produced in the tissues. The thermal perception of the patient is the only safe guide to elevate the optimal temperature in the tissue. It is possible to produce thermal to sub-thermal heating effects with the same intensity in the tissues of different subjects. Therefore; doses cannot be based on the intensity only. Based on the patient perception the doses are[13] divided into four schemes: -

i.   **Dose I:** Lowest – patient does not perceive thermal sensation, however; thermal effects are produced. It is indicated to the patients with an acute inflammatory process.

ii. **Dose II:** Low – mild heating sensation, barely felt. It is advised to the patients with sub-acute, and resolving inflammatory process.

iii. **Dose III:** Medium – patient perceives pleasant medium to moderate heat sensation. It is also advised for the sub acute and resolving inflammatory conditions.

iv. **Dose IV:** Heavy – Vigorous heating that produces a tolerated sensation. It is just below maximal tolerance. Heavy doses are recommended for chronic conditions.

From the research perspective, vigorous heating has commonly been defined as heating tissue to 4 degree Celsius or greater above baseline temperature. For an example, baseline temperature at 2cm depth in the gastrocnemius has been shown to be an average of 35.5 Celsius. A 4 degree increase yields an absolute temperature of 39.5 Celsius, which is well tolerated in human subjects.

Procedure

Preparation of the equipment: - The equipment should have appropriate cables and electrodes and these should be connected to the primary circuit adequately. Check in case of cut in the cable. The cables should not cross each other during the treatment.

Preparation of the patient:- The physiotherapist must ensure that the position of the patient is comfortable throughout the treatment session. The following points should be taken into account -

i. The short wave diathermy chamber or cabin should preferably be made of wood. Metal in the form of stool, chair, plinth or couch should be at least 11 meters away from the chamber.

ii. Take a history of the patient carefully prior the treatment for any contraindications such as metal implants, prosthesis (metal implant) in case of joint replacement, and cardiac pace maker. The patients with metal implant in contra-lateral extremity may be allowed for the exposure of diathermy with caution. However, pregnant women and cardiac pace maker patients must not be allowed into short wave diathermy chamber or cabin.

iii. Remove all clothing, jewelry, and electronic devices from the area to be treated.

iv. Expose and clean the area. There should not be moisture on the skin.

v. Place the patient in a comfortable position with proper back support in case of sitting. The part which is being treated should be in a slacked position. If the goal of treatment is of increasing extensibility of the tissues, then the part which is being treated should be in an extreme lengthened position.

vi. Elevate the part or extremity above the level of heart if the goal of treatment is of reduction of swelling or edema.

vii. Cover the part with one or two layers of the towel to maintain an adequate distance between the electrodes and tissues.

viii. convince the patient for mild to moderate heating sensation. Instruct the patient to inform the therapist in case of any discomfort or excessive heat or press the emergency switch immediately. Instruct the patient that there is no scale for measurement of heat, you only can judge the excessive heat as heat tolerance differs from patient to patient. In case of emergency alarm switch of the equipment and check for any erythema or burn. Use ice for mild burn injuries or refer the patient to the physician for deep burn injuries.

ix. The timer will run out after the completion of the treatment.

x. Remove the towel layer from the treatment area and tell patient to collect the jewellery and other belongings.

xi. The patient is put on the stretching exercises immediately after the exposure of the diathermy if the goal of treatment is of improving range of motion.

Shortwave Diathermy Versus therapeutic ultrasound

Decreased muscle flexibility and joint hypomobility are two common impairements. When electing a deep heating agent prior to stretching or joint mobilization techniques, many clinicians turn to therapeutic ultrasound. However ultrasound is limited to treating relatively small areas that do not exceed two times the size of the sound head, and does not efficiently heat deep muscles. Short wave diathermy effectively heats large areas, while safely heating deep muscle. It matches the depth of penetration and heating rate of 1MHz ultrasound, with the added benefit of heating a large area. Since properly applied SWD can preferentially heat low impedance tissues(skeletal muscle, blood vessels, synovial fluid) it can heat deep muscle more efficiently than therapeutic ultrasound. In addition to that the soft tissues treated with the SWD maintain the tissue temperature increase two to three times longer than an ultrasound treatment. The muscles maintain their peak temperature for 3.3 minutes and tendons maintain up to 5 minutes after the application therapeutic ultrasound. Therefore, short wave diathermy extends these windows, which gives the clinician more time to use passive stretching, joint mobilization and soft tissue mobilization before the tissue temperature receedes to a baseline. Recent researches and clinical experience have shown that joint mobilization techniques and soft tissue mobilization techniques yield better results after reaching therapeutic temperature through preheating with short wave diathermy[14].

References

1. Susan L. Michlovitz, Thomas P. Nolan Jr, Modalities for Therapeutic Intervention, fourth edition, Contemporary Perspective in Rehabilitaiton, pp152.

2. Griffin Je, , Karselis TC, Physical agents for Physical Therapist. Springfield, IL: Charles C Thompson; 1982.

3. Bernadette Hecox, Tsega Andemicael Mehreteab, and Joseph Weisberg, Physical Agents, Comprehensive textbook for Physical Therapist, Appleton and Lange, Norwalk, Connecticut, pp143-146.

4. Klothe L, Morrison MA, Ferguson BH. Therapeutic microwave and short wave diathermy. A review of thermal effectiveness, safe Use, state of the art: 1984, Food and Drug AdministrationUS Departmento f health and Human Services December 1984, HHS Publicaiton FDA 85- 8237. Thom H, Introduction to shortwave and Microwave Therapy. Springfield IL: Charles C Thomas 1966).

5. Vanden Bouwhuijsen F, et al. A manula on pulsed and continuous short wave diathermy. ENRAF-NONIUS, cat no. 1419762, Delft, Holland).

6. Basanta Kumar Nanda, electrotherapy Simplified 2nd edition, pp 297.

7. Ward AR, 1980, Electricity, Fields, and waves in therapy, science press, Marrickville.

8. Millard JB. Effect of high frequency currents and infra red rays on the circulation of the lower limbs in man. Ann Phys Med 6:45, 1961.

9. Mayrovitz, H, & Larsen, P.)1995). A preliminary study to evaluate the effect of pulsed radiofrequency field treatemtn on lower-extremity-peri ulcer skin microcirculation of diabetic patients. Wounds,7, 90-93.

10. Mayrovitz, H. & Larsen, P. (1992). Efects of pulsed electromagnetic fields on skin microvascular blood perfusion. Wounds, 4, 197-202.

11. Brown, M., & Baker, R., (1987). Effect of pulsed short wave diathermy in skeletal muscle injury in rabbits. Physical Therapy, 67(2), 202-214.

12. Bansal B., etal. (1990). Histomorphochemical effectsof short wave diathermy on healing of experimrntal muscularunjury in dogs. India Journal of Experimental Biology, 28, 766-770

13. Susan L. Michlovitz and Thomal P. Nolan, Jr, Modalities for Therapeutic Intervention, 4th edition, Contemporary Perespective in Rehabilitation, pp. 158,

14. A diathermy Comeback? Joseph A. Gallo, Dsc, ATC, PT, and Christopher M. Prouls, DC, MS, ATC, CSCS, Posted on may 22, 2012 on Advance for healthcare Careers Network.

15. Shields N. Gormley J. O'Hare N, 2004: Shortwave diathermy: Current Clinical and Sfety Practice. Physioth Res Int, 7:191-202.

Chapter 03

Microwave Diathermy

Microwave diathermy is used in the management of superficial tumours with conventional radiotherapy and chemotherapy and, its use has been successfully extended to physical medicine and sports traumatology in Central and Southern Europe.[1,2] Microwave radiation is defined as waves having a frequency of 300MHz to 3000MHz, which lies on the electromagnetic spectrum between radio frequency and infrared radiation. This range of frequency is higher than the shortwave diathermy. The microwave radiation is radiated as a beam from an antenna and is absorbed by water rich tissues 7000 times effectively than shortwave radio frequency energy.[2] Tissues of high water contents characteristically absorb microwaves strongly and muscle.[3] fluid filled organs such as the eye, joint effusion and surface water are heated preferentially.[4]

The use of short wave and microwave in clinical practice appears to have declined since the early 1980s, even though it is still extremely popular in physiotherapy department and private practice of several European Union countries, Asutralia, and North America [7-8].

Hyperthermia induced by microwave diathermy into tissue acastimulate repair processes, increase drug activity, allow more efficient relief from pain, help in removal of toxic wastes, increase tendon extensibility and reduce muscle and joint stiffness. In addition to that it improves local tissue fluid drainage, increase metabolic rate and induces alterations in the cell membrane. Hyperthermia induced by microwave diathermy is used in the management of muscle and tendon injuries.[9]

Production

The device which is used for the production of the microwave is called magnetron, a special type of thermionic valve characterized by centrally placed cathode which is surrounded by a circular metal anode. The high electric current is applied on the magnetron which results in generation of oscillating high frequency current which is carried out to the director (applicator) through the co-axial cable. The director also known as transducer is actually an applicator consisting of an antenna and a reflector. The antenna is a piece of wire that is mounted in front of a metal reflector which emits the waves in one direction. The waves produced by the antenna are known as microwaves which are transmitted into the tissues, where, they may be reflected, refracted or absorbed. The depth of penetration of the waves on the tissues depends upon the frequency of the microwaves. The higher the frequency the lower the depth of penetration.

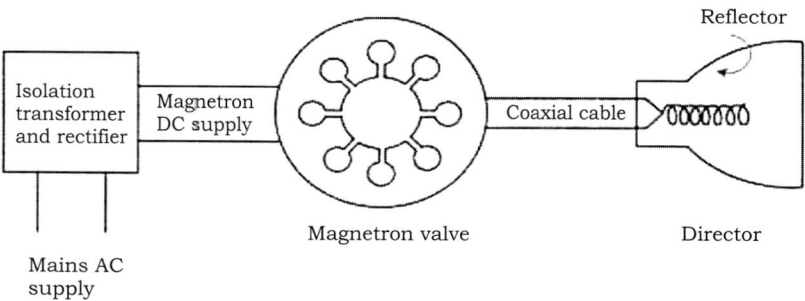

Fig: 3.1 production of Microwaves

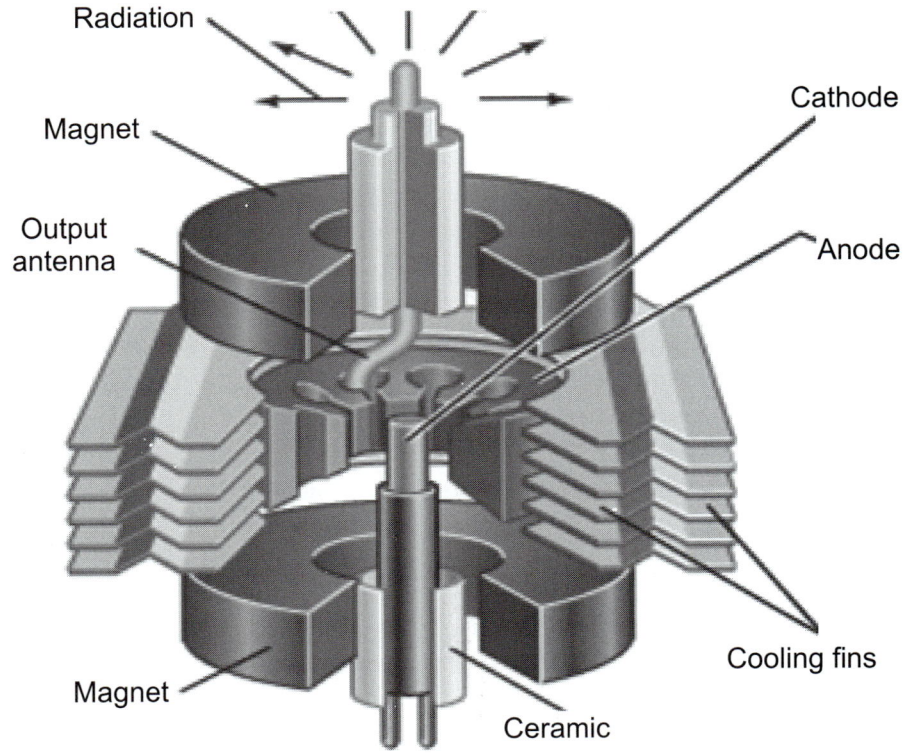

Radiation

Magnet

Output
antenna

Cathode

Anode

Magnet

Ceramic

Cooling fins

Fig: 3.2 Magnetron

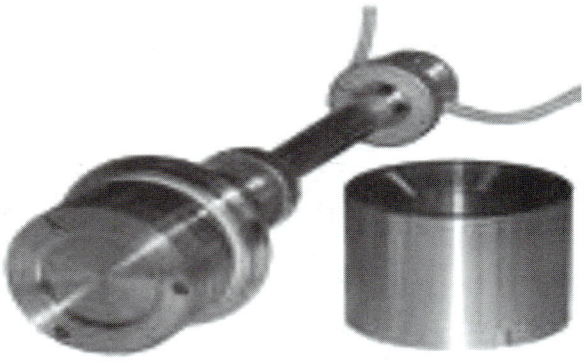

Fig: 3.3 Director

Microwave Diathermy

Characteristics

Microwaves are the form of electromagnetic radiation which lie between the shortwave and infrared waves on the electromagnetic spectrum. The frequency of microwave ranges from 300MHz to 3000MHz, with the wave length of 10mm to 01 meter. The 2450 MHz with the wavelength of 12.24cm is most commonly used for the therapeutic purposes in the physiotherapy practice.

The propagation characteristics of microwaves are first determined by the wavelength and frequency of the energy. The wavelength of the microwave decreases as the frequency increases. The 2450 MHz microwave diathermy has 122.5mm wavelength, whereas, the 915 MHz and 433.9MHz MWD have wavelength of 327mm and 690mm respectively. Hence, the depth of penetration of the microwave diathermy increases as the wave length increases, and frequency decreases. Therefore, the 433.9MHz will have greater depth of penetration than the 915MHz and 2450MHz microwave diathermies.

MWD with various frequencies

Frequency	Wavelength	Depth of penetration
2450MHz	12.24cm	1.85cm
915MHz	32.8cm	5cm
434MHz	69.1cm	Above 5cm still under trial

Table 3.1 MWD with various frequencies and depth of penetration

The microwave diathermy works on the principle of thermionic emission[5]. As soon as the microwave diathermy waves leave the director, they enter into the tissues and may be absorbed, transmitted, refracted or reflected according to the optical laws of radiation[6].

Transmission: - The microwaves are not efficiently transmitted through the subcutaneous tissues into the deep structures like ultrasound and short waves. The transmission depends on the frequency and the wave length of the microwaves. The higher the frequency, the lower the depth of penetration.

Absorption: - The tissues with higher water content absorbs more energy. Water has a high dielectric constant, and higher the dielectric constant, greater the absorption. Muscles contain higher dielectric contents, hence, greater absorption of the microwaves occurs at the muscles. Unlike ultrasound waves, there will be less absorption of microwaves in the periosteum and bone.

Reflection: - Similar to the ultrasound waves the microwaves are also reflected in the body tissues. Reflection occurs at the interfaces. Higher the difference in the density of the two different materials at the interfaces, greater the reflection of the microwaves. The microwaves with the frequency of 2450MHz has 1.85 cm depth of penetration. The waves with this depth of penetration reaches to the muscles but higher heating effects are produced in the subcutaneous tissues than the muscles, this is because reflection of microwaves occurs from the muscles into the subcutaneous tissues.

In microwave ovens, most of metals reflect the microwaves. If it occurs outside the body, the rays may reflect back to the director or transducer or to other people and object in the environment. The metal in the body would reflect the waves to the adjacent area that would cause overheating and tissue burn. The tissue burn is actually not due to heating of the metal similar to the short wave diathermy and ultrasound but it is because of absorption of the higher quantity of the microwave energy by the adjacent tissues.

Physiological Effects

The physiological effect of microwave diathermy such as hyperthermia (rise of tissue temperature) is not as deeper as short wave diathermy and therapeutic ultrasound but essentially the heating effects are deeper to the superficial structure. However the MWD with lower frequency of 915MHz, and 433.9MHz have higher depth of penetration which produce heat in the deep structures similar to the ultrasound and sort wave diathermy. The structures which contain higher concentration of the water molecules such as muscles will absorb greater microwaves and will have higher thermal effects than the other tissues.

The actual ratio of fat : muscle temperature depends on the thickness of the two layers of tissue. However, the MWD with the frequency of 2450MHz would produce less heating effects in the muscles due to lower depth of penetration. Moreover, the microwaves transmitted to the muscles also get reflected to the subcutaneous tissues due to significant difference in the density of the interfaces (fat and muscles). The combined quantities of energy absorbed by the fat lead to a heating pattern in which the temperature of subcutaneous layers may be equal to or even exceed that of muscle when the fatty layer is thicker than 20mm[7]. The higher concentration of microwaves in the subcutaneous tissues results in production of heat in the subcutaneous tissues.

The physiological effects induced by hyperthermia is the regional increase in the blood flow[10-11]. The increase in blood perfusion results from physiological vascular changes such as opening of vessels and contemporary increase in capillary permeability. These two events must be related to the physiological response of the central nervous system, and to the release of vasoactive compounds such as bradikinin and histamine. The release of bradikinin and histamine contributes to vasodilatation that enhances the supply of nutrients and oxygen in the heated region. There is also increase in the extravasion that helps in producing macrophases and granulocytes in the area. This whole process contributes to the removal of necrotic debris and excess fluid.

Hyperthermia improves the contractile performance of muscle, as it increases ATPase activity and changes the mechanical properties of collagen fibers[12]. The microwave diathermy induced hyperthermia decrease pain by altering the sensory nerve response and increasing metabolic rate. The increased metabolic rate washes out the inflammatory mediators from the painful area as the inflammatory mediators interrupt the free ending of the sensory nerve responsible for the pain. The second effect of the hyperthermia in relieving pain is to reduce nerve conduction velocity. The chronic pain is mainly due to hyper-excitability of the nerve especially non-myelinated C type neuronal fibers. The studies conducted on the sciatic nerve have showed that the pain conduction velocity of the sciatic nerve is remarkably reduced for sixty minutes after a hyperthermia session.

Heat shock proteins (HSP), also called stress proteins are a group of proteins present in all cells. Ogura et al. recently reported that HSPs were generated by a rise in the muscle temperature above 41° C induced by microwave diathermy.[13-14] HSPs are also present in cells under normal conditions, acting as 'chaperones', making sure that the cell's proteins are in the right shape and in the right place at the right time. Hence, elevated HSP, level increases protein synthesis and decreases protein degradation. HSPs induced by heat stress preceding eccentric contraction may prevent skeletal muscle breakdown during exercises.[15] This suggests that hyperthermia is not only effective in post traumatic pain and swelling but also effective for exercise preconditioning.

Non Thermal Effects - The normal thermal effects of hyperthermia have not been yet fully documented. These effects may result from an interaction between the imposed electromagnetic field and specific type, or assemblages, of receptors molecules. The sodium and potassium molecules occur within the cell membrane and appear to receive energy directly from an applied electric field. The energy appears subsequently as an enhanced rate of sodium and potassium across the cell membrane. This mechanism is fundamental to many cellular activities, is dependent on both frequency and field intensity and requires that the energy of the weak electric field is amplified at the cell membrane to exert an effect.[48]

Therapeutic Uses

Microwave diathermy is used in the management of various musculoskeletal disorders. The MWD induced hyperthermia produces several physiological effects in the tissues which contributes in increasing range of motion, reducing hematoma, and improving pain associated with tendinopathies.

To increase ROM – Limitation in the range of motion is caused by tightness or shortening of the connective tissues such as ligaments, joint capsule, scarred and thickened synovium and fibrotic muscles. The hyperthermia induced by MWD prior to stretching of the tight connective tissues increases the extensibility. In physiotherapy practice the significant elongation of the short connective tissues can be achieved if stretching is performed along with hyperthermia of the tissues at the therapeutic range between 41°C to 45°C.

The length of the collagenous tissues can be increased under therapeutic range of temperature with a microwave unit at 915MHz.[12] Exclusive use of heat or stretch does not produce elongation of the rat tail tendon, only the application of a sustained tensile load and temperature of 45°C produce significant tendon lengthening.[12] Warren et al. used 915MHz MWD and confirmed that low load, long duration stretching of the tendon performed along with the tissue temperature maintained at the significant therapeutic level results in greatest increase in residual tissue length and produced the least amount of damage[16] when compared with tissue stretching at lower temperatures with higher loads.

Haematoma – Haematoma is the common manifestation in the interstitial space following injury or trauma. There is micro tear of the muscle fibers that allows the blood to enter into the interstitial space to accumulate and form a clot known as haematoma. Haematoma causes functional limitations such as decrease range of motion, difficulty in walking and performing activities of daily living. A study conducted by Lehmann, quantified the resolution of the haematoma produced in the musculature of the experimental animals comparable in size with humans. Haematoma in the biceps femoris muscle were created in pigs by bilateral injecting of blood with chromium (CR) on side of haematoma was treated with the microwave diathermy of 915MHz and other side was used as a control. The tissue temperature was maintained at the therapeutic range between 42°C to 45°C. A decay curve for the radioisotope showed that the time to the half life value was significantly shorter for the treated side. This study supports the use of heat as an adjuct to other therapies aimed for resolution of muscular haematoma[17].

Tendinopathies - Repetitive and overuse of the muscles may cause reactive inflammatory changes in the muscles at the tendon which originates from the periosteum. There is change in the arterial blood flow with resulting local hypoxia and impaired metabolic activity and nutrition may be a key factor[18], together with failed cell matrix adaptation to excessive changes in load.[19-20] A randomized controlled study recruited 42 patients with patellar and tendo achiilis tendinitis. Twenty two patients were treated with the therapeutic ultrasound and rest of twenty were treated with MWD induced hyperthermia. Both groups showed significant improvement in the symptoms. The group treated with the MWD induced hyperthermia, demonstrated better effect on the reduction of VAS score and on subjective overall satisfaction (77% of excellent and good results in comparison with 33% of ultrasound.

Relief of Pain - Microwave diathermy can be used to reduce pain Lehmann[21], although the narrow focus of many commercial applicators may render the treatment of diffuse lesions more difficult than with other methods of diathermy. MWD induced hyperthermia dilates vessels and mobilizes the nocigenic compounds such as bradykinin and histamine from the tissue. The thermal effects on the tissues also stimulate large A beta fibers which stops the pain carrying nociceptors at the substantia gelatinosa in the spinal cord.

2450MHz MWD versus 915MHz MWD

The microwave diathermy with frequency of 2450MHz is less effective than the other lower frequency microwave diathermies like 915MHz. The first reason is that the depth at which 2450MHz microwave penetrates the tissues is slightly deeper to the superficial structures. In addition to that if the subcutaneous layers are thicker than 20mm than the heating effects cannot be produced in the muscles or deeper to the subcutaneous tissues. The 2450MHz microwave is also inconvenient to apply as the director is placed at distance from the body and energy is emitted into the surrounding environment, whereas the power output must be limited so that skin and fat will not be overheated. 434MHz MWD is also introduced and being tried and used in some countries for its deep heating thermal effects.

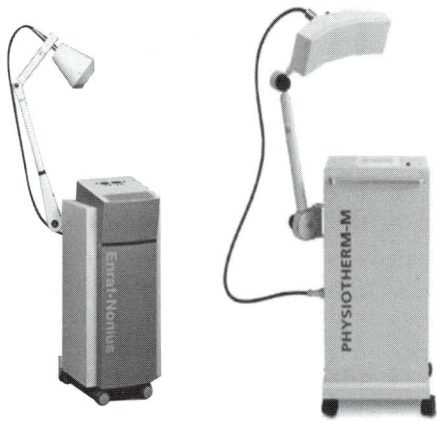

Fig: 3.4 microwave diathermy with circular and rectangular head

MWD induced hyperthermia can be produced at the desired localized areas unlike short wave diathermy by selecting an appropriate shape of director.

Safety

The use of microwave diathermy within the therapeutic range is considered to be safe. The modality is mainly used to produce hyperthermia in the tissues which helps in increasing the extensibility of the connective tissues. To achieve desired effects especially if the aim of treatment is to elongate of the shortened connective tissues the therapeutic temperature must be maintained between $42^{\circ}C$ to $45^{\circ}C$ for at least 10 to 20 minutes. The temperature within the therapeutic range between $42^{\circ}C$ and $45^{\circ}C$ for up to 30minutes does not produce hot spots and thermal injuries to the tissues. This range of temperature and treatment time is tolerated by the patients also. The temperature beyond $45^{\circ}C$ even for a less than one minute can cause hot spots and thermal injury in the tissues and patient experiences it as an intolerable thermal sensation.

Hazards

The use of electromagnetic modalities to produce hyperthermia in the tissues may cause thermal injury such as burn and hot spots, however, these can very well be avoided by adopting a proper procedure of application and by maintaining the temperature within the therapeutic range. Improper application of these modalities can produce the following hazards

i. **Burn** – Improper placement of the director, excessive perspiration over the treatment area, not inspecting the treatment area prior to the treatment for sensory deficit, vascular impairment, metal implants and open wounds are the common reasons of burn. The excessive heat beyond the therapeutic range also causes thermal injury and hot spots in the tissues. The patient must be instructed for warning the therapist or pressing the emergency button in case of excessive or intolerable heat.

ii.   **Symptoms Exaggeration** – Application of MWD to the patients with acute inflammatory conditions such as rheumatoid arthritis; infective conditions, bursitis, where moderate to severe swelling or edema is present can aggravate the symptoms.

Indications

I.   Relief of pain
ii.   Reduction of haematoma
iii.   Musculoskeletal disorders and injuries such as tendinopathies, bursitis, synovitis, tenosynovitis, muscular strain, ligamentous sprain, capsular lesions, shortening or tightness of the connective tissues, chronic rheumatoid arthritis,
iv.   Infected surgical incisions.

Contraindications and Precautions

Contraindications

I.   Eyes – Irradiation to the eyes may develop opacities or cataract
ii.   Malignancy – Application of MWD over the tumor may spread the infection to the other areas
iii.   Cardiac pace maker
iv.   Genital area
v.   Pregnancy
vi.   Metallic implants
vii.   Sensory deficit / impaired thermal sensation
viii. Impaired circulation
ix.   Haemorrhagic or ischemic area
x.   Excessive edema and moderate edema
xi.   Growing bone / epiphysis
xii.   Acute inflammation
xiii. Deep venous thrombosis or phlebitis
xiv.   Acute dermatological conditions
xv.   Blood pressure abnormalities
xvi.   History of recent radiotherapy
xvii. Patients allergic to heat

xviii. Wet dressing and adhesive taps

xix. During menstruation cycle

xx. Tuberculosis

Precautions

I. The area which is being treated with the MWD should not be wet.

ii. The treatment couch should be made of wood.

iii. The patients with cardiac pacemaker should not be allowed into the MWD cabin.

Application Procedure

I. The plinth or couch used for the MWD treatment must not be metallic. It should be made up of wooden. If patient is a wheelchair bound, transfer the patient to the wooden couch. Do not apply MWD to the patient sitting in the wheelchair; doing so can cause unnecessary reflection of the waves to the other areas of the body such as eyes or sexual organs.

ii. Take a lucid history of the patient carefully prior to the treatment for any contraindications such as metal implants, prosthesis (metal implant) in case of joint replacement, and cardiac pace maker. The patients with metal implant in contra-lateral extremity may be allowed for the exposure of diathermy with caution, however, pregnant women and cardiac pace maker patients must not be allowed into the short wave diathermy chamber or cabin.

iii. Inspect the treatment area for circulation, sensation and skin cut or wound.

iv. Remove all the jewelry and metals if any around the area to be treated

v. Clean the area to remove dirt and oils

vi. Place the patient in a comfortable position. Instruct not to change the position during the treatment session.

vii. Selection of Director or transducer - Position the director or applicator over the treatment area with an optimal distance. The selection of the shape of the director or applicator is determined by the treatment area. There are two types of director or applicator of the microwave diathermy circular and rectangular (doughnut shaped) shaped. Both of the directors produce different patterns of heat. The "circular" director produces 100 percent or maximum energy beneath the periphery of the director. Therefore, it used be used over the bony area so that energy can be dissipated to the peripheral parts of the bony area. A "rectangular" director also known as "C" shaped produces maximum microwave energy on the treatment area which lies directly beneath the centre of the director.

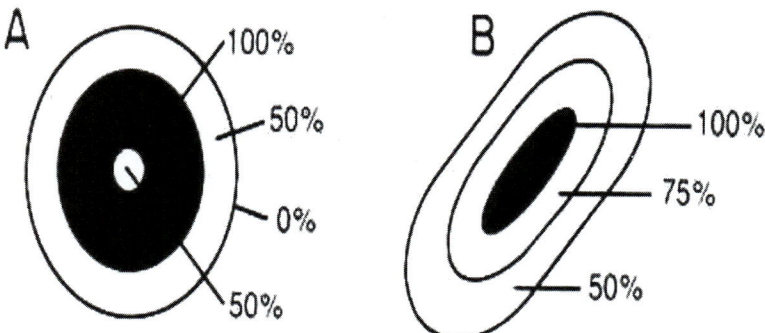

Fig: 3.5 A-Circular Director, B-Rectangular Director

The circular director can be preferred for the superficial bony area which requires less heat in the central part. the rectangular shaped director is preferred for the treatment area which requires more heat in the central part. If the treatment area (skin contour) is uneven the distance from the highest point of the skin to the applicator should be measured. The treatment area which is perpendicular to the applicator or director receives higher MWD rays. The heating effect will be less on the area which is not the perpendicular to the director as it receives less MWD rays.

viii. No towel is required to be placed between the director and the treatment area like short wave diathermy, however, in case of perspiration, it should be watched carefully and removed periodically.

ix. Increase the intensity gradually and wait for the response of the patient. The patient should experience warm that should be comfortable.

x. Treatment time - The treatment time depends on the goal of the physical therapist. If the goal is to increase the extensibility of the connective tissues, the treatment time should be 10-20 minutes. The initial 3 to 8 minute is basically for the tissue temperature to rise to desired levels. Once the temperature reaches to the desired level, an additional 10 to 20 minutes are required to maintain the temperature to gain therapeutic goal[22].

xi. Intensity – There is no scale for determining the intensity. Patient is the best judge to determine the intensity. Patient should experience the sensation of warmth. Increasing beyond the sensation of warmth may cause thermal injury such as burn.

xii. Instruct the patient for heat sensation. Inform the therapist immediately in case of any discomfort or overheating.

xiii. The timer will run out after the treatment is over. Remove the electrode and ask the patient to put on the cloths

References

I. A. Giombini, V. Giovannini, A. Di Cesare, P. Pacetti, Noriko Ichinoseki-Sekinel, M. Shiraishi, Hisashi Naitol and Nicola Maffulli. Hyperthermia induced by mocowave diathermy in the macagement of muscle and tendon injuries. Department of Trauma, and Prthopedic Surgery, Keele University School of Medicine, Stoke on Trent, StaffS, UK, June 2008.

ii. Lehman, J.F. and DeLateur, B.J. Therapeutic Heat, 404-562, 3rd edition, Williams and Wilkins, Baltimore, 1982

iii. Gersten, J.W., Wakim, K.G., Herrick, J.F. and Krusen, F.H. The effect of microwave diathermy on the peripheral circulation and on the tissue temperature in man. Archives OF Ohysical Medicine 1949, 30, 7-25.

iv. Lehman, J.F. and DeLateur, B.J. Therapeutic Heat, 404-562, 3rd edition, Williams and Wilkins, Baltimore, 1982.

v. Virender Kr. Khokhar, electrotherapy for physiotherapy, top publishing company, pp68.

vi. Sheila Kitchen Electrotherapy Evidence Based Practice, 11th edition, pp166.

vii. Brown M, Baker R. Effects of pulsed short wave diathermy on skeletal muscle injury in rabbits. Phys Ther 1987;67:208-214.

viii. Bansal PS, Sobti VK, Roy KS. Histomorphochemical effects of shortwave diathermy on healing of experimental muscular injury in dogs. Indian J Exp Biol 1990;28:766-770.

ix. A. Giombin, V. Giovannini, A. Di Cesare, PPacetti, Noriko Ichinoseki-Sekine, MShiraishi, Hisashi Naito and Nicola Maffulli, institute of sports and medicine and sciene, Rome, Italy, June, 08, 2007.

x. Wiper DJ, McNiven DR. The effect of microwave therapy upon muscle blood flow in man. Br J Sports Med 1976;10:19-21.

xi. Sekins KM, Lehmann JF, Esselman P, et al. Local muscle blood flow and temperature responses to 915 MHz diathermy as simultaneously measured and numerically predicted. Arch Phys Med Rehabil 1984;65:1-7.

xii. Kitchen SS, Partridge CJ. A review of microwave diathermy. Physiotherapy 1980;11:48-53.

xiii. Ogura Y, Naito H, Saga N, et al. Microwave treatment induces heat shock protein 72 in human skeletal muscle. Med Sci Sports Exerc 2006;38 (Suppl).

xiv. Naito H, Powers SK, Demirel HA, Sugiura T, Dodd SL, Aoki J. Heat stress attenuates skeletal muscle atrophy in hindlib-unweighted rats. J Appl Physiol 2000;88:359-363.

xv. Calderwood SK, Theriault JR, Gong J. How is the immune response affected by hyperthermia and heat shock proteins? Int J Hyperthermia 2005;21:713-716.

xvi. Sekins KM, Emery AF, Lehmann JF, Mc Dougall JA. Determination of perfusion field during local hyperthermia with the aid of finite element thermal models. J Biomed Eng 1982;104:272-279.

xvii. Halliwell B, Gutteridge JMC. Free Radicals in Biology and Medicine. Oxford: Clarendon Press; 1985.

xviii. Kannus P, Jòsza L. Histopathological changes preceding spontaneous rupture of a tendon. A controlled study of 891 patients. J Bone Joint Surg (Am) 1991;73:1507-1525.

xix. Laedbetter WBC. Cell-matrix response in tendon injury. Clin Sports Med 1992;11:533-578.

xx. Archambault JM, Preston WJ, Bray RC. Exercise loading of tendons and the development of overuse injuries: a review of current literature. Sports Med 1995;2:77-89.

xxi. Lehman J.F. and DeLateur, B.J. Therapeutic Heat. Third edition, William and Wilkins, Baltimore, 1982

xxii. Bernadette Hecox, Tsega Andemicael Mehreteab, Joseph Weisbeerg, Physical Agents Acomprehensive Text for Physical Therapist, Appleton & Lange Norwalk, Connecticut, pp154.

Chapter 04

Ultrasound Therapy

Ultrasound, a form of acoustic energy is most widely used in the physical therapy practice for its precise deep heating effects. (The sound waves are of mechanical energy, not really electro therapy at all but do fall into the electro physical agents grouping.) The normal sound waves range from 16Hz to 20000 Hz. For the purpose of treatment the sound waves are ranged from 1MHz to 3MHz which are absolutely beyond the capacity of human hearing, therefore, these non audible range of sound waves are known as ultrasound waves.

Therapeutic ultrasound is one of the most widely and frequently used electrophysical agents in the physiotherapy practice. Ultrasound-induced heating is the result of the absorption of ultrasound energy in biological tissues. Therapeutic applications of ultrasonic heating therefore either use longer durations of heating with unfocused beams or use higher-intensity (than diagnostic) focused ultrasound. The use of unfocused heating, for example, in physical therapy to treat highly absorbing tissues such as bone or tendon, can be moderated to produce enhanced healing without injury. Alternatively, the heat can be concentrated by focused beams until tissue is coagulated for the purpose of tissue ablation. Ultrasonic heating, which can lead to irreversible tissue changes, follows an inverse time-temperature relationship. Depending on the temperature gradients, the effects from ultrasound exposure can include mild heating, coagulative or liquefactive necrosis, tissue vaporization, or all three.

For diagnostic ultrasound, temperature elevations and the potential for bioeffects are kept relatively low or negligible[1], by carefully described indications for use, applying the ALARA (as low as reasonably achievable) principal, limited temporal average intensities, and generally short exposure durations.

Production

To produce ultrasound waves the common house current, 60Hz at 110 volts is used. There is a oscillating circuit and a transformer in the ultrasound equipment. The oscillating circuit converts the incoming frequency to the desired frequency i.e. from household frequency to 1MHz or 3MHz. The transformer boosts up the common house current voltage (110V) to the 200-300 volts. This modified energy is carried out by a coaxial cable to the transducer or treatment head.

Transducer – The transducer which contains piezoelectric crystal, converts incoming high frequency into the ultrasound waves through reverse piezoelectric effect. Piezoelectric effect is a phenomenon of developing electric charges on crystal by applying mechanical pressure on the crystal. Reverse Piezoelectric Effect- Following application of the high frequency energy across the crystal there is deformation of the crystal which produces mechanical energy. The crystal deformation changes direction as the flow of current changes direction. The crystal becomes thicker during one half of the alternating current cycle and thinner during the other half of the cycle as the current changes direction. Synthetic ceramic crystals of lead zirconate titanate or barium titanate are used most commonly because of their lower cost and lower voltage requirements. Quartz crystal, which requires 2000-3000 volts for activation, were originally used because of their natural piezoelectric properties. However, the Quartz crystals are not used widely as these are very costlier and require high voltage to get activated.

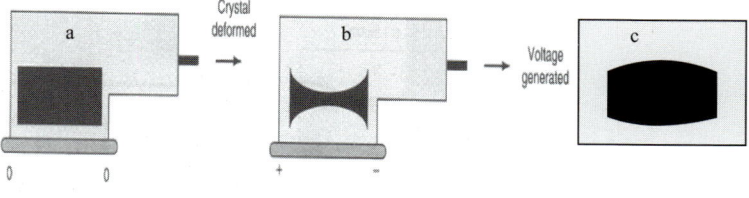

Figure: 4.1 deformation of piezoelectric crystal, a-Normal, b-thinner, c-thicker.

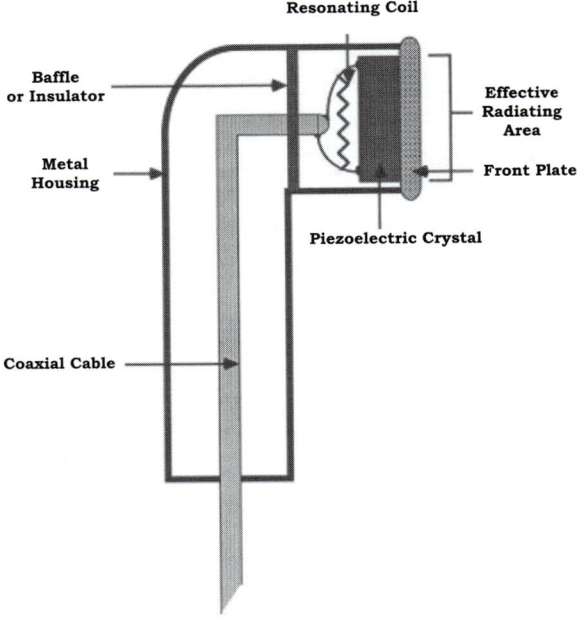

Figure: 4.2 Transducer parts, coaxial cable, metal housing, baffle or insulator, resonating coil, piezoelectric crystal, and front plate

As soon as the ultrasound waves are produced from the transducer they travel in the straight path, as if in a cylinder. The area in which ultrasound waves travel in a straight path from the transducer is known as near field or Fresnel zone. The behavior of the ultrasound waves in this field is far from the regular, with areas of

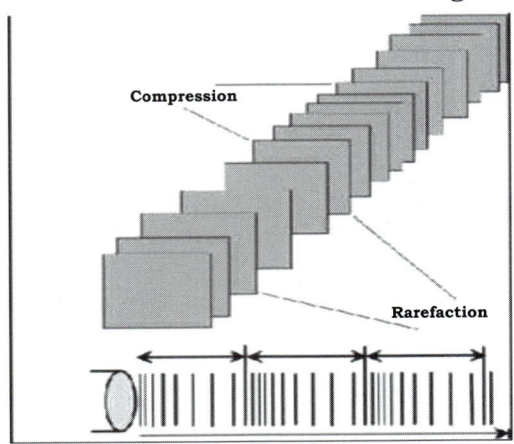

Figure: 4.3 The deformation of the crystal (thinner and thicker) produces longitudinal ultrasound waves which consist compression and rarefaction areas.

significant interference. The intensity of the ultrasound in this field is many times greater than the output set on the machine possibly as much as 12 to 15 times greater. The length of the near field can be calculated using r2/l where r is the radius of the transducer crystal and l is the wave length of the ultrasound. Far field or Fraunhofer Zone- after travelling in straight line, the ultrasound waves start to diverge in the area which is known as Fraunhofer zone. In this area ultrasound waves are more uniform than the near field. For the purpose of therapeutic application, the far field is effectively out of reach.

Physical Characteristics

The waves are eventually transmitted, reflected, refracted, or absorbed in the body. These depend upon the density of the tissue and interfaces between the tissues, through the ultrasound waves transmit. Tissues, when exposed to a sound wave, oscillate about a fixed point rather than move with the wave itself.

Transmission- The impedance to the transmission of the ultrasound waves starts as soon as the waves leave the transducer. Air does not transmit ultrasound waves at all, whereas, a highly homogenous dense medium such as steel will transmit ultrasound waves in a relatively straight pathway at a high velocity.

A less homogenous and low density medium such as water will allow less transmission at a lower velocity. Transmission of waves is directly related to the depth of penetration, whereas, the depth of penetration is inversely related to the frequency of the ultrasound. The effective depth of penetration of the ultrasound is considered to be

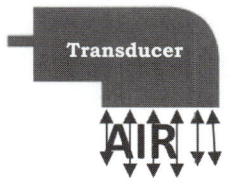 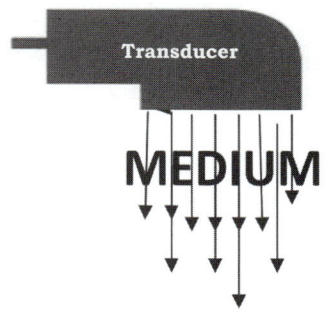

Figure: 4.4 transmission of ultrasound waves, a-reflection at air, b-transmission through coupling medium

from 2.5cm (3MHz) to 5cm (1MHz). As the frequency increases the depth of penetration decreases because attenuation of the ultrasound waves occurs with the increasing frequencies.

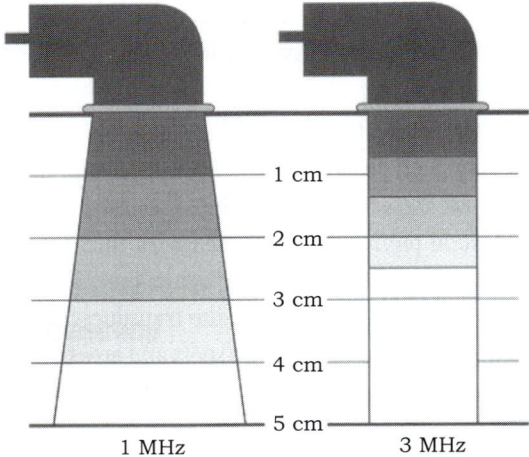

Figure: 4.5 Depth of penetration of the ultrasound waves at tissues, a-1MHz, b-3MHz. Dark to light shadow of the waves shows that as the ultrasound waves pass through various structures its concentration into the deep structures decreases.

Attenuation:- It refers to the combination of absorption and scattering of the waves. Scattering of the ultrasound waves occur in all the living tissues because of non-homogenous composition of different cellular structures. There is production of spherical waves that radiate the reflected waves in all the directions. As the frequency increases, the energy will be scattered in the superficial zone, and will be absorbed in this zone only. Hence, no energy will be available for the deeper structure to penetrate. For the purpose of clinical practice 1MHz ultrasound is most widely used as its deeper depth of penetration (5cm) that allows adequate penetration to treat most of the soft tissue ailments. The depth of penetration of the 3MHz ultrasound is up to 2.5cm which helps in treating most of the superficial soft tissue injuries. 90KHz ultrasound penetrates (10cm) beyond the treatment area is also exposes unwanted soft tissue structures, whereas, 6MHz ultrasound penetrates hardly beyond the skin. Therefore, the depth of penetration increases as the frequency decreases.

Reflection:- Reflection is the returning of the ultrasound waves following imposing on the particular medium. Air reflects all the ultrasound waves (100% reflection) back to the transducer, whereas, water reflects only 0.3% of the ultrasound waves rest of 99.7% waves are transmitted effectively. If even a small air gap exists between the transducer and the skin the proportion of ultrasound that will be reflected approaches 99.998% which means that there will be no transmission of the waves.

Reflection in the body occurs largely at the tissue interfaces, these interfaces include fat to muscles, muscles to fascia, tendon to periosteum, and ligament to periosteum. The greater the difference in the density of the tissues at the interfaces, the larger is the reflection such as at the ligament to periosteum interface. The lesser the difference in the density of the materials at the interface, smaller the reflection such as at the interface of muscle to fascia, and fat to muscles. The angle of reflection, equals the angle of incidence. If the angle of incidence is perpendicular to the tissues, the ultrasound waves will reflect to the transducer (90^0). If the angle of incidence is 45 degree, the wave will reflect at the 60 degree to the opposite side.

Refraction – Refraction is the deflection of the waves when transmitted from one medium to the other medium (from fat to muscles, muscles to fascia, tendon to periosteum, and ligament to periosteum). The angle of refraction depends on the velocity and wavelength of the ultrasound wave. When the ultrasound wave is transmitted from high density medium to a lower density medium, the velocity and wavelength decreases while the angle of refraction becomes less than the angle of incidence.

Absorption – Tissues with highest protein and collagen contents show the greatest amount of absorption of the ultrasound waves. The tissues with their ability of absorption from higher to lower are arranged as follows- bone, peripheral nerves, skeletal muscles, fat, and blood. Water does not absorb the ultrasound waves, it transmits all the waves effectively. The importance of this arrangements is that the skin, fascia, and fat will not significantly absorb the ultrasound waves and therefore, these allow effective transmission of the ultrasound waves to be available into the deeper structures. Thermal effects in the deep structures were not possible if ultrasound waves would have been adsorbed in the skin, face and fat

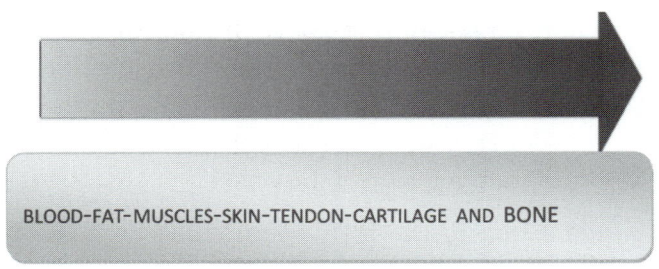

BLOOD-FAT-MUSCLES-SKIN-TENDON-CARTILAGE AND BONE

Fig: 4.6 Arrangement of connective tissues in increasing order of absorption of ultrasound waves. Increasing protein contents in the tissues give increasing absorption

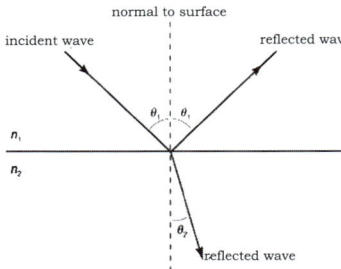

Fig:4.7 ultrasond transmission, reflection, angle of incidence from the transducer

Shear Waves- During mode conversion, a percentage of reflected incident energy is converted from a longitudinal wave form into a transverse or shear wave form which cannot propagate on to the soft tissue side of the interfaces and is therefore absorbed rapidly, causing heat rise at the interfaces mostly between periosteum and the soft tissues. This is extremely hazardous for the tissues as the excessive heat is not dissipated to the non sonated areas easily and can result in periosteum burn. Sometimes symptoms are not observed by either the patient or therapist until the systemic manifestations such as pain and fever are exhibited.[2] The transformation of the longitudinal wave form into the transverse wave form at the periosteum is called the shearing effect and is to be avoided by keeping the transducer at the perpendicular to the treatment area. Shear waves are common at the periosteal region because of high acoustic impedence between the periosteum and other soft tissues that reflect 20% to30% ultrasound waves which become transverse waves. Therapist should ensure that the treatment head at the bony prominences should not be oblique especially during the conversion. Solids have strong three dimensional intramolecular bonding; which allows transverse waves to be transmitted whereas liquids with their weaker intramolecular bonds, ineffective of transmission of shear waves. Hence, the shear waves in the tissues accumulate, and eventually get absorbed by the tissues that leads to excessive heat.

Standing Waves- if the ultrasound head is not moved continuously over the treatment area, ultrasound waves can cyclically be transmitted and reflected to and fro the treatment head. There is overlapping of the reflected and transmitted waves in the tissues. Summation of the waves occurs. When the overlapping ultrasound waves reach equilibrium, they become standing waves. Standing waves are potentially hazardous to biological tissues because high concentration of energy is produced during multiple waves are in phase. In order to avoid standing waves the ultrasound head must be moved constantly over the treatment areas throughout the treatment session.

Physiological Effects

The therapeutic ultrasound is most widely used for its deep thermal effects and non thermal effects. A key element of therapeutic applications of ultrasonic energy is the capability to focus energy several millimeters to centimeters away from the transducer plate. It is, therefore, very important to accurately determine the location of the treatment zone with ultrasound systems. It is too simplistic to assume that with a particular treatment application there will either be thermal or non thermal effects. It is almost inevitable that both will occur, but it is furthermore reasonable to argue that the dominant effect will be influenced by treatment parameters, especially the mode of application i.e. pulsed or continuous.

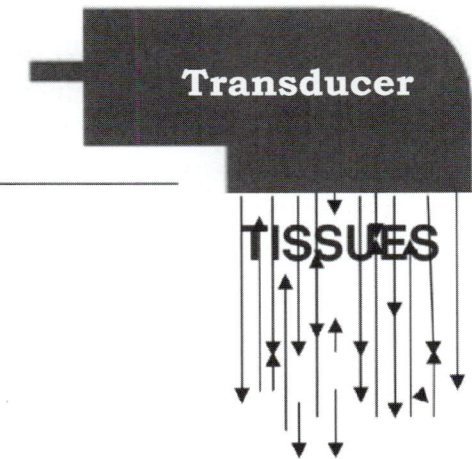

Fig: 4.8 standing waves

Thermal Effects:- Ultrasound-induced heating is the result of the absorption of ultrasonic energy in biological tissues. A biologically significant thermal effect can be achieved if the temperature of the tissues is raised to between 40 and 45 degree centigrade for at least five minutes.[1] The controlled heating in the tissues can produce desirable effects such as relief in pain, decrease in joint stiffness, increase blood flow, increase extensibility of the collagen fibers and scar tissues. The energy produced with 3 MHz ultrasound is absorbed three times faster than that produced from 1 MHz ultrasound although the thermal effects of 1MHz ultrasound last longer. Preheating the treatment area for 15 minutes using a moist heat pack will decrease the treatment time required to reach vigorous heating level by 2-3 minutes in deep (3-cm) tissue using a 1MHz output.[3] Draper at al.[4] found that 3MHz ultrasound at 1.5w/cm2 heated at a rate of .9degree/minute and 1MHz ultrasound heated at a rate of .3degree/minute. These findings make perfect sense because the crystal of 3 MHz ultrasound is deforming three times faster, thus, the energy should be absorbed three times faster[4]. Contrary to the above study, Bradley at al.[55] stated that 3 MHz ultrasound heated at a rate of 1.19degree/min (close to, yet faster than, the Draper at al. 3MHz ultrasound data), whereas, 1MHz heated at a rate of only .13degree centigrade/minute (much slower than the Draper at al 1MHz data). This finding is more than ten times lower and slower than over 3MHz data. They determined, however, that three MHz ultrasound penetrates deeper into tissues than originally theorized, and that alone is new finding.[55]

To produce heating effects in the body the energy must be absorbed by the tissues. The rise of temperature in the tissues depends upon the intensity of the energy, length of time, thermal conductivity, degree of vascularization, and the frequency.

The Factors Affects the Thermal Effects

Intensity- The intensity of the ultrasound should be adequate to produce heating effects in the tissues. Low intensity ultrasound will produce less energy in the tissues that will be inadequate to produce heat in the tissues. On the other hand if the intensity of ultrasound is applied at an extremely high rate, the higher tissue temperature rise will produce pain. In addition to that overheating of the tissues will stimulate thermal nocicepters which may require a withdrawal of the treatment before producing significant tissue temperature rise. Therefore, to produce significant heat in the tissues the intensity of the ultrasound should be between .5w/cm^2 to 2w/cm^2. Therapeutic ultrasound could increase the tissue temperature at a rate of .86degree C per minute with 1W/cm2 intensity.[17]

Treatment Duration- The treatment time should also be considered for heating effects in the tissues. Tissue temperature rise cannot be achieved if the treatment duration is short with low intensity. However, short duration with extremely high intensity will also not allow tissue temperature rise due to stimulation thermal nociceptors (pain). For heating the tissue the optimal duration of between 5 minutes to 10 minutes with intensity of 1.5w/cm^2 to .5w/cm^2 should be used.

Thermal conductivity- the structure which has higher thermal conductivity cannot be heated as the energy is dissipated to the cooler, non sonated surrounding area. Bone has a higher absorption coefficient despite of that it does not become proportionately hotter than the muscles and tendons lying next to it as the heat produced in the bone is quickly dissipated to the cooler nonsonated areas. Moreover, bone reflects 30 percent ultrasound waves to the tendons and ligaments due to greater acoustic difference. The structures with impaired blood circulation is heated excessively as it does not dissipate the heat to the non sonated area. Therefore, thermal injury to these structures is always greater than the tissues which have intact blood circulation.

The amount of temperature increase may also be generator dependant, with some brands potentially producing more heating than other brands. A treatment area two times the effective radiation area can raise the subcutaneous tissue temperature by 6.3F (3.5^0 C) using 1 MHz ultrasound and 14.9.F (8.3^{0}C) using 3MHz ultrasound. Using the same output parameters but increasing the treatment area six times the effective area(much larger than the effective treatment area) results in only 2.3.F (1.3^{0}C) temperature increase.[5]

Non-thermal Effects:- There is a common, widespread belief that heating alone cannot account for the therapeutic effects. Ultrasound can induce effects not only through heating but also through non-thermal mechanisms, including micro-massage, acoustic streaming, ultrasonic cavitation, gas body activation, and other undetermined non-thermal processes.

Micromassage- The term micromassage was used as early as 1942 to describe the action of the ultrasound. The micromassage is referred to the microscopic movements or oscillations of the body fluid as a result of exposure to the therapeutic ultrasound. Ultrasound waves transmitted into a tissue have compression and rarefactional pressure amplitudes of several mega-pascals which help in producing a form of micromassage. The other non thermal effects of the ultrasound are probably as a result of micromassage to the body tissues.

Acoustic streaming- It is defined as the physical forces of the sound waves that provide a driving force capable of displacing ions and small molecules.[24] At the cellular level, organelles and molecules of different molecular weight exist. While many of these structure are stationary, many other are free floating and may be driven to move around more stationary structures. This mechanical pressure applied by the wave produce unidirectional movement of fluid along and around cell membranes.

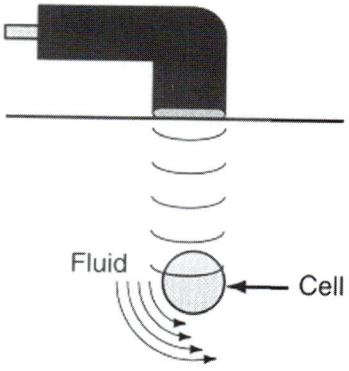

Fig: 4.9 acoustic streaming

Ultrasound causes a stirring effect in the fluid near a biological membrane. This agitation of the ions increases the ionic concentration gradient, thereby accelerating the diffusion rate.[53] The increased membrane permeability could result in therapeutically advantageous changes such as increase secretion form mast cells, increased protein synthesis, increased fibroblast mobility changes, increased uptake of second messenger calcium and increased production of growth factors by macrophases.

Cavitation- Cavitation is defined as the formation of the tiny gas bubbles in the tissues as a result of physical force of the sound waves on micro-environmental gases within fluid. As the sound waves propagate through the tissues, the characteristic compression and rarefaction (microscopic movement) causes formation of microscopic gas bubbles in the tissue fluid to contract and expand. There are two types of the cavitations- stable and transient. Stable Cavitation- These bubbles oscillate to and fro within the pressure waves and remain intact. The stable cavitation, associated with acoustic streaming is considered to have therapeutic values. These types of cavitations are formed at lower intensities. Transient Cavitations- The transient cavitations increase in size over the time with the pressure waves of the ultrasound. When the volume of the bubbles changes rapidly, they collapse and produce high pressure and temperature at the local tissues. It is generally thought that the rapid changes in pressure (caused by the leading and lagging edges of the wave), both in and around the cell, may cause gross damage to the cell. Substantial injury to the cell can occur when microscopic gas bubbles expand and then collapse rapidly, causing a microexplosion. The transient cavitations are the result of high pressure and intensity at the high rate

Ultrasonic cavitation and gas body activation are closely related mechanisms, which depend on the rarefactional pressure amplitude of ultrasound waves. Ultrasound transmitted into the tissues may have rarefactional pressure amplitudes of several megapascals. Cavitation and gas body activation primarily cause local tissue injury in the immediate vicinity of the cavitational activity, including cell death and hemorrhage of blood vessels.

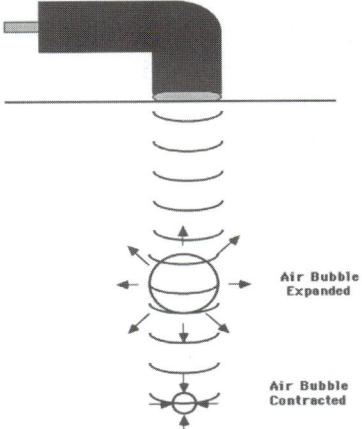

Fig. 4.10 cavitations

Ultrasound Therapy

Other effects: In addition to direct physical mechanisms for bio-effects, there are secondary physical, biological, and physiologic mechanisms that cause further impact on the organism. Alves EM et al., Hundt W at al., and Silberstein J at al.[6-8] state that some effects of vasoconstriction, ischemia, extravasation, reperfusion injury, and immune responses are also achieved through the ultrasound application. Some-times these secondary effects are greater than the direct insult from the ultrasound.

Ultrasound in Tissue Repair

The process of tissue repair is a complex series of cascaded, chemically mediated events that lead to the production of scar tissue that constitutes an effective material to restore the continuity of the damaged tissue.

The application of ultrasound during the inflammatory, proliferative and repair phases is not of value because it changes the normal sequence of events, but because it has the capacity to stimulate or enhance these normal events and thus increase the efficiency of the repair phase.[9] It would appear that if a tissue is repairing in a compromised or inhibited fashion, the application of therapeutic ultrasound at an appropriate dose will enhance this activity. If the tissue is healing 'normally', the application will, speed the process and thus enable the tissue to reach its endpoint faster than would otherwise be the case. The effective application of ultrasound to achieve these aims is dose dependent.

Inflammation - Following an acute injury there is rupture of muscle fibers and micro vessels, resulting in an active bleeding in the tissues (swelling). The area of damaged becomes walled off, and the flow of fluid into the extracellular space eventually ceases. The tissues remain swollen because the excessive extracellular fluid and waste products have not been reabsorbed by the body. In the next process of inflammation tissue scarring occurs as a result of uncontrolled edema. Frequently, the collagen tissue, commonly called scar tissue, is distributed in a manner that impairs the normal function of the tissue. Eventually there is a chronic condition resulting from a periodic microtearing and further scarring.

Inflammation, the early, dynamic phase of repair is characterized initially by clot formation. The blood platelet is a major constituent of the blood clot and, addition to its activities associated with clotting, platelets also contains numerous biologically active substances including prostaglandins, serotonin, and platelet-derived growth factor. During inflammatory phase, the ultrasound has a stimulating effect on the platelets, mast cells, white cells with phagocytic roles and macrophages.[10-13] One of the major chemicals that modifies the wound environment at this stage after injury is the histamine. The application of ultrasound causes stirring effect on the biological membrane of the cell which increases the permeability of the cell membrane. The calcium ions permeability into the mast cells increases. In this process, the membrane of the cell, in response to increased levels of intracellular calcium, ruptures and releases histamine and other products into the wound site, the process of releasing of histamine from the mast cells is known as degranulation of the mast cell.[14-15] By increasing the activity of these cells, the overall influence of therapeutic ultrasound is certainly pro-inflammatory rather than anti-inflammatory. The benefit of this mode of action is not to 'increase' the inflammatory response as such (though if applied with too greater intensity at this stage), it is a possible outcome[16], but rather to act as an 'inflammatory optimiser. The ultrasound encourages edema formation to occur more rapidly.[17-18] Reversible membrane permeability changes to calcium have also been demonstrated by Dino et. al., 1989, Mortimer and Dyson 1988, and Mummery, 1978, by using therapeutic levels of ultrasound.[19-21] The inflammatory response is essential to the effective repair of tissue, and the more efficiently the process can complete, the more effectively the tissue can progress to the next phase to the proliferation.

Proliferation - During the proliferative phase (scar production) ultrasound also has a stimulative effect (cellular up regulation), though the primary active targets are now the fibroblasts, endothelial cells and myofibroblasts.[22-23]

Ultrasound in this stage too pro-proliferative in the same way that it is pro-inflammatory. The application of ultrasound during this stage does not change the normal proliferative phase, but maximizes its efficiency by producing the required scar tissue in an optimal fashion. Harvey et al[52] demonstrated that low dose pulsed ultrasound increases protein synthesis and several research groups have demonstrated enhanced fibroplasia and collagen synthesis. Recent studies have identified the critical role of numerous growth factors in relation to tissue repair, and some accumulating evidence has identified that therapeutic ultrasound has a positive role in producing the scar tissues and maximizing the proliferative phase.

Remodeling - During the remodeling phase of repair, the somewhat generic scar that is produced in the initial stages is refined such that it adopts functional characteristics of the tissue that it is repairing. A scar in ligament will not 'become' ligament, but will behave more like a ligamentous tissue. The application of therapeutic ultrasound can influence the remodeling of the scar tissue in that it appears to be capable of enhancing the appropriate orientation of the newly formed collagen fibers and also to the collagen profile change from mainly Type III to a more dominant Type I construction, thus increasing tensile strength and enhancing scar mobility. Ultrasound applied to tissues enhances the functional capacity of the scar tissues.[24] The role of ultrasound in this phase may also have the capacity to influence collagen fiber orientation.

Precautions

i.   The transducer head should be kept perpendicular to the treatment area, especially, over the bony prominences to prevent formation of shear waves.

ii. The pressure on the treatment area of the ultrasound head should be an optimal to prevent formation of transient cavitations.

iii. While purchasing ultrasound unit the therapist should ensure that the beam nonuniformity ratio (BNR) should be as low as possible preferably 1:2 to prevent formation of hot spots in the tissues.

iv. The intensity of the ultrasound should be carefully calculated for the acute injuries. The use of continuous mode with high intensity for the acute injuries can cause adverse effects in the tissues.

v.   Therapist should be cautious while applying ultrasound over the Bony prominences, decreased sensitivity area, decreased circulation area, peripheral part of the wound and skin cut.

Contraindications

Cancerous lesions, metal implants, pregnant uterus, eyes, heart, reproductive organs, over the spinal column, head, deep vein thrombosis, fractures, tissue under therapy with radiation, growing epiphyseal junction.

Methods of Application

There are several methods of application of ultrasound but moving sound head method is used most widely. The following methods are explained as under:

Stationary Method - The stationary method is generally not used because of its potential thermal injury to the tissues. The cyclical transmission of the ultrasound waves to the tissues increases the energy gradually and produces heat. If the ultrasound head is not moved, the increased heat may cause thermal injury to the underlying tissues which are exposed to the ultrasound waves. Some equipments have high beam non-uniformity ratio (BNR). BNR is the ratio of peak intensity to spatial average intensity. The higher difference in the peak intensity and spatial average intensity produces hot spots especially if the head is stationed. However, some manufacturers are designing stationary mode ultrasound equipments. These equipments have auto switch that runs out if the intensity of the ultrasound is turned higher to the $.5w/cm^2$. If the ultrasound waves transmit parallel to the underlying vessels this may cause impairing of the blood flow. This mechanism is believed to be associated with the production of standing waves that accompany the stationary technique.

Moving Sound Head Method - The transducer must be moved over the treatment area in a smooth rhythmical pattern. It is important to keep the rhythm constant throughout the treatment session. If the ultrasound head moves slowly the tissues will receive high amount of energy, whereas movement of transducer with the high speed will transmit less energy to the tissues. Therefore, a consistent movement of the transducer is required to ensure the even distribution of the ultrasound energy. The speed limit for moving the sound head is approximately 4 cm per second, but the slower, the better. The transducer may be moved in a small overlapping circles and small overlapping strokes.

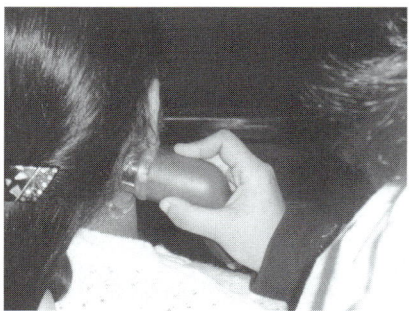

Fig. 4.11 moving sound head method

It is important for the therapist to determine the treatment area. If the treatment area is larger than the transducer, the area should be divided into the parts equivalent to the size of the transducer. The first part is treated for thirty seconds and the head is moved to the second area which is also treated for thirty seconds. This procedure is repeated over the entire treatment area until the total prescribed treatment time is reached or the first two parts should be treated for an appropriate time and then the next two parts. The following steps should be taken while performing the moving sound head method

I.   Explain the procedure

ii.   Place the patient in a comfortable relaxed position.

iii.   Expose the treatment area adequately

iv.   Spread the coupling agent over the treatment area, it should cover the entire area with a thin film.

v.   Select the desired mode- pulsed or continuous.

vi.   Check the meter to ensure that the intensity is at zero

vii.   Place the sound head firmly on the treatment area and glide it smoothly over the treatment area. Increase the intensity gradually with maintaining total contact with the skin. The sound head must be moved smoothly in a rhythmical manner.

viii.   At the end of treatment the timer should run out and stop the output of the power. Turn the intensity control to zero before removing the sound head from the treatment area. Remove the couplant from patients skin and the transducer and place the head in its holder.

Immersion Method - The treatment area, especially peripheral distal joints are exposed to the ultrasound waves in the degassed water. The method is used for irregular surfaces such as joint of the hands and feet, and area that are too sensitive to touch or have broken skin. **Precaution**-the ultrasound generator should be plugged into a receptacle that is protected by a ground fault interrupter (GFI). This will protect both the patient and the therapist from a potential shock associated with leakage of low level current that would not trip a standard circuit breaker. The therapist must put on surgical gloves. The ultrasound head is directed to the skin surface to reduce surface reflection. The head is moved over the treatment area approximately ½ to 1 inches distance from the skin. The Intensity is increased gradually. The therapist must ensure that the head should be perpendicular to the treatment area because the angle of incidence increases the less energy will be transmitted to the area.

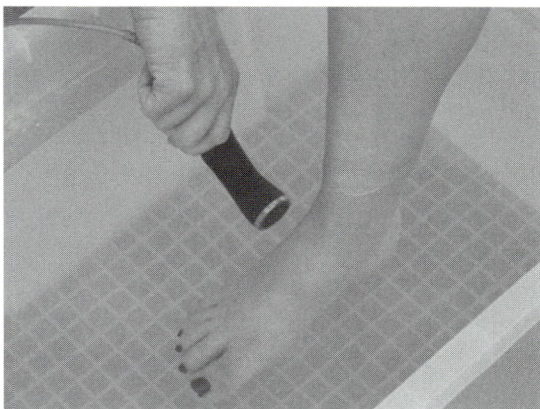

Fig:4.12 Immersion Method

Fluid Filled Method - This method is not used widely but it may be an alternative for treating areas that have irregular contours. Fluid filled method requires a thin membrane bag such as surgical glove or condom and a coupling medium such as degassed water, mineral oil or glycerin. The surgical glove is filled with the degassed water. The transducer head is placed inside the surgical glove and then the mouth of glove is sealed with a rubber band. Spread the coupling agent on the treatment area and place the surgical glove over the area with the firm contact and the ultrasound head is moved within the surgical glove in a smooth rhythmical manner till the prescribed time.

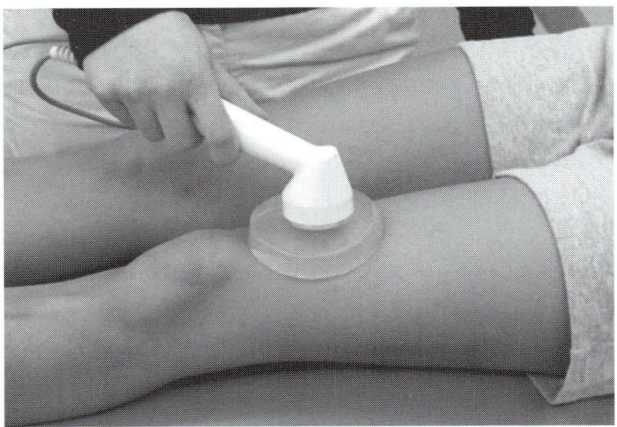

Fig: 4.13 Fluid filled method

Application Parameters

The therapist must ensure following parameters before application of therapeutic ultrasound as ignoring these can be hazardous to the living tissues.

Coupling Medium- Coupling medium is the medium between the transducer and treatment area. Transmission of ultrasound waves depends upon the acoustic impedance of the medium through which they pass. Greater the difference in the acoustic impedence between two mediums, larger the reflection of the ultrasound waves. There is higher difference in the acoustic impedance between the skin and air, hence majority of the ultrasound waves reflect back to the transducer. Therefore, in order to avoid reflection of the ultrasound waves, the acoustic impedance of the coupling medium should be as low as possible or equivalent to the tissues (skin). The best coupling medium in terms of acoustic properties is water as it transmits 99.7% waves because acoustic impedance between water and soft tissues is small.[25] The disadvantage of water is that it cannot be held between the transducer and skin for long time, however, it is the choice of medium especially for peripheral joints such as hand and ankle joints, using immersion method. On the other hand the acoustic impedance between air and skin is very high; hence, air does not transmit the ultrasound waves at all. Aqueous Gels, Oils and Emulsions have similar acoustic properties to water with the advantage that their higher viscosities makes them more users friendly.

The ultrasound can also be used on the wound and cut for accelerating the healing process. The cut or wound cavity is filled with sterile saline up to the edge of cut. Polyurethane film dressing or polyacrylamide agar gel dressing is placed over the wound or cut. A coupling medium is spread covering the dressing including the peripheral part of the wound and cut. The ultrasound head is placed over the dressing and moved continuously in a smooth rhythmical manner till the treatment time is over.

Frequency: For therapeutic purposes 1MHz and 3MHz ultrasounds are commonly used. The effective depth of penetration and rate of heating is based on the output frequency of therapeutic ultrasound. The depth of penetration of ultrasound energy is decreased as the frequency of the ultrasound increases because attenuation occurs in all the living tissues. 1MHz ultrasound targets up to 5cm deep structures, whereas, 3MHz ultrasound targets up to 2.5cm. Therefore, 1MHz ultrasound is advised for the deep soft tissue injuries and 3MHz ultrasound for the superficial soft tissue injuries. The energy produced with 3 MHz ultrasound is absorbed three times faster than that produced from 1 MHz ultrasound although the thermal effects of 1MHz ultrasound last longer. 90 KHz penetrates up to 10cm deep structures whereas; 6MHz ultrasound does not penetrate beyond the skin. Hence 90 KHz and 6 MHz ultrasounds are not used in the physiotherapy practice because of their unwanted exposure and non significant effects to the tissues.

Intensity: The intensity is measured in watts. The output intensity is spread over the transducer of different sizes (centimeters). Therefore, the output intensity (W) is divided by the size of the transducer (centimeter) and represented as W/cm^2. The more accurate term for therapeutic ultrasound intensity is spatial (area) average intensity. If 15W of output intensity is spread over the transducer of 10 square centimeters, the spatial average intensity would be $1.5W/cm^2$ (15W/10sqcm), which is shown by the meter of the equipment. The output intensity emitted by the ultrasound generator may not be spread uniformly on the transducer. The some part especially center, may produce higher energy than the peripheral part of the transducer. The greatest energy produced by the transducer at the center is known as Peak Intensity.

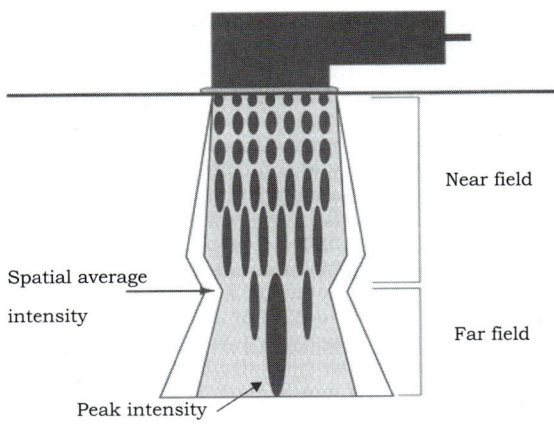

Fig : 4.14 distribution of energy, spatial average and peak intensity

When the pulsed mode is advised, **Spatial Average Temporal Average (SATA)** is used to describe the average intensity over the whole treatment time (average over both on time and off time of the pulse) for a specified area expressed as W/cm^2. SATA = SATP x Duty cycle. **Spatial Average Temporal Peak** is the, spatial average intensity during the on time of the pulse.

Although estimates of treatment intensities are based on a scale of .1 to $2W/cm^2$, the key rule is to rely on the patients response and clinical signs. If the patient experiences pain during the treatment, reduce the intensity immediately. A sharp, stabbing pain is usually a sign of periosteal overheating. A prickling, tingling, stinging, or vibrating sensation under the sound head may indicate an inadequate amount of couplant or inadequate contact with the skin.[53]

Generally for acute conditions, the intensity used should be no higher than $.5W/cm^2$ (SATA).[25] For sub acute conditions $.5W/cm^2$ to $1W/cm^2$ intensity with pulsed mode should be used to produce minimal thermal effects. For chronic conditions 1W/cm2 to 2W/cm2 intensity with continuous mode is advised to produce significant thermal effects in the tissues. The patient should be instructed to warn the therapist if there is any complaint of discomfort.[53] The higher intensities may produce shear waves and unstable cavitation in the tissues; therefore, the ultrasound head shall be kept perpendicular to the treatment surface especially during the conversion and moved continuously over the treatment area with minimal pressure.

Ultrasound Therapy

Continuous and Pulse Modes - Continuous mode of the ultrasound allows transmission of the ultrasound waves continuously into the tissues till the treatment time is over.

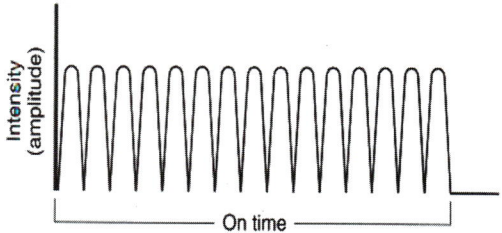

Fig: 4.15a intensity showing on time

Continuous mode is recommended for the chronic conditions to produce significant thermal effects in the tissues. Pulsed mode of the ultrasound is the transmission of the acoustic energy in a brief cyclical breaks into the tissues. The breaks or brief intervals in the transmission reduces acoustic energy concentration in the tissues.

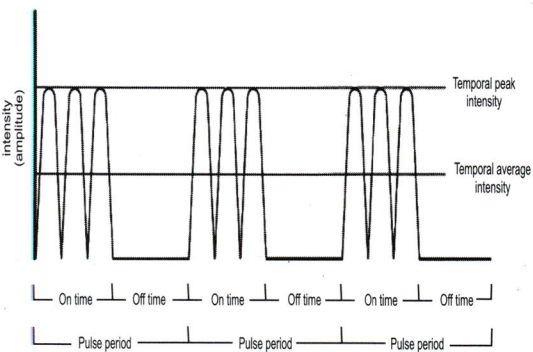

Fig:4.15b pulse ultrasound interruption in the pulses, on time and off time

There is a common belief among the physiotherapy practitioners that the pulsed mode of therapeutic ultrasound is used for the non-thermal effects in the tissues. The fact is that both continuous and pulsed ultrasound will produce thermal effects in the tissues if the intensity is high or non-thermal effects are always accompanied by thermal effects or vice versa. It would be better to say that pulsed ultrasound would transmit less energy than the continuous ultrasound at the same intensity and time. If $1W/cm^2$ of pulsed ultrasound is used for 1minute, the patient receives less energy than if continuous ultrasound is used at $1W/cm^2$ for 1minute.

Because of less transmission of the acoustic energy compared with the continuous ultrasound the pulsed ultrasound is preferred for the acute soft tissue repair.

The depth of penetration is a factor when selecting pulsed or continuous mode. To treat the deep structures like menisci or rotator cuff tendon acute injuries, pulsed mode with high intensity ultrasound should be selected. Unfortunately ultrasound waves cannot be transmitted to the deep structure if the intensity is low with the pulsed mode. To produce energy in the deep structure with the minimal thermal effects, the higher intensity with low duty cycle will allow the energy to penetrate to the deep structure. For example, to treat the supraspinatus tendon in the acute stage, the intensity may be kept high at $2w/cm^2$ with the low duty cycle approximately 25%. High intensity will push the ultrasound waves into the deep structures whereas; low duty cycle would reduce the concentration of the energy which helps in reducing significant thermal effects in the tissues.

Duty Cycle - The duty cycle must be considered to determine the overall energy the patient receives during the pulsed ultrasound. Duty cycle is the percentage or ratio of the pulse duration (on time) to the pulse period (the sum of the on and off time of the pulse) during each cycle. It can be adjusted according to the conditions. The duty cycle should be kept low for the acute conditions. 100 percent duty cycle means no intervals in the transmission of the acoustic energy hence, it is considered continuous mode of ultrasound.

Effective Radiation Area- The effective area of the transducer represents the portion of the transducer's surface area that actually produces ultrasound waves. The effective area is always of lesser area than the actual size of the transducer's face, because most of the energy is concentrated at the center, with less energy produced to the peripheral part of the head.

Beam Non-uniformity Ration (BNR)

Beam nonuniformity ratio is a numerical value that represents the ratio of peak intensity to the spatial average intensity. The acoustic energy is not distributed evenly on the beam (transducer). There will be much higher energy in the center of the beam than the adjacent area of the beam. The higher difference in the peak intensity and spatial average intensity is considered unsafe for the living tissues. The peak intensity is not shown by the meter. If the peak intensity is 12W/cm2 and an average spatial average intensity is 2W/cm^2, the ratio of peak intensity to spatial average (BNR) would be 6:1. Hence, the peak intensity is 6 times greater that the spatial average intensity and if the ultrasound transducer remains stationed this may create hot spot in the tissues. The lower the ratio, the more uniform the beam. The BNR must be considered while purchasing the ultrasound equipment; the company must show the graph of the BNR on the equipment.

Irradiation Time and Surface Area

The treatment time depends upon the stage of the conditions. The first treatment should be shorter than the subsequent treatments. The acute conditions require shorter periods than the chronic conditions. The larger area require more time than the smaller areas. For example the effective area of the transducer is 5cm^2 (transducer) and the treatment area is of 20cm^2. The treatment area is four times larger than the effective area. Therefore, if this area is treated for four minutes, the each area will be irradiated only for one minute. To treat each area for three minutes the treatment time should be 12 minutes in this case. The therapist must divide the treatment area by the effective radiation area before considering the treatment time.

Half Layer Value

There is no depth at which entire ultrasound energy is absorbed, therefore it is common to specify the half value depth or half layer value i.e. - the depth at which half of the initial energy is absorbed[54]. The half layer value indicates the depth at which 50 percent energy is absorbed by the tissues. If ultrasound is applied at 1W/cm^2 and loses 50 percent of its energy at a depth of 2.3 cm, the beam intensity beyond this range is 0.5W/cm^2. At twice this depth (4.6cm, the ultrasound intensity is reduced to 0.25W/cm^2.

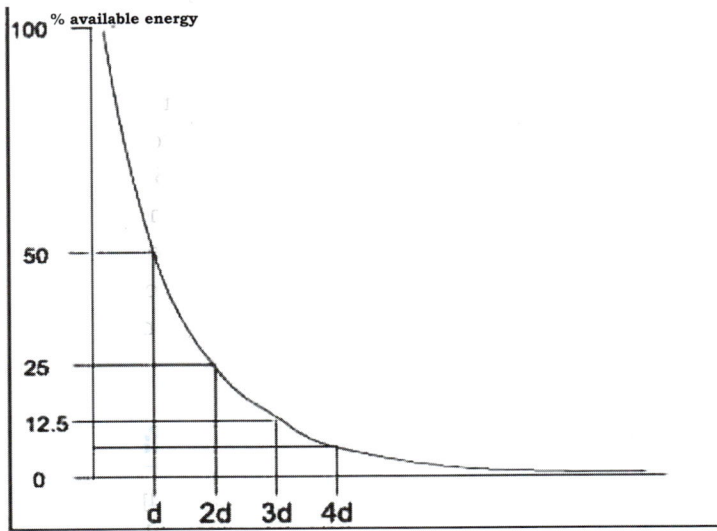

Fig: 4.16 half value depth or half layer value and. The availability of the ultrasound energy from skin to the deeper structures. 100% energy is avalable in the skin and it decreases in the amount as it passes through various structures into the deepeer tissues. As depicted in the figure hundred percent energy is available in the skin, 5o % energy is availabel upto d, 25% energy is available at depth 2d, and no energy availabe at the depth of 4d and beyond 4d.

The energy as it passes deeper to the tissues it decreases exponentially with distance from the source, because a proportion of it is absorbed, at each unit distance so that the remaining amount becomes smaller in percentage of the initial energy. The absorption of the ultrasound energy depends upon the composition of the soft tissue structures, therefore, the half value distance will be different for all the tissues for any given ultrasound frequency.

One of the important parameters of the ultrasound is frequency. Frequency is selected based on the depth of the tissues to be treated. Depth of the ultrasound penetration is usually decreases in terms of the half value depth for the specific ultrasound frequency.

Ultrasound devices have been described for producing therapeutic heating of depth between 1 and $2^{1/2}$ value depth. Therefore, 1MHz continuous ultrasound with a half value depth of approximately 2.3cm is frequently used to treat deep tissues that are approximately 2.3 to 5 cm deep. With its smaller half value depth, 3MHz ultrasound is frequently used to heat the tissues that are more superficial from .8 to 1.6 cm deep.

Phonophoresis

Phonophoresis is defined as the migration of drug molecules through the skin under the influence of ultrasound. However, it is debatable whether these forces are strong enough to produce a net forward movement capable of pushing all drugs through the skin to their target tissue.[25] Hydrocortisone, dexamethasone, and lidocaine are the medications commonly administered through Phonophoresis.[53] Williams described the Phonophoretic effect as a synergistic interaction of ultrasound and drugs.[53] For Phonophoresis, pre heating of the area to be treated is recommended to decrease skin resistance and increase the absorption of the medication.[26] The hydrocortisone should be combined with an aqueous base to form 10 percent concentration is placed immediately on the target area. The transducer is placed on the drug and moved in rhythmical manner throughout the treatment session. Phonophoresis of low intensity and long duration proved to be more effective in deriving cortisol into pig muscles and nerve in a study involving 10 subjects[53], however some studies have shown that to produce effective results, the Phonophoresis should be used at the intensities mid to higher range of $1W/cm^2$ to $2W/cm^2$.

Combination Therapy

The therapeutic ultrasound and electrical stimulation of the muscles may be combined to produce thermal effects in the association with muscle contraction. The ultrasound head serves as an electrode for electrical stimulation current. The combination

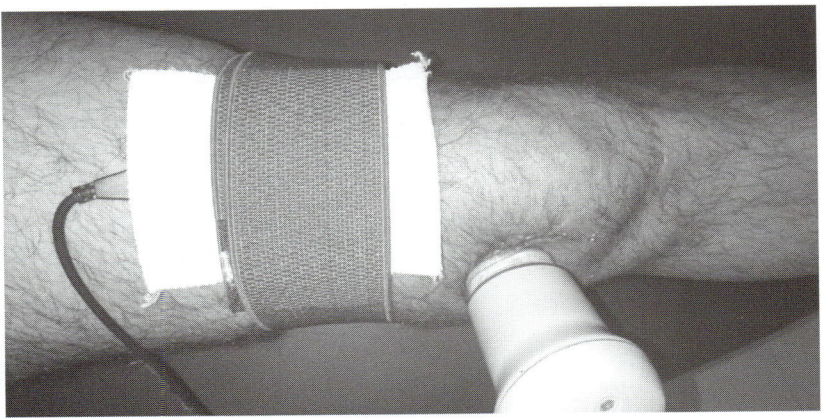

Fig; 4.17 combination therapy

therapy may help in relieving pain of trigger points, muscle spasm, can break adhesions of scar tissues, and increase the blood circulation. When a moderate pulse duration and moderate pulse frequency are applied at an intensity sufficient to produce a strong muscle contraction, the muscle fibers within the trigger point may fatigue to the point where they no longer have the biochemical ability to spasm.

Recent Trends In Ultrasound Application

It has been suggested that an increase of 1^{0}C mild heating over the base line of muscle temperature of 36 to 37 ^{0}C accelerate the metabolic rate in the tissues. An increase of temperature 2^{0}C to 3^{0}C (moderate heating) reduces muscle spasm, pain, and increase blood flow. Vigorous heating, over an increase 4^{0}C or more has been suggested to alter the viscoelastic properties of collagen and inhibit sympathetic activity.

Ultrasound in Fracture Healing

Between 5 and 10% of fractures are complicated by delayed healing.[27] Common causes include inadequate fixation of the fracture, distraction of fracture fragments by fixation devices or traction, repeated manipulations or excessive early motion at the fracture site or excessive periosteal stripping and damage to other soft tissues during operative exposure[28]. Various biological, mechanical and physical interventions have been implemented to improve fracture healing. Low-intensity (energy) pulsed ultrasound (LIPUS) has been used in patients with abnormal fracture healing to enhance fracture recovery and improve functional outcome.

Duarte[29] and Xavier were the first to report acceleration of healing, both radiographically and histologically, with a LIPUS device, at the site of a controlled fibular osteotomy and in a femoral drill-hole defect in a rabbit model. Pilla et al.[31] investigated the effect of LIPUS on the rate of healing of fresh fractures in 139 mature New Zealand white rabbits, which had received a bilateral mid-shaft fibular osteotomy : one limb was subjected to 20 min of LIPUS stimulation a day. The ultrasonic stimulation significantly enhanced fracture healing. Wang et al.[32] reported similar findings in an experiment involving 22 rats with bilateral closed femoral fractures. The fracture in one limb was treated with LIPUS, and the contralateral limb served as the untreated control. Sixteen of the 22 rats were treated with either 0.5 or 1.5 MHz of LIPUS. The remaining six received sham treatment with the ultrasound device to control the effects of anaesthesia and handling. LIPUS at either 0.5 or 1.5 MHz enhanced fracture-healing radiographically, histologically and biomechanically. The average maximum torque and torsional stiffness were significantly greater in the LIPUS-treated limbs than in the control limbs.[33ands56]

Several clinical investigations involving LIPUS[34-37] have shown successful healing of acute fractures, delayed unions and non-unions, including non-unions of fractures fixed with metallic implants. In two different trials of fresh fractures of tibia[38] and the distal radius[39] LIPUS significantly accelerated radiographic healing.

The mechanisms by which ultrasound accelerates bone healing are unknown. In terms of physical mechanism, ultrasounds impart mechanical forces at the cellular level. Mechanical force modulates bone formation both in vitro and in vivo.[40-41] Low-intensity ultrasound produces increased blood flow in an animal fracture model. New blood vessels formed during the inflammatory stage of repair, and in vitro cell studies have demonstrated that exposure to LIPUS increases nitric oxide production and activation of hypoxia-inducible factor-1α, thus leading to increased expression of vascular endothelial growth factor-A levels in osteoblasts. This may stimulate angiogenesis, which is crucial in early bone repair and a necessary precursor to endochondral ossification.[42-43] LIPUS also increases the production of cytokines, such as vascular endothelial growth factor, fibroblast growth factor and interleukin-8 in osteoblasts and periosteal cells[44] all of which are necessary for angiogenesis.[45] Rawool et al. used Doppler sonography to study blood flow around mid-shaft fractures of the ulna in dogs, and found a 3-fold increase in blood flow after 1 week of 20 min daily LIPUS treatment.

Wang et al[46] suggested that the primary effect of LIPUS is on the chondrocyte population in the healing fracture, as LIPUS increases soft-callus formation, advances endochondral ossification of the callus and increases stiffness and strength of the fracture site. Chondrocytes exhibit an increase in aggrecan gene expression [47] and proteoglycan synthesis after LIPUS exposure. Further, Parvizi et al.[48] showed that this stimulation is a result of an increase of LIPUS-induced intracellular Ca^{2+} that occurs within seconds after LIPUS stimulation. The link between LIPUS and intracellular Ca^{2+} does not seem to be unique to chondrocytes. Li et al.[49] demonstrated an increase in osteoblast proliferation after LIPUS exposure. The mechanism for this proliferation was related to an increase in cytosolic calcium.

There is evidence from randomized trials that LIPUS treatment may significantly reduce the time-of-fracture healing for fractures treated non-operatively.[50-51] Simple fractures managed with proper reduction and immobilization should not be the target of the LIPUS therapy. Its function may be more useful for some comminuted and open fractures involving risk patients with associated comorbidities, including elderly, smokers, DM, malnourished. LIPUS also may reduce healing time, and could produce substantial cost savings and decreases in disability associated with delayed union, non-union fractures, and long periods of limb lengthening.

Extensor Carpi Radialis Brevis Tendinitis

Lateral Epicondylitis of elbow also known as tennis elbow is more commoner in the tennis players. Extensor carpi radialis tendon is most frequently (100%) involved in the tennis elbow. The incidence of lateral epiconylitis in recreational and professional tennis players is 39% to 50%.[57] However it occurs in the individuals who are not associated with tennis sport. Any individual using hand tools for work or an avocation are susceptible to developing symptoms. The combination of continuous grip along with repeated wrist and elbow activity precipitates symptoms. The activities such as gripping and lifting that put stress on the ECRB tendon aggravate the symptoms.

The management of lateral epicondilytis involves various therapeutic approaches ranging from non steroidal anti inflammatory drugs to rest, deep transverse friction massage, ultrasound, low energy laser, mobilization, mills manipulation, splint, brace and local steroid injections. Despite of wide range of therapeutic approaches the patients do not report significant improvement in the sign and symptoms, and some time need surgical removal of the proximal calcified tendon of the ECRB. Thus tennis elbow is often associated with prolonged disability. This disability is not necessarily recognized by their medical practitioners as patients frequently, do not return for further treatment. The effects of ultrasound therapy on the lateral epicondylitis on literature are not consistent. There are the studies who claim the results of ultrasound superior than the steroidal injections, however some studies claim just a placebo effects. Ultrasound is a modality that physiotherapist use daily in their clinical practice. There is strong evidence that ultrasound has positive effects on the tendon healing. This strong evidence is supported by animal studies. Stasinopoulos Dimitrious and et al. reviewed the parameters of the therapeutic ultrasound.[58] The effectiveness of ultrasound on tennis elbow is based on its parameters.

Frequency – The most common frequency used in the physiotherapy practice is 1 MHz and 3 MHz. higher the frequency the superficial is the depth of penetration. The LET a superficial condition and the ideal frequency for it is 3 MHz.[59] The studies show negative effects of the ultrasound in the management of lateral elbow tendinopathy because they have used 1 MHz frequency. . Therefore, the negative effects of ultrasound in these studies were expected as one of the most important ultrasound parameter, the frequency, was in wrong direction.

Mode – The mode of ultrasound is based on the progression of the disease. The acute conditions are managed with the pulsed mode and chronic conditions are treated with the continuous mode. The aim of ultrasound on LET should be of non – thermal. The more acute the presentation, the more pulsed the machine output should be used. The pulse ratio should be 1:4 for acute lesion, whereas pulsed ration for chronic conditions should be 1:1.[60]

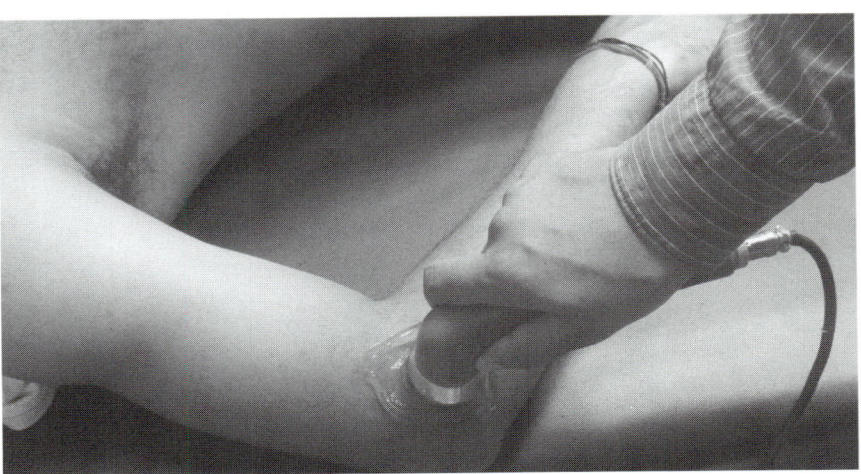

Fig. 4.18 application of ultrasound on tennis elbow

Intensity – The intensity should be between 0.1 and .3 W/cm^2 and should not be higher than 0.5W/cm^2 for acute conditions, where as for chronic conditions it should be between 0.5 and 0.8 W/cm^2 and should be no higher than 1W/cm^2.

Duration - For acute LET the treatment duration should be of 2 minutes and for chronic LET it should be of five minutes.[61] The acute LET requires daily session of ultrasound therapy or sometimes twice daily with the interval of six hours. The chronic LET needs ultrasound session on alternative days.[60] The total treatment sessions are not documented scientifically. Today, ultrasound treatment can occur for several weeks.[59]

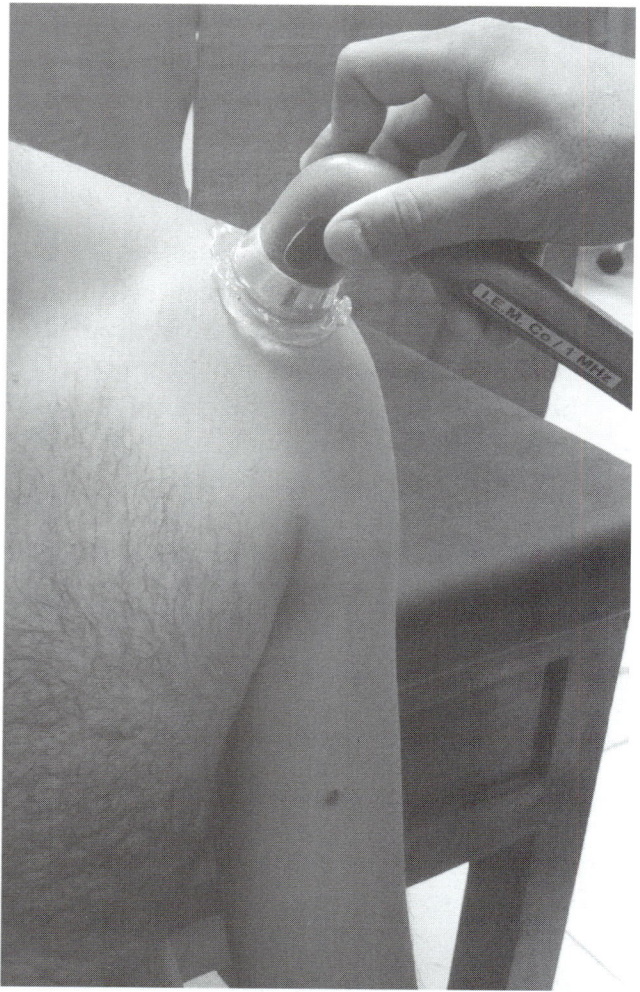

Fig. 4.19 application of ultrasound on subacromial bursa

Ultrasound Therapy

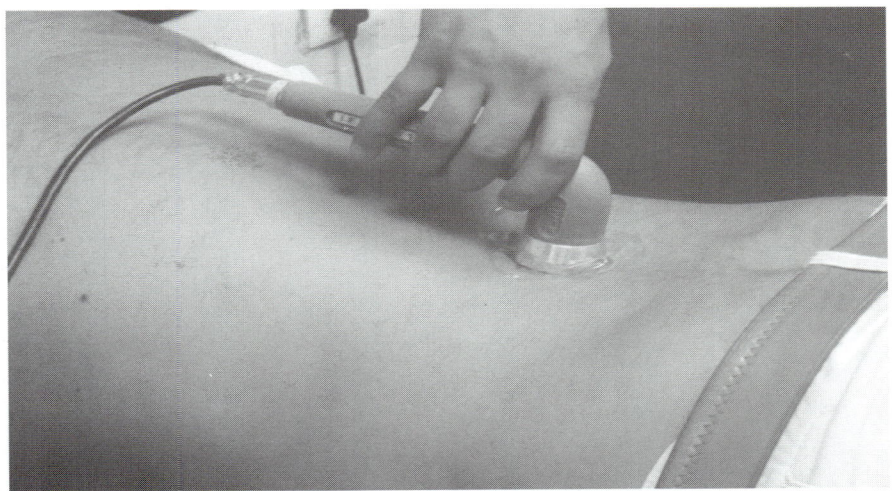

Fig. 20a Application of ultrasound on lumbar spine

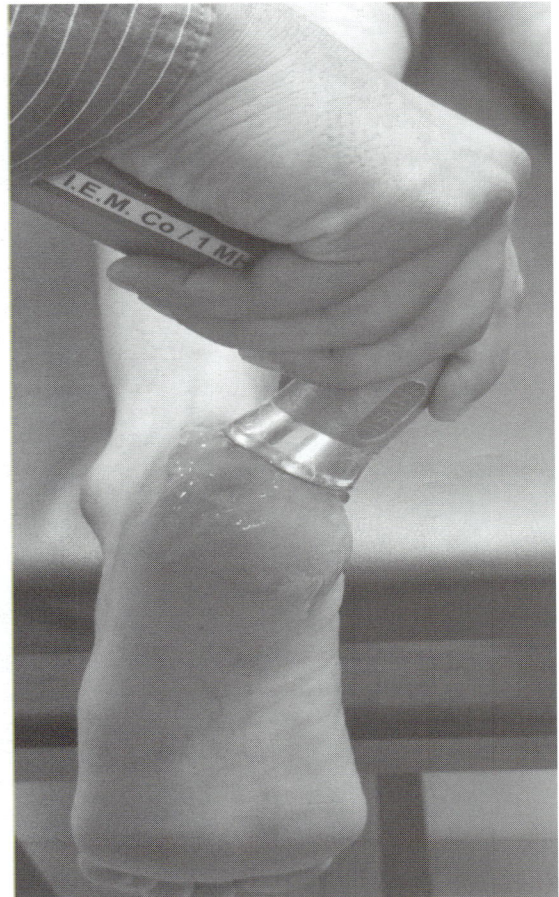

Fig. 20b application of Ultrasound on heel

Ultrasound Therapy

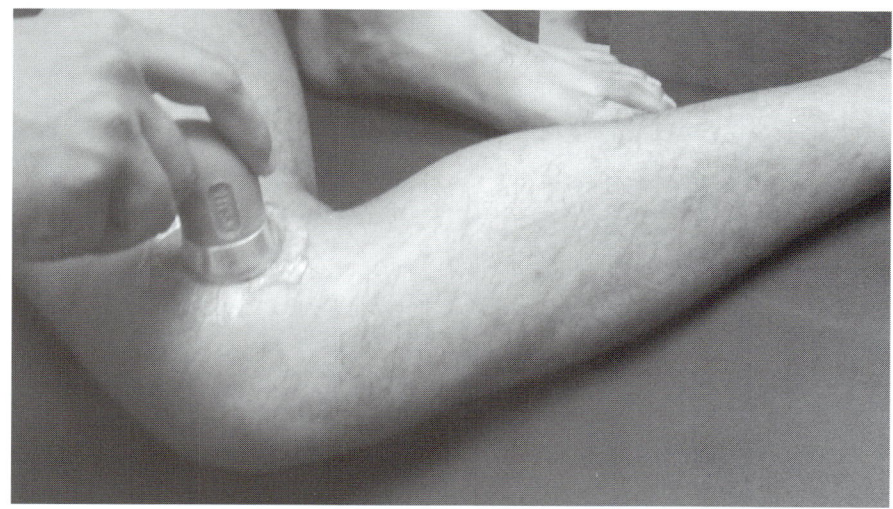

fig. 4.20c application of ultrasound on medial joint space of knee joint

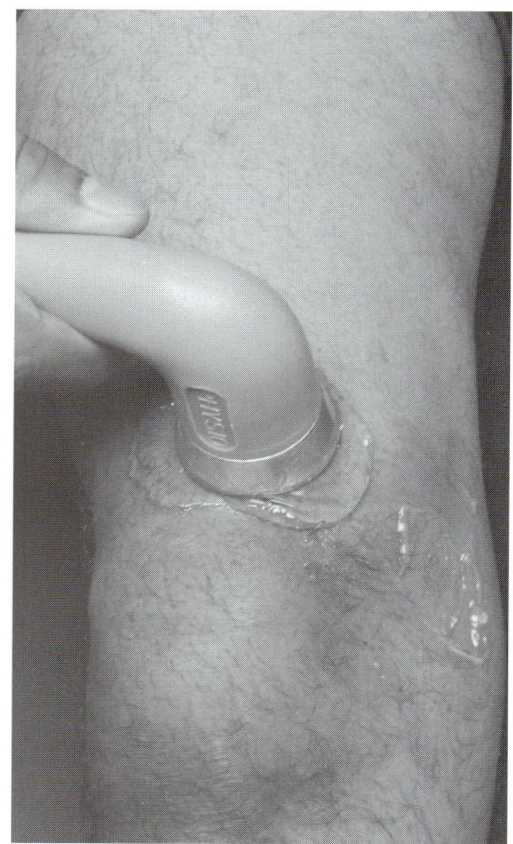

fig. 4.20d application of ultrasound on suprapetaller region of patellofemoral joint

Ultrasound Therapy

References

1. Fowlkes JB. Bioeffects Committee of the American Institute of Ultrasound in Medicine. American Institute of Ultrasound in Medicine consensus report on potential bioeffects of diagnostic ultrasound: executive summary. J Ultrasound Med 2008; 27:503–515

2. Joseph Khan, PH.D., PT. Principles and practice of electrotherapy second edition

3. Draper, DO, et al: Hot pack and 1MHz ultrasound treatment have an additive effect on muscle temperature increase. 33:21, 1998.

4. Draper DO, Castel JC, Castel D. Rate of temperature increase in human muscle during 1MHz and 3MHz continuous ultrasound. J Orthop Sports Phy Ther. 1995; 22;142-150.

5. Garrett, CL, et al. Heat distribution in the lower leg from pulse short wave diathermy and ultrasound treatment. J Athletic Training35:50, 2000.

6. Alves EM, Angrisani AT, Santiago MB. The use of extracorporeal shock waves in the treatment of osteonecrosis of the femoral head: A systematic review. Clin Rheumatol 2009; 28:1247–1251.

7. Hundt W, Yuh EL, Bednarski MD, Guccione S. Gene expression profiles, histologic analysis, and imaging of squamous cell carcinoma model treated with focused ultrasound beams. Am J Radiol 2007; 189:726–736.

8. Silberstein J, Lakin CM, Parsons JK. Shock wave lithotripsy and renal hemorrhage. Rev Urol 2008; 10:236–241

9. Ter Haar, G. "Therapeutic Ultrsound." Eur J Ultrasound 9: 3-9. Watson, T. (2008). "Ultrasound in contemporary physiotherapy practice." Ultrasonics 1874-9968 (Electronic).1999, Vol 48 ; 321-329.

10. Nussbaum, E. "The influence of ultrasound on healing tissues." Journal of Hand Therapy. 1998, 11(2): 140-7.

11. Ter Haar, G. "Therapeutic Ultrsound." Eur J Ultrasound. 1999, 9: 3-9.

12. Fyfe, M. C. and L. A. Chahl (1982). "Mast cell

degranulation: A possible mechanism of action of therapeutic ultrasound (Abstract)." Ultrasound in Med & Biol 8(Suppl 1): 62.,

13. Maxwell L. "Therapeutic ultrasound: Its effects on the cellular & mollecular mechanisms of inflammation and repair." Physiotherapy. 1992, 78(6): 421-426.

14. Mortimer, A. J. and M. Dyson. "The effect of therapeutic ultrasound on calcium uptake in fibroblasts." Ultrasound in Med & Biol. 1998, 14(6): 499-506.

15. Leung, M. C., et al. "Effect of ultrasound on acute inflammation of transected medial collateral ligaments." Arch-Phys-Med-Rehabil. 2004,85(6): 963-6.)

16. Ciccone et al , Ciccone, C. D., et al. (1991). "Effects of ultrasound and trolamine salicylate phonophoresis on delayed-onset muscle soreness." Phys Ther 1991,71(9): 666-75; discussion 675-8.

17. Fyme MC, Chahl LA. The effect of single or repeated application of therapeutic ultrasound on plasma extravasation during silver nitrate induce inflammation of the rate hindpaw and ankle joint in vivo. Ultrasound in medicine and Biology. 1985, 11: 273-283)

18. Watson, T. and S. Young. Therapeutic Ultrasound. Electrotherapy : Evidence Based Practice. Edinburgh, Churchill Livingstone – Elsevier,2008.

19. Dinno et. al. The significance of membrane changes in the safe and effective use of therapeutic and diagnostic ultrasound. Physics in Medicine and Biology,1989, 34: 1543-1552,

20. Mortimer and Dyson. The effect of therapeutic ultrasound on calcium uptake in fibroblast. Ultrasound in Medicine and Biology. 1988 14:499-506

21. Mummery. The effect of ultrasound on fibroblast in Vitro. PhD Thesis, University of Londan, 1978.

22. Ramirez et al 1997, Mortimer, A. J. and M. Dyson (1988). "The effect of therapeutic ultrasound on calcium uptake in fibroblasts." Ultrasound in Med & Biol. 1997, 14(6): 499-506.,

23. Watson, T. and S. Young. Therapeutic Ultrasound. Electrotherapy : Evidence Based Practice. Edinburgh, Churchill Livingstone. 2008.

24. Klucinec, B, et al. The transducer Pressure Variable: its influence on acoustic energy transmission. J Athletic Training 35:417, 2000.

25. Sheila Kitchen. Electrotherapy Evidence Based Practice, 11th edition.

26. Quillen WS. Phonophoresis: A review of the literature and technique. Athletic Training15 : 109, 1980.

27. Praemer A, Furner S, Rice DP. Musculoskeletal Conditions in the United States. Park Ridge, IL: The American Academy of Orthopaedic Surgeons; 1992. p.85-124.

28. Einhorn TA . Enhancement of fracture-healing. J Bone Joint Surg Am 1995;77-A:940-56.

29. Duarte LR. The stimulation of bone growth by ultrasound. Arch Orthop Trauma Surg 1983;101:153-159.

30. Xavier CAM, Duarte LR. Treatment of non-unions by ultrasound stimulation: first clinical applications. Read at the Annual Meeting of the American Academy of Orthopaedic Surgeons, San Francisco, California, 25 January. 1987.

31. Pilla AA, Mont MA, Nasser PR, et al. Non-invasive low-intensity pulsed ultrasound accelerates bone healing in the rabbit. J Orthop Trauma 1990;4:246-253

32. Wang SJ, Lewallen DG, Bolander ME, et al. Low intensity ultrasound treatment increases strength in a rat femoral fracture model. J Orthop Res 1994;12:40-7.

33. Wang SJ, Lewallen DG, Bolander ME, et al. Low intensity ultrasound treatment increases strength in a rat femoral fracture model. J Orthop Res 1994;12:40-7.

34. hoffie M, Duarte LR. Low-intensity pulsed ultrasound and effects on ununited fractures. Read at the Orthopaedic Health Conference, University Hospital, University of Sao Paulo, Brazil, June 15. 1994.

35. Knoch GH, Klug W. Stimulation of Fracture Healing with Ultrasound. Telger TC, editor. New York: Springer; 1991. Dijkman BG, Sprague S, Bhandari M. Low-intensity pulsed ultrasound: nonunions.Indian J Orthop 2009;43:141-8.

36. Griffin XL, Costello I, Costa ML. The role of low intensity pulsed ultrasound therapy in the management of acute fractures: a systematic review. J Trauma2008;65:1446-52.

37. Walker NA, Denegar CR, Preische J. Low-intensity pulsed ultrasound and pulsed electromagnetic field in the treatment of tibial fractures: a systematic review. J Athl Train 2007;42:530-5.)

38. Heckman JD, Ryaby JP, McCabe J, et al. Acceleration of tibial fracture-healing by non-invasive, low-intensity pulsed ultrasound. J Bone Joint Surg Am 1994;76-A:26-34.

39. Kristiansen TK, Ryaby JP, McCabe J, et al. Accelerated healing of distal radial fractures with the use of specific, low-intensity ultrasound. A multicenter, prospective, randomized, double-blind, placebo-controlled study. J Bone Joint Surg Am 1997;79-A:961-73.

40. Binderman I, Zor U, Kaye AM, et al. The transduction of mechanical force into biochemical events in bone cells may involve activation of phospholipase A2.Calcif Tissue Internat 1988;42:261-66.

41. Rubin C, Gross T, Qin YX, et al . Differentiation of the bone-tissue remodeling response to axial and torsional loading in the turkey ulna. J Bone Joint Surg1996;78-A:1523-33.

42. Reher P, Harris M, Whiteman M, et al. Ultrasound stimulates nitric oxide and prostaglandin E2 production by human osteoblasts. Bone 2002;31:236-41.

43. Wang FS, Kuo YR, Wang CJ, et al. Nitric oxide mediates ultrasound-induced hypoxia-inducible factor-1a activation and vascular endothelial growth factor-A expression in human osteoblasts. Bone 2004;35:114-23.

44. Leung KS, Lee WS, Tsui HF, et al. Complex tibial fracture outcomes following treatment with low-intensity pulsed ultrasound. Ultrasound Med Biol2004;30:389-95.

45. Reher P, Harris M, Whiteman M, et al. Ultrasound

stimulates nitric oxide and prostaglandin E2 production by human osteoblasts. Bone 2002;31:236-41.

46. Wang FS, Kuo YR, Wang CJ, et al. Nitric oxide mediates ultrasound-induced hypoxia-inducible factor-1a activation and vascular endothelial growth factor-A expression in human osteoblasts. Bone 2004;35:114-23.

47. Yang KH, Parvizi J, Wang SJ, et al. Exposure to low intensity ultrasound increases aggrecan gene expression in a rat femur fracture model. J Orthop Res1996;14:802-9.

48. Parvizi J, Parpura V, Greenleaf JF, et al. Calcium signaling is required for ultrasound-stimulated aggrecan synthesis by rat chondrocytes. J Orthop Res2002;20:51-7.

49. Reher P, Harris M, Whiteman M, et al. Ultrasound stimulates nitric oxide and prostaglandin E2 production by human osteoblasts. Bone 2002;31:236-41.

50. Heckman JD, Ryaby JP, McCabe J, et al. Acceleration of tibial fracture-healing by non-invasive, low-intensity pulsed ultrasound. J Bone Joint Surg Am 1994;76-A:26-34.

51. Kristiansen TK, Ryaby JP, McCabe J, et al. Accelerated healing of distal radial fractures with the use of specific, low-intensity ultrasound. A multicenter, prospective, randomized, double-blind, placebo-controlled study. J Bone Joint Surg Am 1997;79-A:961-73.

52. Harvey W, Dyson M, Pond JB and Grahame R(1975), The in vitro stimulation of protein synthesisin human fibroblasts by therapeutic levelsof ultrasound, Proceedings 2nd European Congresson Ultrasonics In MediCine. Excerpta medica International Congress Series. 363, 10-21.

53. Bernadette Hecox, Tsega Andemicael Mehreteab, and Joseph Weisberg, Physical Agents, Comprehensive textbook for Physical Therapist, Appleton and Lange, Norwalk, Connecticut

54. Basanta Kumar Nanda, electrotherapy Simplified 2nd

edition.

55. Bradley T. Hayes, Mark A, Merrick and Mitchell L. Cordova, J Athl Train, 2004 July-Sep, 39(3):230-234

56. Azuma Y, Ito M, Harada Y, et al . Low-intensity pulsed ultrasound accelerates rat femoral fracture healing by acting on the various cellular reactions in the fracture callus. J Bone Miner Res 2001;16:671-80

57. Nirschel RP. Soft tissue injuries about the elbow. Clin Sports Med. 1986;5:637-652.

58. Stasinopoulos Dimitrious, Cheimonidou Areti-Zoe and ChatzidamianosTheodoros. Are there Effective Ultrasound Parameters in the Management of lateral Elbo Tendinopathy? A systematic Review of the Literature. Int J Phy Med Rehabil 2013,1:3.

59. Prentice W 2009. Therapeutic modalities for sports medicine and athletic training 6th edition, McGrawHill.

60. Watson T 200. Electrotherapy evidence based therapy, 12th edition, Churchill Livingstone Elsevier.

61. Watson T 2000. The role of electrotherapy in contemporary physiotherapy practice. Man Ther 5:132-141.

Chapter 05

Superficial Heating Modalities

Clinicians have been using the thermal agents for last thousands of years for various ailments. The therapeutic superficial heating modalities are primarily used for elevating the temperature of the skin, subcutaneous tissues, superficial joints, muscles (through reflex mechanism) and the collagen tissues to increase their flexibility.

Increased local tissue temperature accelerates the healing process by dilating blood vessels and shifts the oxy-hemoglobin dissociation curve to increase the oxygen and nutrient supply to the tissues[1] as well as fibroblast proliferation[2], accelerating endothelial cell proliferation[17], and improve phagocytic activity of inflammatory cells.[3] The superficial heating agents must be capable of increasing the skin temperature within the range of 104°F TO 113°F to produce therapeutic effects.[18]

The basic principle of any thermal modality is the transfer of heat across a temperature gradient. The temperature is transferred from the hot object to the cold object. Application of hot pack causes transfer of the temperature to the body, whereas, the application of cold pack causes transfer of heat from the body to the cold pack. If the temperature of both the object is same no heat transfer takes place. The application of the heat to the body causes heat exchange due to the temperature gradient, the larger the temperature gradient, the greater the heat exchange between the modality and the tissues.

The temperature of the skin is approximately 33°C which is easily influenced by the ambient temperature, humidity, exercise, food and alcohol consumption. The deeper the tissue within the body, the higher the temperature. The modalities like paraffin wax bath, moist hot packs, contrast bath, and infrared rays produce heating effect on the skin which is absorbed by the skin. As per the law of Grothus-Draper which states that heat energy absorbed by one tissue layer cannot be transmitted to the deeper layers. Most of the energy is absorbed by the superficial structures and less energy or very minimum energy is transferred to the deeper structure. To produce therapeutic temperature in the muscle or deeper structures the temperature must be raised between $42^{\circ}C$ and $45^{\circ}C$, therefore, the temperature of the skin should be raised from $33^{\circ}C$ to $45^{\circ}C$ which is not allowed by thermo-receptors. Hence, there modalities have more heating effects in the superficial structures. On the other hand, the ultrasound and short wave diathermy energy is not significantly absorbed by the superficial structures. The energy is transferred to the deeper structures, where it is absorbed. This is the reason that shortwave and ultrasound modalities produce deep heating effects.

Heat Transfer Methods

There are three methods of transfer of heat namely conduction, convection and radiation. The superficial heating modalities transfer the heat by conduction and convection method whereas; deep heating modalities such as short wave diathermy and ultrasound transfer the heat by radiation method. The difference between the superficial heating modalities and deep heating modalities is that the deep heating modalities transfer the heat to the deep structures without heating up the skin and subcutaneous tissues significantly . Whereas; the superficial modalities heat up the skin and subcutaneous tissues first and then heat is transferred to the deeper structures if the patient tolerates, therefore; there would be more heat in the superficial tissues than the deeper tissue.

Conduction – The heat energy is transferred by direct contact. When hot packs of higher temperature are placed on body the tissues would come in contact with the hot source. Therefore, the heat from hot packs would be transferred to the tissues. The tissues close to hot packs would heat up first and then heat would be transferred to the next tissues (cooler part). Therefore, the kinetic motion atoms and molecules of one object is passed on to another object is often described as "atoms jostling one another". Similarly when the ice pack is placed on tissues heat is transferred to the ice pack. The tissues closest to the ice pack looses its temperature first and then the adjacent tissues. The process of conduction of heat from tissues to the ice pack continues till both the mediums have equal temperature.

The grater the temperature gradient between the skin and the hot packs greater, the resulting tissue temperature change. The change in the temperature of the skin occurs immediately of the hot pack application; however; deeper tissue structures require longer time and more intense heating agents to elevate the temperature.

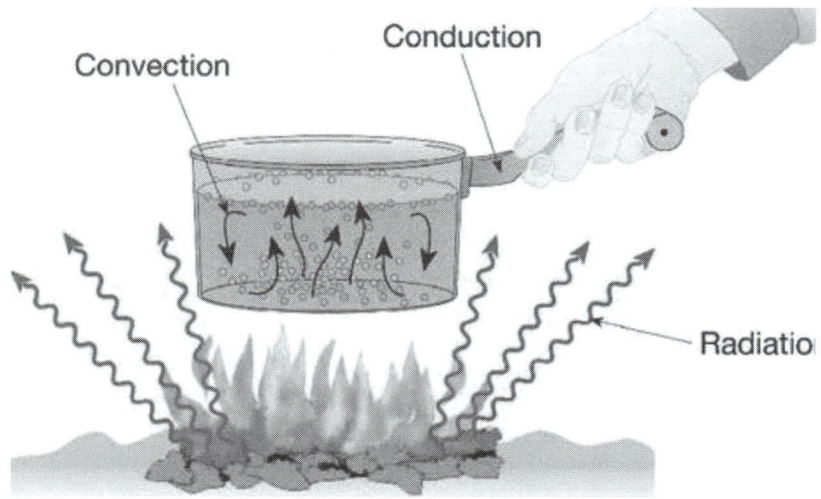

Figure 5.1 Methods of heat transfer

Convection – Convection is the transfer of heat by mass motion of a fluid such as air or water when heated fluid is caused to move away from a source of heat, carrying energy with it. This method of heat transfer is more rapid than conduction and occurs in liquids and gases.[4] Heating of a pot of eating vessel over a flame expands the water. The heated water becomes more buoyant. The molecules move further apart and the fluid becomes less dense. In consequence, the part of the fluid rises and displaces the more dense fluid above, which in turn descends to take its place, and the pattern of circulation is formed. Similarly, when the baseboard heater heats up the air adjacent to it, the warmer air will expand and rise to the ceiling which descends the cooler air towards baseboard heater. There will be circulation of the warmer air (less dense/lighter) towards ceiling and cooler air (high dense/heavier) towards baseboard heater. The process would be continued till the temperature of the room is equivalent to the temperature of the air emitted by the baseboard heater. The rising warmer air molecules collide with the descending cooling resulting some heat is conducted.

Radiation – The objects receive or transfer the heat through the process of radiation. Radiation is the transfer of heat in the form of waves through space. Dull black surfaces are better than white shinning ones at absorbing radiated heat. The transmission of the sun rays to the earth is through the process of radiation. The objects emit energy at infra red frequencies will radiate from the hot objects and be absorbed in a cooler object. The molecules of hot object are in a state of rapid vibration, or are at the centre of rapid periodic disturbances, producing electromagnetic waves, and that there waves travel between the hot body and the receiving body causing a similar motion in the molecules. The heat is produced as the result of kinetic motion of the tissues and absorption of the waves.

Physiological Effects of Heat

The application of heat to the body is aimed to achieve certain physiological effects in order to decrease pain and muscle spasm. Elevation of the temperature of the tissues should be within the therapeutic range. Lehman and deLateur stated the therapeutic range of tissue temperature should be between $40^{\circ}C$ and $45^{\circ}C$. Excessive temperature above $45^{\circ}C$ can unnecessarily heat up and damage the tissues. The elevation of the temperature of the local area increases blood circulation. The cooler blood circulates into the heated area and removes some of the heat. If the rate of temperature increase is very slow the amount of heat could be balanced out by the convective effect of cooler blood, and therapeutic effects may not be achieved.

The physiological effects of the temperature on the tissues depend upon the rate at which heat is being applied to the tissues, duration of the treatment, and the area of tissue exposed to the heating modality. The common physiological effects produced by the temperature rise are – increase metabolic activity, hemodynamic function, neural response, skeletal muscle activity, and collagen tissue physical properties.

Metabolic Response – Temperature elevation within the therapeutic range increases the metabolic activity and chemical reactions in the cells of the body. The leucocytes and phagocytes of white cells play important role in accelerating heating process. The increase metabolic rate following tissue temperature rise increase the activity of leucocytes and phagocytes of white cell which in turn hasten the healing process and restore the damaged tissues. Furthermore, increased blood circulation would increase oxygen uptake, therefore, more nutrients will be available to promote tissue healing[6]. The cellular activity and metabolic rate increases two to three times for each 10^0C temperature.

Vascular Response – Skin blood flow has an important role both in nutrition and in the maintenance of constant core body temperature of 37^0C, and is primarily under the control of sympathetic adrenergic nerve.[7] Application of heat to the body elevates temperature, produces vasodilatation, decreases viscosity of the blood and increases blood circulation of a local area. The temperature elevation causes sweat secretion and the enzyme kallikrein is released from sweat glands which acts on the globulin, and kininogen, to release bradykinin.[8] These chemical mediators act on the smooth muscle tone and endothelial cell contractility which in turn increase capillary and post capillary venule permeability. The increase capillary hydrostatic pressure allows outward fluid filtration from vascular to extra-vascular spaces that results increase in interstitial fluid. There is increase nutrients, leucocytes (enhances tissue healing) and rate of clearing of metabolites. All these contribute in relieving pain and muscle spasm.

Reflex Vasodilatation – Following application of heat to the body, there is elevation of temperature of a local area, that results in vasodilatation. This vasodilatation is not limited to the area where the heat is applied directly but also occurs in areas that are not directly heated. For example application of heat to the lower back area can increase the cutaneous blood flow at the feet. Reflex vasodilatation may be beneficial for the patient with peripheral vascular diseases.

Neuromuscular Response – Superficial heating therapy modalities raise tissue temperature which may elevate pain threshold, alter nerve conduction velocity and change muscle spindle firing rates. Muscle spasm is mainly of protective type which results from overuse during exercise, injury, trauma or pathological changes in the tissues. Muscles guard the joint to prevent the movement and pain, therefore, sustain contraction of the muscle in order to prevent movement in the joint, further contributes to the pain. The muscle spindle (afferent) that alter their rate of firing, primarily in response to tonic or static stretch, are the type II afferents. Superficial heating modalities do not raise the temperature of the muscle at the therapeutic level so do not alter type II afferent directly. The elevation of the skin temperature at the therapeutic level demonstrated to produce a decrease in gamma efferent activity which reduces the stretch on the muscle spindle and afferent firing from the spindles.

PARAFFIN WAX BATH

Paraffin wax bath therapy is a superficial heating method of the soft tissues used to treat chronic joint disorders and to reduce secondary muscle guarding. It is most commonly used for the treatment of the distal joint such as ankle, foot, knee, hands, wrist and elbow of the extremities. The heat is transferred to the tissues through the conduction. The paraffin wax has three important physical characteristics that makes it an efficient source of heat –

I. The melting temperature of the paraffin wax is 54^0C. The melting temperature is lowered to 42^0C by adding paraffin oil or mineral oil to it. The ratio of paraffin wax and paraffin oil should be 6:1.[8] Petroleum jelly may also be added to the bath for an adequate lubrication effect that helps in suppling and easy removal from the body. The ratio of solid wax, paraffin oil (mineral oil) and petroleum jelly should be 2:1:1.[10]

ii. The specific heat of the paraffin wax is 2.72kj/kg/^{0}C which is lower than the specific heat of water 4.2kj/kg/^{0}C. Low specific heat allows for application at a higher temperature than water without the risk of burn. It means that it does not feel as hot as water at the same temperature; therefore, there is much less risk of a burn with the treatment of paraffin wax bath.

iii. The paraffin wax conducts heat more slowly than the water at the same temperature. Low thermal conductivity allows for heating of tissues to occur more slowly, thus reducing the risk of overheating the tissues. This helps in preventing burn as tissues are heated up more slowly.

These, three aforementioned physical characters low melting temperature, low specific heat and slow conduction make the paraffin wax more user friendly in the physiotherapy clinical practice.

Therapeutic Uses

The paraffin wax bath therapy is commonly used to reduce the secondary muscle spasm or guarding following arthritic conditions such as rheumatoid arthritis, osteoarthritis, and post fracture stiffness of the joints. The application of wax does not increase inflammation as it is a superficial heating modality; hence, it is the safest modality in reduction of pain and spasm of the patients with arthritis. However; wax is used in non-flare phases to decrease pain and increase flexibility of the tissues. Restriction of range of motion due to lightnes of the joint capsule, ligaments and muscles as a result of post fracture cast application can also be improved by application of paraffin wax bath. Wax helps in increasing the local blood circulation of the tight structures. Stretching exercises following wax therapy increases the flexibility of the tight structures and the range of motion of the joint. To improve skin pliability over healed areas, a temperature of $47^{\circ}C$ has been suggested.[11] stretching following application of wax demonstrated a maintainable average range, and increase range of motion of 7° to 10° in the joints of patients with burn scars.[12]

Paraffin Wax Bath Unit

There are several types of paraffin wax bath units which are made up of stainless steel. The equipment should have electric heating element with thermostat control between $35^{\circ}C$ and $85^{\circ}C$. The unit should have a protective earth connection and must be connected to a wall socket with protective earth. Ideally the tank for the clinical practice should have wax capacity of 25 to 30 litters. As soon as the temperature of the tank reaches to the upper limit ($85^{\circ}C$) the power should cut off automatically, this mechanism prevents overheating of the unit.

The wax is molten directly by using the filament or indirectly with the help of water. The later method of wax bath heating is known as Bain Marie in which water is filled in the tank below the wax compartment. The boiled water transfers the heat to the wax to melt it. This method is safe, and heats up wax quickly and provides even distribution of heat. It is the latest method of melting wax and is being used in the physiotherapy practice.

108

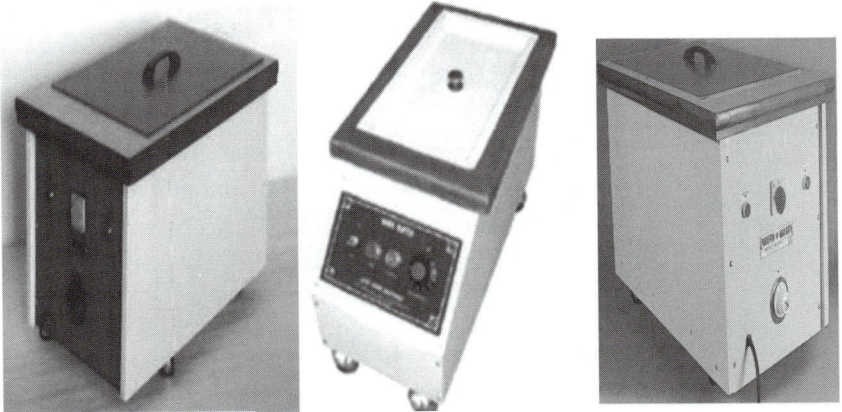

Figure 5.2 Paraffin Wax Bath Unit of different sizes.

Contraindications

    i.   Open wounds

    ii. Skin infections

    iii. Sensory deficit

    iv. Vascular and arterial insufficiency

    v.   Over the jewellery or ornament

    vi. Acute swelling

Application

The part which is being treated with the paraffin wax bath should be examined for any contraindications such as sensory deficit, open wound, circulatory impairments, and thermal sensitivity. When contagious skin conditions or warts are present, the area is covered with a bandage or some form of plastic skin film, prior to immersion in bath as the wax bath could become contaminated. The treatment part must be exposed adequately and cleaned with the soap to remove dirt from the part. The paraffin bath tank is checked for the therapeutic range of temperature, excessive temperature can cause the burn; therefore, a thermometer should be installed in the tank.

There are four major methods of application of paraffin wax bath. The selection of the method depends upon the parts of the extremity and the underlying condition.

A. **Dip and Wrap** – There are two versions of dip immersion methods – dip and wrap, and dip and immersion. Dip and wrap is used for the distal part of the extremity such as hand, feet or fingers. The part is dip into the paraffin wax for 2-3 seconds and taken out. The hand or foot is kept out of the wax bath unit for 2-3 seconds till the wax stops dripping. The hand or foot is dip again into the wax. The procedure is repeated for eight to ten time until a solid wax glove of 3-4mm thick layer is formed around the fingers, hand or wrist. The treatment part is secured in a plastic bag and wrapped with a towel to retain the heat for at least ten more minutes.

B. **Dip and Immersion** – The technique is similar to the dip and wrap. The hand or foot is immersed into the wax and kept for 2-3 seconds. The part is removed from the wax and held out of the wax for few seconds until the wax stops dipping usually for 2-3 seconds. The part is dipped again into the wax for 2-3 seconds and taken out of the wax bath. The process is repeated at least for eight to ten times until a solid wax glove of 3-4mm thick is formed around the part. The part with solid wax glove is dip into the wax and kept for the period of another ten minutes. The patient is instructed not to move the hand or feet or treatment part during the procedure to avoid breaking of the glove or thick layer of the wax.

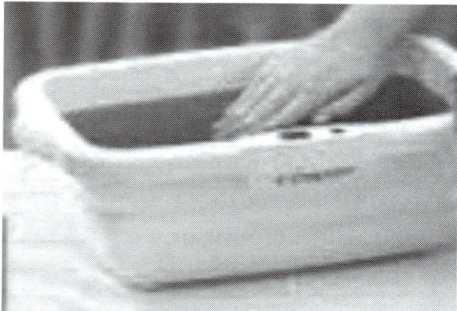

Figure 5.3 Dip and Immersion Method

C. **Direct Pouring Method** - The hand or foot is placed directly over the paraffin wax bath and the molten wax is poured by a mug or utensil on the part. Four to six layers of wax are made on the treatment part and then the part is secured in a plastic bag and then wrapped in a towel to prevent heat loss and kept for ten to twenty minutes. After twenty minutes the wax is removed from the part and put into the bath for reuse.

Superficial Heating Modalities

D. Brushing or Painting Method – The method is commonly used for the knee and elbow joints. The treatment part is placed directly over the paraffin wax bath and eight to ten coats of wax are applied on the part to be treated with the help of paint brush. The treatment part is then secured in a plastic bag and then wrapped in a towel for ten to twenty minutes to prevent heat loss. The wax is removed from the treatment part after twenty minutes. The method can also be used for the other distal joints

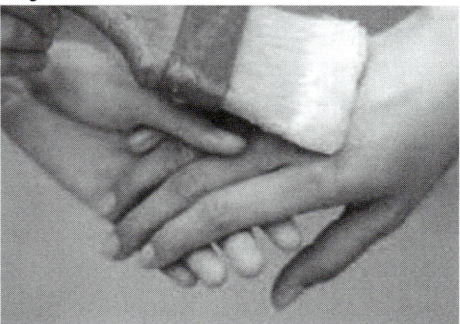

Figure 5.4 Brushing Method

E. Toweling or Bandaging Method – A roll of bandage is immersed in molten paraffin wax and then wrapped around the body part. This method is preferably used for treating proximal joints such as elbow and shoulder.

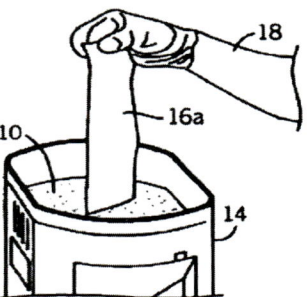

Figure 5.5 Toweling or Bandaging method

Purification of Wax

The water is added to the paraffin wax bath container and heated till the wax is molten. The power is cut off to allow the molten wax to cool. All the dirt and other material will deposit at the bottom, whereas; the wax solidifies above it. The top layer of the wax is removed carefully for reuse. The tank is cleaned and all the dirt and other material is removed from a container.

MOIST HEAT THERAPY

Moist heat therapy has been believed to be more effective at warming tissues than dry heat, because water transfers heat more quickly than air. Moist heat is less likely to cause skin dehydration. In addition to that the skin is less irritant to the moist heat therapy. These are the reasons that the moist heat is preferred over the dry heat for the reduction of muscle spasm, pain associated with musculoskeletal disorders, dilatation for the vessels and increase local blood circulation.

Mechanism of heat transfer – When the hot packs of higher temperature are placed on the body the tissues would come in contact with the hot source. Therefore, the heat from the hot packs would be transferred to the tissues. The tissues close to the hot packs would heat up first and then the heat would be transferred to the next tissues. Therefore, the kinetic motion of atoms and molecules of one object is passed on to another object is often described as "atom jostling on one another".

Physiological effects

The physiological effects of the moist heat therapy such as metabolic response, vascular response, reflexive vasodilatation, and neuromuscular are same as described earlier in the chapter.

Indications

  i.   Muscle spasm
 ii.   Musculoskeletal pain
iii.   Post fracture joint stiffness
 iv.   Adhesive capsulitis
  v.   Chronic inflammation
 vi.   Post burn contractures
vii.   In conjunction with other technique to achieve muscle realaxation and improve range of motion

Contraindications

i.   Impaired skin sensation
ii.   Circulatory dysfunction
iii. Analgesic drugs
iv.   infections and open wounds
v.   Cancer and tuberculosis
vi.   Gross (generalized) edema
vii. Lack of comprehension
viii. Deep X-Ray Therapy

Dangers

i. **Burn –** The moist therapy induced heat in the tissues cannot be quantified by the equipment, the patient is the best judge to tell about the sensation of temperature. Sometimes patients do not inform the therapist as they feel more heat can be beneficial for their symptoms. The excessive temperature in the tissues can lead to tissue burn. Proper instructions to the patient and screening of contraindications prior to the treatment can decrease the chance of burn.

ii. **Exaggeration of Symptoms –** The application of heat to acute inflammation, acute injuries, and edema can aggravate the symptoms.

Moist heat Unit

The moist heat unit is made up of heavy gauge stainless steel sheet double walled well insulated in between the walls. The average size of the unit may be 38cm (width) x 30cm (breadth) x 45cm (height). The unit is fitted with the 1000 watts immersion heater, two pilot lights green and red and a thermostat for temperature control. The temperature may range from 30^0C to 110^0C, but for therapeutic purposes the temperature is maintained between 70^0C and 75^0C.[13] The unit has multiple chambers which hold the hot packs in vertical position.

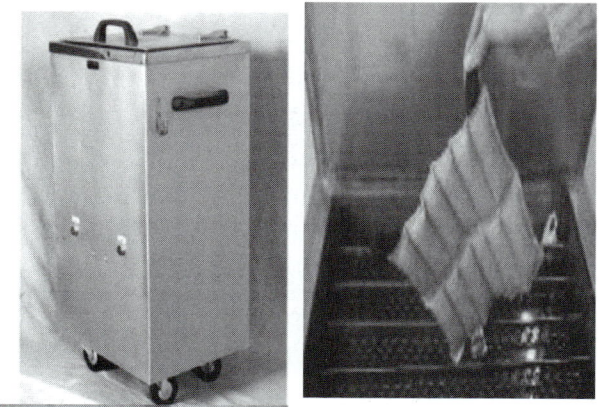

Figure 5.6 Moist Heat Therapy Units

Moist hot packs

Moist heat is transmitted through the hot packs to the tissues. Moist hot packs are made up of canvas or nylon cases filled with a hydrophilic silicate, bentonite or some other hydrophilic substances or sand. Bentonite is preferred as it strongly absorbs the water and holds the heat for a longer period of time. The moist hot packs are of different sizes and shapes for different parts of the body. Water from the hot packs comes out during treatment if there is a leakage in the packs. Old and worn packs may leak the paste like material within them. These should be discarded and replaced with good ones which have no leakage of water.

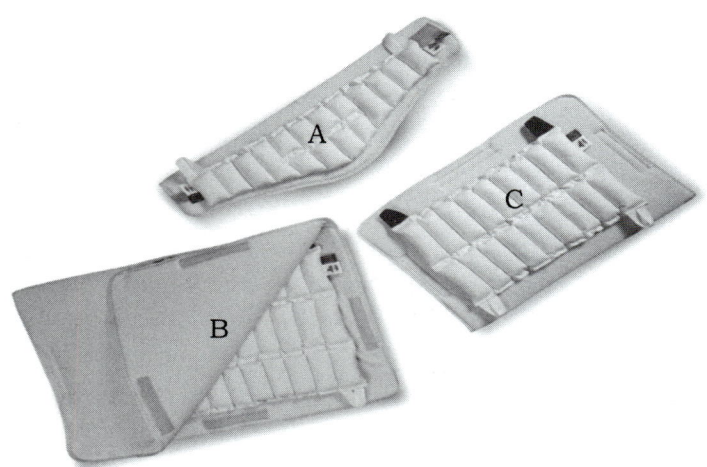

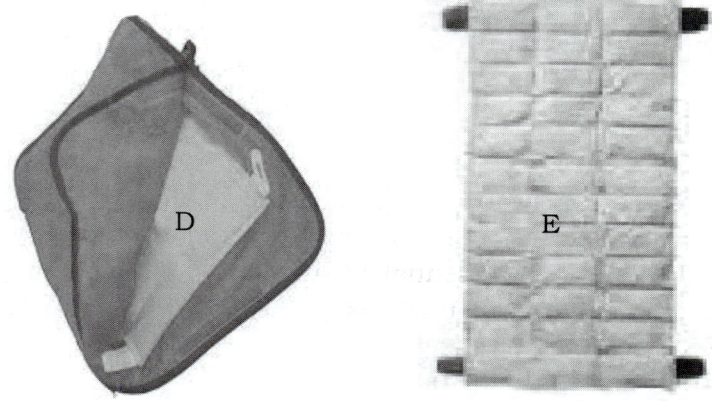

Figure 5.7 hot packs of different sizes (A-E)

Application

The hot packs are stored in a thermostatically controlled unit at a temperature between 70°C and 75°C. An appropriate sized pack is removed from the unit with the help of tongs. The pack may be held over the unit or shaken for the moment to remove the excess water out of the pack. This removes the chances of getting patient wet and leakage of water during the application. The hot pack is wrapped in a Macintosh or plastic sheet and then into the towel or hot pack bag. The hot pack Macintosh or bag is placed over the treatment area. The patient should experience mild to moderate heat within the tolerable range during the treatment period. The old adage "the hotter the better" could result in skin burn.[8] An appropriate layers of towel between the treatment area and hot pack is placed in case of discomfort or excessive heat. The patient is instructed to warn the therapist immediately in case of excessive heat. The therapist should monitor the patient every five minutes especially in the first visit to avoid any adverse effect of hot pack on the body such as burn. Significant change in the color of the skin is the indication of the burn. Use more layers of towel between the hot packs and treatment area if there is a sign of burn.

CONTRAST BATH

Contrast bath is most commonly used for the athletic injuries. It involves placing of one or both the extremities into the hot and cold water. The use of hot and cold alternately produces dilatation and contraction of the vessels in the superficial region, increasing local blood circulation. Therefore, the contrast bath is considered to be the vascular exercise as alternate vasodilatation and constriction hunts the vessels and help in reducing edema, pain and hastening healing in the extremity.

The lymph system, unlike the circulatory system, lacks a central pump. Alternative hot and cold, lymph vessel dilate and contract to essentially "pump" and move stagnant fluid out of the area. The contrast bath can also significantly improve muscle recovery following exercise by reducing the levels of blood lactate concentration. The studies suggest that the contrast bath treatments are superior than using passive recovery or rest after exercise.

Contrast bath Unit

The unit has two chambers of hot and cold water constructed of double walled, well insulated, stainless steel sheet of heavy gauge. The standard size of each chamber should be 56cm width x 25cm breadth with 30cmdepth. The hot chamber should be fitted with special heating elements and the other cold chamber with heavy duty compression unit. Each chamber is provided with digital temperature control cum indicator, pilot lights and water outlet.

The extremity which is being treated with the contrast bath should adequately be exposed. The temperature of the contrast bath unit should be maintained for hot and cold chambers between 40.6^0C to 43^0C and 15^0C to 20^0C respectively[14]. The extremity is immersed into the hot bath first for three minutes and then into cold chamber for one minute. Three minute warm and one minute in cold significantly increase the blood flow of the foot than placing the limb continuously in hot water or using the ratio of 6:2 warm to cold bath time.[19] The extremity is alternately placed from hot to cold for 20-25 minutes.

Indications

Contrast baths are most commonly used for athletic injuries to improve muscle recovery following exercise by reducing the level of blood lactate concentration. The modality also helps in reducing the edema as the alternate vasodilatation and vasoconstriction produce pumping action and drains the collected fluid. The conditions such as rheumatoid arthritis, osteoarthritis, diabetic foot, muscle strain,

Superficial Heating Modalities

ligament sprain, and other musculoskeletal disorders are treated with the contrast bath. The acute inuries should be treated carefully as contrast bath induced vasodilatation can increase swelling and the symptoms.

Contraindications

The patients with peripheral vascular disease, sensory deficit, open wounds, hypersensitivity to the temperature should not be considered for the contrast bath therapy.

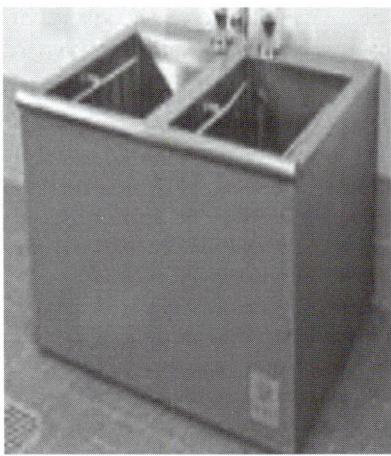 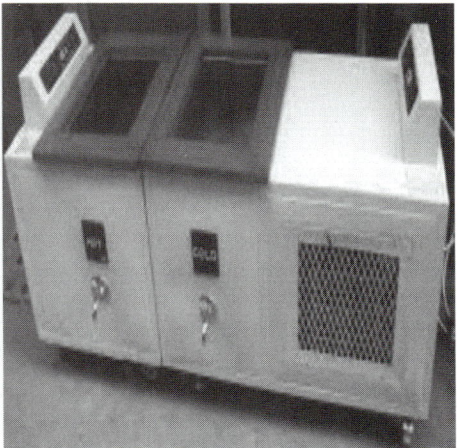

Figure 5.8 Contrast Bath Units contain hot and cold chambers

FLUIDOTHERAPY

Fluidotherapy is a form of dry heating involving a suspension of cellulose particles which are kept in motion by air movement.[15] The heat energy is transferred to the tissues by convection. Extremely small solid particles are heated and suspended by circulating area, thus producing an effect similar to circulating warm liquid. The thermal conductivity and specific heat of the particles and air allows the temperature of the unit to be higher than that of water used therapeutically.[16]

The equipment consists a heating element, an air compressor, tiny silicon or corn-cob particles in an enclosed see through container into which the limb is inserted. The unit consists timer, a temperature gauge, and a mesh sleeve. Heated air is circulated through the particles so that the particles can move like fluid.

Superficial Heating Modalities

To prevent edema formation in the hand the temperature may be set low. However, if there is no history of formation of edema (gravity dependant due to weakness of the muscles) the temperature may be set between 41.1°C and 50.6°C. The patient with hypersensitivity of the fingertips from the traumatic amputations, patient in the stage of reflex sympathetic dystrophy, and patient with scar hypersensitivity may all benefit from fluidotherapy.

The patient is screened for all the contraindications to fluidotherapy. The part which is being treated is exposed adequately and placed into the sleeve and closed snugly around the more proximal portion of the limb so that particles do not come into the room once the blower is turned on. The temperature is set between 46.1°C and 50.6°C and timer usually at 15 minutes. The patient is instructed to perform the exercises as explained before starting the treatment with the fluidotherapy. The therapist can also insert his or her hand through the separate access sleeve to perform passive stretching exercises.

References

1. Rabkin JM, Hunt TK. Local heat increasesblood flow and oxygen tension in the wouds. Arch Surg.1987;122(2):225.
2. Xia Z, Sato A , Hughes MA, cherry GW. Stimulation of fibroblast growth in vitro by intermittent radiant warming. Wound repair Regen . 2001;8(2):138-144.
3. Price P, Bale S, Crook H, Harding KG. The effect of radiant heat dressing on pressure ulcers. J Wound Care.2000;9(4):201-205
4. Bernadette Hecox, Tsega Andemicael Mehreteab Joseph Weisberg. Physical agents, A comprehensive text for physical therapist, pp68
5. Lehmann JF, deLateur BJ, therapeutic heat. In Lehmann JF (ed), therapeutic heat and cold, 4th ed. Baltimore : Williams and Wilkins, 1990
6. Halvorsen, GA. Therapeutic heat and cold for athletic injuries. Phys sports med 18:87,1990
7. Low j, reed a. electrotherapy explained : principles and practice . Oxford, UK:Utterworth-Heinemann, 1990.
8. Susan L. Michlovitz, Thomas P. Nolan, jr. modalities for therapeutic intervention, fourth edition, contemporary perspective in rehabilitation , Jaypee, pp. 64-69.
9. Abramson DL, Bell Y, Tuck S, et al. changes in blood flow. O^2 uptake and tissue temperature produced by therapeutic physical agents. III. Effects of indirect or reflex vasodilatation Am j Phys Med 404:5, 1961.
10. Basant Kumar Nanda, Electrotherapy simplified, second edition, Jaypee,pp263.
11. Burns S, Conin T. the use of paraffin wax bath I the intercention of burns. Physiother Can 39:258,1987
12. Head MD,Helms PA, Paraffin and sustained stretching in the treatment of burn contractures. Burns 4 : 136,1977.
13. Lehmann JF ,Delateur BJ. Therapeutic heat in Lehmann JF (ed), therapeutic heat and cold. 4th ed. Baltimore : Williams and Wilkins,1980.
14. Bernadette Hecox Tsega Andemicael Mehreteab Joseph Weisberg. Physical agents, a comprehensive text for physical therapist, pp246.
15. Sheila Kitchen, Electrotherapy evidence based practice, eleventh edition, previous edition entitled Clayton's Electrotherapy, Churchill Livingstone, pp132.
16. Bernadette Hecox, Tsega Andemicael Mehreteab Joseph Weisberg. Physical agents, a comprehensive text for physical therapist, pp133
17. Hughes MA, Tang C, Herry GW . effect of intermittent radiant warming on proliferation of human dermal endothelial cell in vitro. J wound care. 2003;12(4) :135-137.
18. Lehman,JFf, et al : Therapeutic heat and cold. Clin Orthop 99:207,1974.
19. Petrofsky J, Lohman E 3rd, Lee S, de la Cuesta Z, Labial L, Iouciulescu R, Moseley B, Korson R, Al Malty A. Effects of contrast bath on skin flow on the dorsal and planter foot in people with type 2 diabetes and aged match controls. Physoither Theory Pract. 2007 Jul-Aug: 23 (4): 189-97).

Chapter 06

Ultraviolet Rays

The therapeutic application of radiant energy from the ultraviolet portion of the electromagnetic spectrum has been used for the treatment of a variety of skin disorders.[1] The ultraviolet part of the spectrum corresponds to electromagnetic radiation with a wavelength 100-400nm) shorter compared with visible light (400-700nm), but longer than X- rays (greater than 100nm).[2] ultraviolet radiation is used for the treatment of various conditions such as psoriasis, acne, folliculitis, pressure sores and wound healing but its use in physiotherapy practice has largely dropped due to advancement in the pharmacological agents.

Ultraviolet irradiation is divided into four distinct spectral areas, including vacuum ultraviolet from 100 to 200nm, ultraviolet C from 200-280nm, ultraviolet B from 280 to 315nm, and ultraviolet A from 315 to 400nm. This division allows the distinction between the effects of solar and artificial ultraviolet exposure on living species. Wavelengths < 290nm are blocked by stratospheric ozone; so there is no natural exposure to UVC. UVB penetrates the ozone layer and constitutes 5% to 10% of the terrestrial solar ultraviolet radiation. Radiation in the UVA range is by far the most abundant solar ultraviolet radiation (>90%).

Ultraviolet A penetrates human skin more efficiently than UVB.[3] Ultraviolet radiation has both beneficial and harmful effects depending upon the type of organism, wavelength range (UVA,UVB, or UVC), and irradiation dose(intensity X duration).[4]

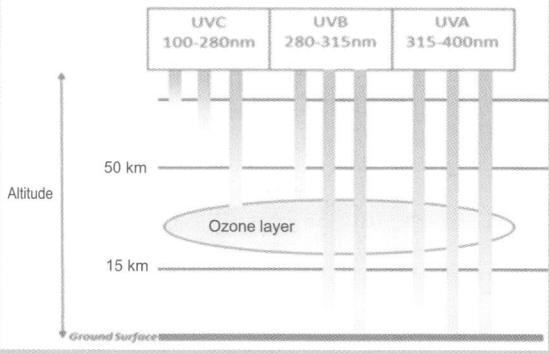

Fig. 6.1 Distribution of UVR A,B and C in the atmosphere

Wavelength	Electromagnetic spectrum	frequency
↓	Electrical Stimulating Currents	↑
	Commercial Radio and Television	
	Shortwave Diathermy	
	Microwave Diathermy	
	Infrared Rays	
	Visible Light	
	Ultraviolet	
	Ionizing Radiation	

Table 6.1 Electromagnetic Spectrums with their respective wavlength in descending order and frequency increasing order

Production

Sun is the natural source of the ultraviolet rays. Ozone, (a layer of the atmosphere) filters most of the harmful ultraviolet rays and sends only the spectrum of 180nm to 400nm. Thus scientists got engaged in the production of artificial ultraviolet and it was first developed in the 19th centaury. In 1983, Niels Finsen introduced the use of artificial ultraviolet light from a carbon arc to treat skin disorders such as lupus vulgaris, for which he received the Nobel Prize.[4] the following artificial generators can produce ultraviolet rays –

1. **Mercury Vapor Lamp –** The mercury vapor lamp was first developed early in the 20th century. There are two types of mercury lamps which produce ultraviolet rays used in the physical therapy practice to manage various skin disorders.

   a. Medium Pressure Mercury Arc Lamp – The lamp consists U shaped glass tube which contains argon gas at a low pressure and small amount of mercury. The tube is sealed at both the ends. Both the ends are connected with the electrodes (negative and positive). The high voltage current (400V) is applied to the tube to ionize the argon gas. The flow of current through the argon gas in the tube produces heat which results in vaporization of the mercury atom. The mercury atoms become excited by collision with the electron flowing between the lamp and electrodes. The excited electrons return to their particular state in the mercury atom and doing so release some of the energy they have absorbed in the form of radiation (UVR)

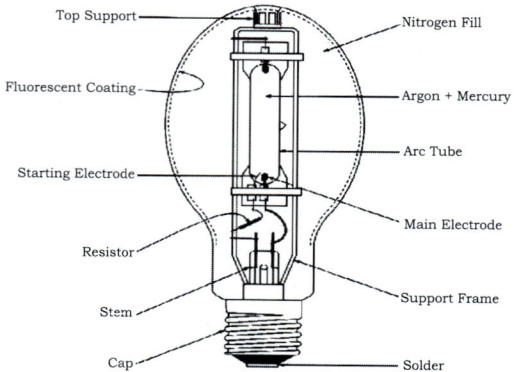

Figure 6.2a Diagram of Medium Pressure Mercury Arc Lamp

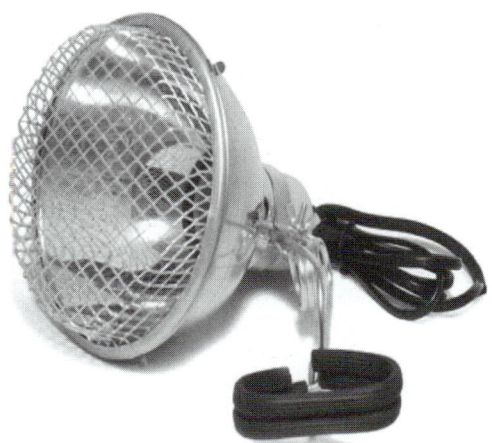

Figure 6.2b Medium Pressure Mercury Arc Lamp

b. Kromayer – The kromayer is a medium pressure mercury vapor ultraviolet lamp. It is enclosed or surrounded by the water jacket. The cooled water circulated over the lamp absorbs infrared rays, this advantage of absorbing infrared rays by circulating makes kromayer lamp tissue friendly, hence the lamp can be placed over the tissues as there is no damage or no tissue burn occurs. The water circulation should be continued for five minutes after the treatment to let the lamp cool and to avoid damage. Kromayer lamp's, wavelength at 366nm gives both UVA and UVB, used for treating localized lesions such as pressure sores areas, ulcers and sinuses in open areas. The wavelength of the rays produced are concentrated at 366nm but a wide range of both UVA and UVB are produced.

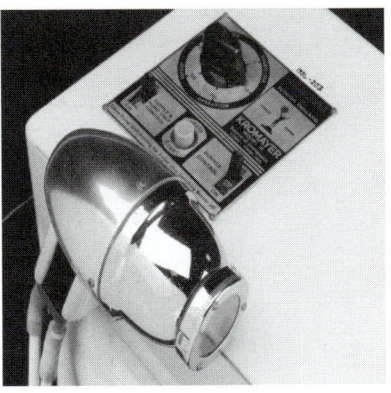

Figure 6.3 Kromayer Lamp

Ultraviolet Rays

2. **Fluorescent Lamp** – It is a low pressure mercury vapor lamp which has a phosphor coating inside the glass tube. The phosphor coating of the glass tube is also known as enveloping. The phosphor at low pressure in mercury vapor absorbs the short ultraviolet rays spectral line at a wavelength of 253.7nm. This results in emission of the long wave length UVR by the phenomenon of fluorescent . The spectrum of each tube depends upon the type of phosphor coating.

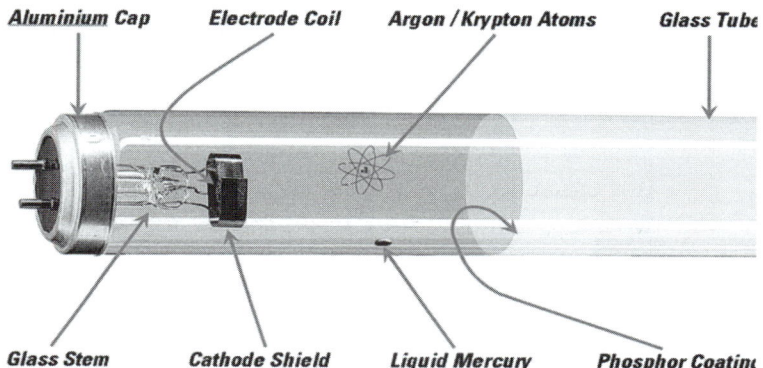

Figure 6.4 Fluorescent Lamp

3. **Theraktin Tunnel** - Theraktin tunnel is a semi-cylindrical frame in which four fluorescent tubes each are mounted on its own parabolic reflector. The length of each fluorescent tube is usually 120cm, but that can be increased or decreased for even irradiation. The Theraktin tunnel produces ultraviolet rays with spectrum of 280nm to 400nm. A narrow band output fluorescent tube is also used to produce specific range of wavelength. One of tubes produces wavelength of around 311nm.

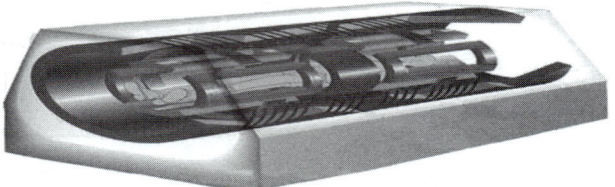

Figure 6.5 Theraktin Tunnel

Ultraviolet Rays

4. **PUVA –** The patients with psoriasis are treated with the wavelength of 315 nm to 400nm (UVRA). The special type of fluorescent tubes usually 48 are required and are mounted on a wall of vertical battery or on the four sides of box. The patient is surrounded by four sides of vertical box and the box may contain as many as 48 tubes. The treatment lasts for two hours.

Physiological Effects

The effects of ultraviolet irradiation in tissues include a consecutive series of events starting with the absorption of the photons by chromospheres in the skin (photo-excitation), followed by photochemical reactions, which induce molecular changes in cell and tissue biology and affect signaling networks. Ultraviolet irradiation my cause both beneficial and damaging effects, which depend on wavelength, radiation exposure, and the ultraviolet source. Following physiological effects of ultraviolet may be observed in the tissues –

Erythema–The mechanism of erythema production following ultraviolet radiation is understood poorly. It is believed that the vasodilatation is caused by liberation of histamine like substance and bradykinin. Increased blood circulation in the superficial skin occurs following application of the ultraviolet rays. However, in case of superficial vessels, following low doses of both 250 and 300nm wavelength there is a slight increase in blood flow, and following higher doses, a marked reduction in blood flow can be observed. This reduction was attributed to the stasis in these superficial vessels, perhaps, secondary to vascular damage.[5]

There is enlargement and engorgement of minute blood vessels in the corium (the superficial layer of the dermis) that results in erythema. This process helps in formation of granulation tissues that contributes to the tissue repair. Not all the ultraviolet radiation produce erythema equally. The erythema produced by ultraviolet C is differ from the erythema produced by ultraviolet B. The erythema usually   occurs when the skin is exposed to ultraviolet B. The skin is thousand times less sensitive to the ultraviolet A and ultraviolet C.

The therapeutic significance of erythema is to accelerate the tissue healing and also to calculate the doses of the ultraviolet rays. The ultraviolet rays induced erythema reaches to its maximum intensity between 8 and 24 hours of the exposure but takes several days to resolve completely. There is a latent period two hours before development of erythema.

Pigmentation – It is the production of melanin in the deeper strata of the epidermis, which ascends to the more superficial zones. The production and then migration (ascending) of melanin to the superficial layer of skin results in darkening of the skin and thickening of the corneum. The darkening of the skin following pigmentation is called tanning. Tanning protects the skin from excessive exposure of UVR by partially blocking the UVR to penetrate into the skin. Tanning is best achieved with the wavelength of between 254nm and 299nm. The pigmentation takes place within two days of exposure of ultraviolet light. There is also formation of hyperplacia, thickening of both the epidermis and stratum corneum due to division of epidermal cells. The hyperplacia begins to occur around 72 hours of the exposure of UVR, it also limits the damage of skin to further ultraviolet rays.

Vitamin D Production – Low dose UVB 280nm-300nm exposure induces the production of vitamin D in the skin.[6] Ultraviolet B converts sterols present in the skin as 7 dehydrocholestrol into vitamin D (calciferol, cholecalciferol). Infected wounds – It has been known for the last 100 years that ultraviolet light (particularly UVC in the range of 250nm-280nm) is highly germicidal; however; its use to treat wound infections remain at an early stage of development. Most of the studies are confined to in vitro and ex vitro levels, while in vivo animal studies and clinical studies are rarer.[7] The high dose of ultraviolet C or ultraviolet B, can cause direct damage to nucleic acids and proteins that can lead to genetic mutation or cell death.[8] The mechanism of ultraviolet inactivation of microorganisms is to cause cellular damage by inducing changes in the chemical structure of DNA chains.[9] The consequence is the production of CPD causing damage and distortion of the DNA molecule which causes malfunctions in cell replication and rapidly leads to cell death.

Wound Healing – Exposure of the skin to ultraviolet produces erythema, epidermal hyperplasia, increased blood flow in the microcirculation, and also has bactericidal effects.[10] The ultraviolet radiation induced erythema initiates the first phase of healing (inflammatory phase) by creating an inflammatory response via the mechanism of vasodilatation. This may be partially explained by the effects of ultraviolet light on the arachidonic acid pathway.[11] In addition, ultraviolet light exposure induces cellular proliferation in the stratum corneum.[12] This proliferation or thickening of the skin is a protective mechanism against further sunlight damage. Ultraviolet avoidance and use of sunscreen are commonly advised during the re-epithelialization process as well as after wound closure. However, it is possible that the currently accepted practice of ultraviolet protection prevents the normal cutaneous response to injury, with melanocyte redistribution and pigmentation creating hypo-pigmented scars.[13]

Determining Minimal Erythemal Dose (MED)

The smallest dose of UVR to result in erythema that is just detectable by eye at between 8 and 24 hours after exposure is termed the minimal erythema dose (MED).[14] First of all an erythrometer is prepared. The following steps should be followed to determine the MED –

i. The erythrometer can be made from a piece of paper, card board, exposed x-ray film, or fabric measuring four inches by eight inches (4"x8").

ii. Six holes erythrometer are made on the paper or card board. Each hole should be of ¾ inches and the distance between of the holes should be of same (¾ inches).

iii. Clean and dry the tested area which has not been exposed to the ultraviolet radiation before this. The suitable area for determining the minimal erythemal dose is flexor aspect of the forearm and lower abdomen.

iv. Place the erythrometer over the area to be tested. Cover all the holes of the erythrometer.

v. Drape the patient completely. Ask the patient to close the eyes or wear a pair of goggles. The examiner or therapist should also wear the goggles to protect the eyes from ultraviolet radiation.

vi.   Ask the patient regarding photosensitization drugs.

vii. Switch on the lamp for five minutes prior to an MED testing. Position the ultraviolet lamp perpendicular over the tested area with a distance of 30 inches.

viii. Uncover the first hole for ultraviolet radiation while keeping all the remaining holes covered. Uncover the second hole after the fifteen seconds for the ultraviolet radiation. Continue uncovering each subsequent hole at the interval of fifteen seconds in this way all the six holes get uncovered.

ix.   Uncover all the holes after exposing each hole to the ultraviolet rays. In the testing process of MED the first hole has received ultraviolet rays throughout the testing time or for 90 seconds, whereas, the last hole has received only fifteen seconds of ultraviolet rays. Hence, each hole has been exposed with different times in increasing order.

x.   After completing the testing process of MED the patient is asked not to wash the area but to observe all the holes carefully every two hours in the next 24 to 48 hours.

Doses Calculation

i.   Exposure time needed to produce a faint erythema of the skin is 24 hours after exposure

ii.   Area of skin to be tested should have pigmentation similar to area to be treated

iii. Patient returns in 24 hours and a visual inspection determines MED

iv.   Suberythemal Dose – Area tested that reveal no erythema 24 hours after testing.

v.   Minimal Erythemal Dose – Area showing erythema lasting 24 hours.

vi.   First Degree Erythema Dose – (E1 = 2.5 X MED or it corresponds 2.5 times of minimal erythemal dose) evidence of erythema lasting as long as 48 hours

vii. Second Degree Erythema Dose – (E2 = 5 x MED or it corresponds five times of minimal erythemal dose). Evidence of intense erythema with edema, peeling and pigmentation that will last as long as 72 hours is present.

viii. Third Degree Erythema Dose – (E3 = 10 x MED or it corresponds ten times minimal erythemal dose). Erythema with severe blistering and exudation limited to an area no larger than 25sq cm.

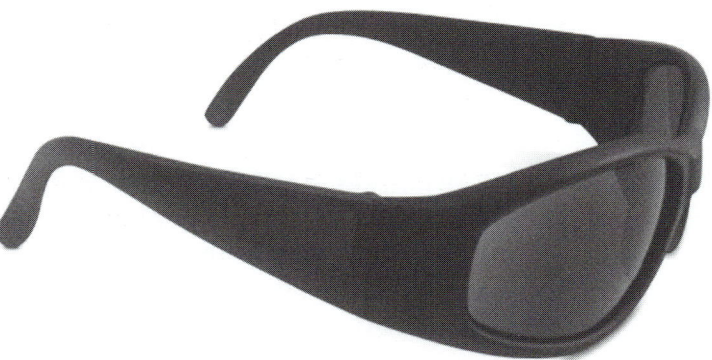

Figure 6.6 Goggles to protect the eyes of patient as well as therapist from ultraviolet rays

Treatment Procedure

i. The room should be well ventilated to eliminate the accumulation of poisonous ozone gas from warm up as the short ultraviolet wavelengths are absorbed by the oxygen in the air to form ozone and nitrogen oxides. The patient and therapist should wear goggles especially designed for the ultraviolet radiation. If the eyes are not protected the UVR energy is absorbed in the superficial structure of the eyes that may damage the area of eye. The area which is being treated should be cleaned. Cover all the area of the patient till the involved area is exposed to ultraviolet rays for the prescribed time of period. The treatment is given either to the local area or generalized area.

ii. **For local area** – The therapist should make a chart of the area with reference to the bony land marks so that overexposure of the area can be prevented. The patient is positioned properly. The lamp is positioned at distance of 30 inches perpendicularly. The therapist should never decrease the distance of the lamp lower than the 15 inches. The exposure time should be calculated according to the formula given below -

$$T2 = T1 [(D2)^2 / (D1)^2]$$

Where T2 = new exposure time, T1 = initial exposure time, D1 = initial distance, D2 = new distance

iii. **For generalized area** – Both the dorsum and ventral part can be treated separately. Focus should be made on the proper exposure to the UVR and measures should be taken to avoid overexposure. For the exposure of the ventral part to the ultraviolet radiation, place the patient in supine position with the head turned to one side with the palms up. Body is divided into two parts upper and lower using the anterior superior iliac spine as the borderline. Cover the patient, provide an extra protective covering over the nipples, umbilicus, genitalia, hair and eyes. Position the UVR lamp over the superior half of the patient's body with the distance of 30 inches away from the sternum. The lower area of the body is exposed by covering the upper body parts above an anterior superior iliac spine and by positioning the lamp over the lower part of the body. The same is repeated for the back in prone position by exposing upper and lower parts in the same manner. Duplication of the exposure should be avoided during the exposure of ventral surface followed by dorsal surface carefully covering the body parts adequately.

Switch on the lamp five minutes prior to the exposure and then open the shutters and direct the ultraviolet radiation to the treatment area for the prescribed time. The time and the distance will be same as it was used to determine the MED. Turn off the lamp at the end of the treatment and cover the exposed area immediately after the treatment. Since human skin adapts to ultraviolet exposure, MED will gradually increase with repeated treatments. It is necessary to gradually increase exposure time to achieve the same reaction; usually it is increased by five seconds per treatment session. When the total exposure for each area reaches three times, the distance can then be reduced to avoid increasing the exposure time further. Height of lamp remains constant throughout entire process.

iv. **Local treatment by cold Quartz –** The cold quartz is commonly used to treat decubitus ulcers for the bacterial healing effects.[4] The determination of minimum erythemal dose is not required. The lamp is placed directly over the treatment area with the distance of one inch. Exposure time for the different doses is predetermined. For the distance of one inch an MED would be 12-15 seconds, E1 = 36-45 seconds, E2 = 72-90 seconds, E3 = 135-180 seconds. For the deeper penetration 55 percent energy of the cold quartz should be used. The procedure remains same as above. The wound area is cleaned with soap and water and left to dry. The area is covered with sterile drape. The cold quartz is turned on for 1-3 minutes for warm up. Direct the lamp over the treatment area with the distance of one inch. Turn off the lamp at the end of the treatment.

Indications

i. Acne

ii. Aseptic wounds

iii. Septic wounds

iv. Sinusitis

v. Psoriasis

vi. Pressure sores

vii. Osteomalacia

viii. Increase vitamin D production

ix. Sterilization

x. Tanning

xi. Hyperplasia

xii. folliculitis

xiii. Pityriasis rosea

xiv. Tinea capitum

xv. Diagnosis of skin disorders

Contraindications

i. Prophysis

ii. Pellagra

iii. Lupus erythematosus

iv. Sarcoidosis

v. Xeroderma pigmentosus

vi. Acute psoriasis

vii. Acute aczema

viii. Herpes Simplex

ix. Renal and hepatic insufficiencies

x. Diabetes

xi. Hyperthyroidism

xii. Generalized dermatitis

xiii. Advanced arteriosclerosis

xiv. Active and progressive pulmonary tuberculosis

Infrared Radiation

Sir Frederick William Herschel had discovered infrared rays in 1800. The German astronomer, split light using a prism (an object that can split white light into a spectrum or rainbow) and used three thermometers with blackened bulbs to measure heat of different colors. He concluded that colors are associated with the heat. Sir Frederick studied beyond red light and discovered below red, infrared and light red radiation. Today infrared rays are used for heating food, TV remote control, consumer goods, in the space, and heating the superficial tissues. The infrared lamp is now primarily limited to drying seeping open wound or sedating superficial sensory nerve. Infrared rays lie between the visible and microwaves.

Infrared rays are electromagnetic waves which are invisible to the human eyes, unless reflected off an object. The wavelength is ranged from 760nm to 1mm (10^6).[16] The frequency of infrared rays lies between 4×10^{14} Hz and 7.5×10^{11} Hz

Production

The infrared rays can be produced by any hot body like sun electric bulb, coal fire, gas fire, etc however; sun is the natural source of the infrared rays. The infrared rays used in the physiotherapy clinical practice for producing superficial heating effect can either be produced by the non luminous or luminous generators.

Non luminous generator: These generators are also known as infrared radiation generators as these produce nearly infrared rays. The non luminous generators consists of simple type of element or metal spiral coil around a non conducting material (cylinder of some insulating material) such as fireclay or porcelain. As the electricity flows through the coil, it encounters resistance, thus producing heat. All the nonluminous generators require five to ten minutes to heat up and reach to the peak intensity, hence, these lamps should be switched on before 5-10 minutes of the application.

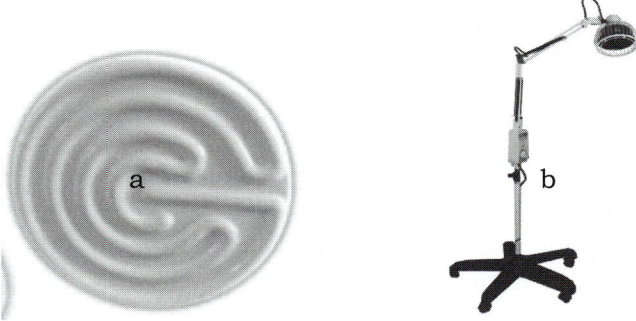

Figure 6.7 a. Non Luminous Filaments and b. Lamp with stand

Luminous infrared lamp- These lamps are the incandescent lamps consisting of a wire filament with an inert gas at low pressure within the glass. The filament is made up of tungsten which is a coil of fine wire. The inner layer of the glass is often silvered to reflect the rays. The filters are used to limit the output to particular wave band. Red filter is used to filter out the blue and green light waves. The tungsten filament is heated up to 3000°C which emits 70% near infrared rays, 24% long infrared rays, and 1% ultraviolet rays. The glass absorbs the ultraviolet rays, therefore, these rays are not emitted from the lamp.

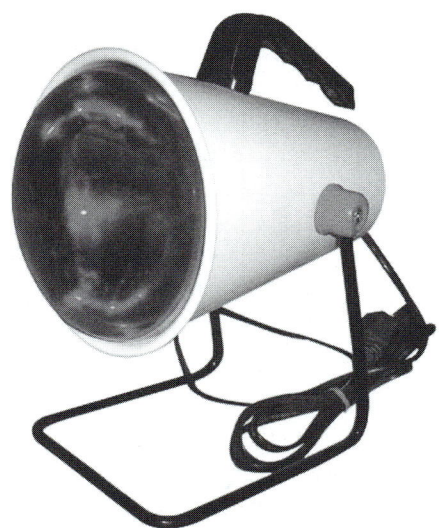

Figure 6.7c Luminous Lamp.

Physical characteristics

The infrared rays follow the rule of cosine law. As soon as the rays strike the body they may reflect, transmit or absorbed in the tissues.

Reflection - The reflection depends upon the angle of incidence and composition of the soft tissues. Larger the angle of incidence, greater the reflection of the rays. If the angle of incidence is perpendicular to the treatment area it reduces reflection of the rays. **Transmission –** the infrared rays are transmitted into the tissues where there are either absorbed or reflected. The transmission of infrared rays depends upon the composition of the tissues. If the difference in the density of two medium through which the rays are transmitted is high, that would cause more reflection of the ways. The depth of penetration also depends upon the wavelength. The luminous infrared rays (wavelength between 350 and 4000nm) are transmitted into the deeper structure than the nonluminous (wavelength between 750 and 15000nm) infrared rays. **Absorption –** The structures which contain water and protein contents absorb infrared rays effectively. The infrared rays energy transmission decreases exponentially with the depth, as most of the energy is absorbed in epidermis and dermis, therefore, the most of heating due to infrared rays will occur superficially. The maximum depth of penetration of the shorter wavelengths would be 3 mm, for the long infrared wavelength would be 1mm.

Physiological Effects

The physiological effects of the infrared rays would be similar to the other superficial thermal agent such as cutaneous vasodilatation (due to secretion of the chemical such as histamine) and due to axon reflex mechanism. Infrared rays increases the activity of sweat gland that results in sweating. This absorbs the infrared rays which helps in surface cooling as it evaporated the sweat. There is increased metabolic rate and demand of oxygen and food stuff following application of infrared rays. The increased blood flow removes waste metabolites.

Therapeutic Uses

Relief of pain and muscle spasm – There is no direct effect of infrared rays on the muscle spam. Spasm in the muscles is secondary due to any injury or pathological changes in the epidermis or dermis. Due to pain in the superficial structure, muscles guard the joint to avoid movement, Limitation in the range of motion further contributes to pain and spasm. Infrared rays produce superficial thermal effect in the subcutaneous tissues, which results in increase in the blood flow. The exudates and metabolites which are responsible for the pain are removed from the area. This process helps in decreasing pain and reduction in pain eventually reduces muscle spasm. Skin lesions skin fungal infection such as paronychia, and psoriasis may be resoved by the therapeutic infrared rays. The increased superficial temperature helps in reduction of the plaques associated with psoriasis. The superficial pressure sores or ulcers in the epidermis and dermis are resolved with the infrared rays radiation as it enhances the healing by increasing blood circulation, and retarding bacterial growth.

Contraindications and dangers

The infrared rays produce thermal effects in the superficial structures and have minimal effect in the deep structures such as muscles, ligaments and joint capsule as maximum heat is absorbed in the superficial structures. However, patient should be screened for the following before irradiation.

i.   Impaired arterial blood supply

ii.   Sensory deficit

iii.   Over the eyes

iv.   Active infective diseases or tumors

v.   Active bleeding or hemorrhage

vi.   Metal or jewelry over the superficial tissues

Dangers

i.   Burn – The infrared rays can raise the temperature of the superficial structures to therapeutic temperature 44.5°C. The patient receives it comfortably. If the distance between the lamp and the treatment area is shorten or the intensity of the heat is higher it can raise the temperature above the therapeutic range which can cause burn. The patient with sensory deficit and vascular impairment also prone to the burn injuries during the exposure of the infrared rays.

ii.   Gangrene – Prolong exposure of the treatment area to the infrared can cause gangrene especially if there is arterial circulation of the area is compromised.

iii.   Dehydration, faintness, and low blood Pressure-The exposure of large area for prolog period of time can cause excessive sweating of the fluid. If the fluid is not replaced with water it can cause dehydration. The excessive loss of the water also lead to hypoxia. The blood pressure decreases. The patient feels of fainting especially when he or she gets up or stands suddenly from the lying after the end of the treatment .

Application

i.   The patient is screened for the contraindications such as sensory deficit, vascular impairment , infection , and sensitivity to heat.

ii.   Patient is placed in a comfortable and relaxed position

iii.   The part which is being treated is exposed appropriately. All the jewelry and metal like chain should be taken off the treatment area. If jewelry is not removable it should be covered with reflecting tape to avoid heating up of the metal and burn.

iv. Select the infrared rays lamp- The luminous infrared rays lamp is the choice for chronic conditions and deeper heating effects in the subcutaneous tissues. The nonluminous infrared rays lamp is used for the acute inflammatory and recent injuries and for more superficial thermal effects.

v. Place the infrared lamp at the appropriate distance of the treatment area. The infrared rays should strike the body at the right angle (90°) to avoid reflection and to maximize the absorption of the rays. Ideally the nonluminous lamp are placed at the distance of 18-24 inches. The distance from the treatment area can be increased or decreased as per the tolerance of the patient. To treat the patient with decubitus ulcers or to produce minimal heating effect for prong period of time the distance between the patient and treatment area can be increased to 40 inches.

vi. Switch on the nonluminous infrared rays lamp fifteen minutes prior to the treatment as the generators takes 5-10 minutes to reach the peak intensity. Luminous lamps do not require much time to get heated.

vii. The treatment area should be inspected regularly during the treatment session. The therapist should observe for any unwanted signs such as mottling, red and white patches, erythema and skin pigmentation may occur due to over exposure.

viii. Stop the treatment in case of any discomfort or allergy to the radiation

ix. Switch off the lamp at the end of treatment

References

I. K.S. Suh, J.S.Kang, J.W.Baek, T.K. Kim, J.W.Lee, Y.S.Jeon, et al. efficacy of ultraviolet A1 phototherapy in recalcitrant skin diseases Ann Dermatol, 22 (2010),pp. 1-8 kai CKY, Wee LKS. Phototherapeutic regime : a synopsis.singapore : national skin centre.

ii. Asheesh gupta, Avci, tianhong dai, ying-ying huang, and ,Michael R.Adv Would care (new Rochelle). 2013 oct. 2 (8) : 422-437.

iii. Vazquez M.Hanslmeir A Ultraviolet radiation in the solar system. Berlin, germany ; springer; 2006.

iv. Bernadette hecox, tsega andemicael mehreteab, joseph weisbeerg, physical agents a comprehensive text for phy sical therapist, Appleton & lange Norwalk, Connecticut, pp377.

v. Ramsay CA. challoner A V. Vascular changes in human skin after ultraviolet irradiation. Br J Dermatol . 1976;94:487 (PubMed)

vi. Mason RS.Reichrath J. Sunlight, vitamin D, and skin cancer. Anticancer agents Med Chem. 2013; 13:83 (PubMed)

vii. Dai T. Vrahas MS. Murray CK. Hamblin MR. Ultraviolet C irradiation: an alternative antimicrobial approach to localized infections? Expert Rev Anti Infect Ther. 2012; 10:185. (PubMed).

viii. Hockberger PE. A history of ultraviolet photobiology for humans, animals and microorganisms. Photochem. Photobiol. 2002;76:561. (PubMed)

ix. Chang JC. Ossoff SF. Lobe DC. Dorfman MH. Dumais CM. Qualls RG. Johnson JD. UV inactivation of pathogenic and indicator microorganisms. Appl Environ Microbiol. 1985;49:1361. (PubMed).

x. Eaglstein WH. Weinstein GD. Prostaglandin and DNA synthesis in human skin: possible relationship to ultraviolet light effects. J Invest Dermotol. 1975;64:386. (PubMed)

xi. Camp RD. Greaves MW. Hensby CN. Plummer NA. Warin AP. Irradiation of human skin by short wavelength ultraviolet radiation (100-290nm – UVC): Increased concentrations of arachidonic acid and prostaglandines E2 and F2 alpha. Br J Clin Pharmacol. 1978;6:145. (PubMed).

xii. Sauder DN. Stanulis-Praeger BM. Gilchrest BA. Autocrine growth stimulation of huma keratinocytes by epidural cell-derived thymocyte-activating factor: Implication for skin aging. Arch Dermatol Res. 1988;280:71. (PubMed).

xiii. Rennekampff HO. Buche MN, Knobloch K. Tenenhaus M. Is Ultraviolet radiation beneficial in postburn wound healing? Med Hypotheses. 210;75:436. PubMed).

xiv. Sheila Kitchen, Electrotherapy Evidence Based Practice, 11th Edition, Previous edition titled Clayton's Electrotherapy, Churchill Livingstone, pp193.

xv. Chad Strakey, Therapeutic Modalities, 3rd edition, FA Davis Company, Philadelphia.

xvi. Basant Kumar Nanda, Electrotherapy Simplified, Second edition, the health science publishers, pp407.

Chapter 07

Therapeutic Currents

Therapeutic currents can broadly be defined as electrical currents, produced by electrotherapeutic devices, induced to the body tissues to elicit certain physiological and clinical effects or the currents which are used to treat various musculoskeletal, neurological, and other sports conditions are termed as therapeutic currents. The therapeutic currents are classified on the basis of direction of flow, frequency, and voltage.

I.   Direction of flow
   a.   Alternating current
   b.   Direct current

ii.   Frequency
   a.   Low frequency currents - between 50 and 100 Hz.
   b.   Medium frequency currents - between 100 and 4000 Hz.
   c.   High frequency currents above 1 MHz

iii.   Voltage
   a.   Low voltage currents less than 100 volts
   b.   High voltage current greater than 100 volts

Direct current

Direct current has a single phase of impulse which flows in a unidirectional towards positive or negative poles; therefore, it is also called as mono-phasic current. The pattern seen on the oscilloscope for direct current would be straight line, so especially direct current has no wave form (an oscilloscope is device for amplifying, measuring and visually observing an electrical signal).

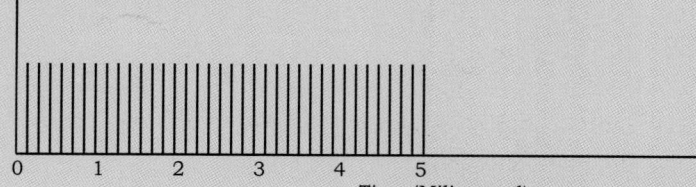

Fig. 7.1 aDirect Current (DC) with no wave form

The direct current is modulated for the clinical applications by interrupting the current flow after one second, reversing the polarity, and gradually increasing or decreasing the amplitude(ramped DC). Interruption is the most useful modification of the direct current. Interruption makes the flow of current commence and cease at regular intervals.

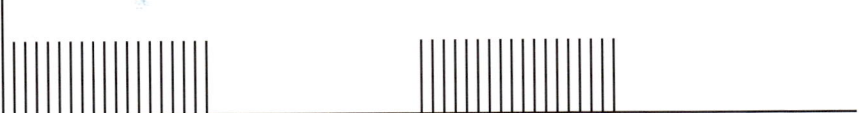

Fig. 7.1b Direct Current with interruptions (rectangular wave forms)

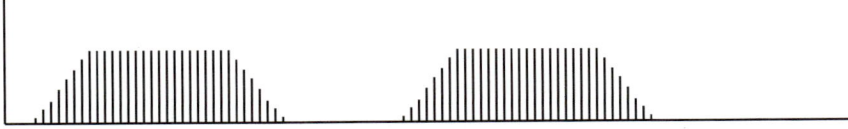

Fig.7.1c Direct Current with interruptions (saw tooth wave forms)

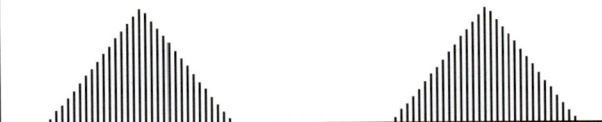

Fig. 7.1d Direct Current with interruptions (triangular wave forms)

Alternating Current

Alternating current is a biphasic current, which flows in the bidirectional. This current may have symmetrical and asymmetrical wave forms. Wave form shape could be of rectangular, triangular, depends on the capabilities of the generator. The square wave is characterized by a fast rising leading edge of the pulse, flat plateau at peak, and rapid return to zero. The symmetrical biphasic square wave allows selective treatment of smaller muscles by allowing the clinicians to identify the anode and cathode and choose the effective direction of flow for depolarization. The symmetrical biphasic square wave dictates that the current flows equally "hard and fast" in both phases, thus allowing both electrodes to act as active electrodes. This wave form is preferred for stimulation of the large muscle groups. Symmetric biphasic waveform is preferred over the asymmetric biphasic waveforms.

Therapeutic Currents

For therapeutic uses there are two modulated forms of the alternating currents- time modulated AC (Russian current) and amplitude modulated AC (interferential current). The time modulated current is mostly used for the stimulation of innervated muscles and control over the pain gate (Neuromuscular electrical stimulation).

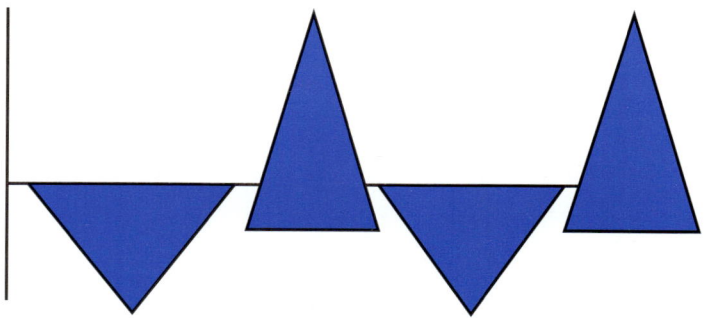

Fig.7.1e Alternating Current with two unequal (asymmetrical) phases

The frequency of cycles of AC is measured in cycles per second or hertz. There is an inverse relationship between frequency and phase duration. As the frequency of AC increases, phase duration automatically decreases.

Low Frequency Currents

Electrical muscle stimulation is the method of stimulating nerve and producing involuntary contraction of the muscles through the currents. Luigi Galvani (1791) provided the first scientific evidence that current can activate muscle. He stimulated frog nerves and muscles with electrical charges from lightning and recorded that the animals spontaneously developed electricity. However, Alessandro Volta in 1976 proved that the electrical changes in Galvani's experiment were the result between dissimilar metals that were in contact with each other and not spontaneously produced by the animals. During the 19th and 20th centuries, researchers studied and documented the exact electrical properties that generate muscle movement.[1-2] It was discovered that the body functions induced by electrical stimulation caused long-term changes in the muscles.[3,4] Faradic and Galvanic currents are usually used to stimulate the nerves and muscles.

Faradic Current

In 1930s Faraday discovered that bidirectional electrical current could be induced by moving magnet. He called this a faradic current. Faradic type of current is short duration interrupted direct current with pulse duration of .1 millisecond to 01 millisecond and frequency of 50-100 Hz. Frequency is the rate at which the individual pulses are delivered to the nerve and is measured in pulses per second or Hz. The faradic type of current was initially produced by the induction coil (faradic coil) which consists of two unequal phases, first of low intensity, long duration and second phase of high intensity and short duration.

The faradic coil is now replaced with electronic stimulators. The faradic current produced by the electronic stimulators and induction coil has same physiological effects on the tissues but differ from the wave forms. The plane faradic current has insufficient time between the pulses that lead to fatigue of the muscles easily in a short period of time. Therefore, in order to avoid fatigue faradic current has been modified into surges.

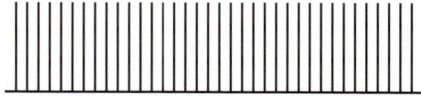

Fig. 7.2a Unmodified or plane faradic current, no relaxation period between the pulses

The modified faradic current is interrupted at regular intervals to provide sufficient time to the muscle to get ready for the next contraction. The regular intervals between the pulses can be increased or decreased according to the conditions of the muscles. Each pulse of the modified current has a series of contractions which may increase either gradually or suddenly and fall gradually or suddenly after reaching to the peak points. The pulse of a series of contractions is termed as "surge". The surges can be modified into various durations, frequencies and wave forms.

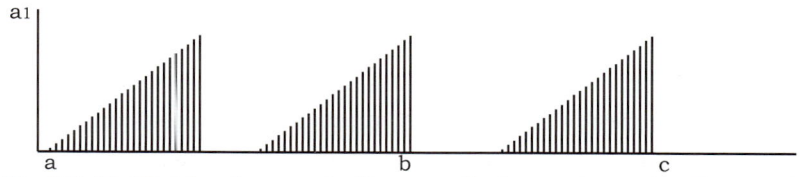

Fig. 7.2b Modified faradic current with surges. Each surge has series of contractions which may increase gradually and fall suddenly after reaching to the peak. There is a distance between two surges which is known as relaxation period, that can be increased

or decreased. a-a₁ (amplitude) strength of impulse, a-d pulse width with various relaxation period between the phases, the relaxation period between a and b is smaller than the b and c. it is therefore, the relaxation period between the pulsed can be modified according to the status of the nerve and muscles.

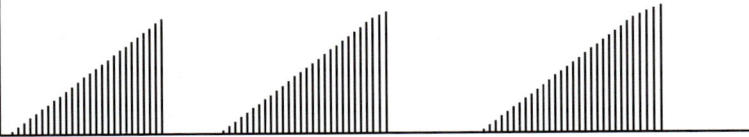

Fig. 7.2c Surges of various pulse widths. The pulse width of the surge can be increased or decreased. the pulse width of c is greater than the a and b.

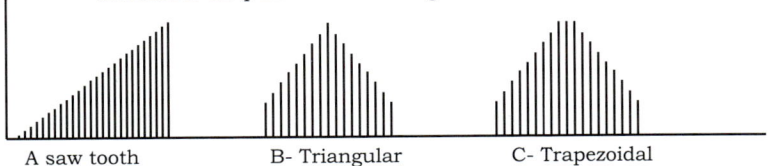

| A saw tooth | B- Triangular | C- Trapezoidal |

Fig. 7.2d Surges of various wave forms. A. Saw tooth- the contraction increases gradually and falls suddenly after reaching the peak. B-Triangular- the contraction increases gradually and falls gradually after reaching the peak. C- Trapezoidal- The contraction increases gradually and sustains at the peak for some time and then falls gradually.

Interrupted Galvanic Current

Interrupted galvanic current is a long duration of (1 millisecond to 600 millisecond) monophasic direct current with a frequency between 1Hz and 6Hz. The impulses rise and fall gradually followed by a brief period of relaxation. The rise and fall of the impulses with relaxation do not allow accommodation of the nerve. These impulses are often termed as selective because a contraction of denervated muscle can often be produced with an intensity of current that is insufficient to stimulate the motor nerve as accommodation occurs[5]. Galvanic is a long duration current that can be adjusted according to the conditions of the muscles. To stimulate denervated muscles the pulse duration should be 600ms initially, however; as soon as patient shows improvement in the strength of the contraction that muscle can be stimulated at the short pulse current. An impulse of 100millisecond with frequency of 30 per minute is commonly practiced. If the duration of the current is increased from 100ms the frequency of impulses must be decreased, on the other hand if the pulse duration of the current is decreased from 100ms the frequency must be increased. This is to avoid fatigue of the muscles. The ratio of contraction (impulse) and relaxation (interval between the pulses) period should be 1:1 or preferably 1:2.

Physiological Effects of faradic and Galvanic

The stimulus with an adequate strength and enough duration can produce following physiological effects in the tissues-

Nerve Depolarization – In the resting state there are the positive ions outside and negative ions inside of the nerve membrane. If there is no transmission of ions across the membrane then it can be said that the nerve is at the state of polarization. This is also known as resting membrane potential. Nerve at rest has a membrane potential of -60 milli volt secondary to the selective permeability of the membrane to potassium and sodium ions (a higher concentration of sodium ions results extracellularly, leaving intracellular space more electrically negative.)

When a stimulus of sufficient strength is applied over a sufficient length of time, sodium channels in the cell membrane open rapidly, while potassium channel open slowly. The sodium ions rush into the cell through the membrane. This makes the cell more positive inside the membrane and as soon as membrane potential reaches to +30 milli volt, the permeability to sodium ions decreases. Now the potassium channels open rapidly. The membrane permits potassium ions outside of it. The reduction of negative charges, which also represents a reduction of the membrane potential of the cell, is known as depolarization phase. The abrupt change of the resting potential, leading to the development of an action potential or excitation of cell. The transmission of ions from sodium (outside) to potassium (inside) and potassium to sodium causes nerve depolarization.

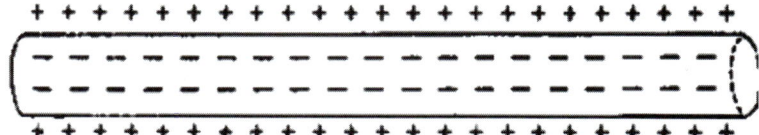

Fig. 7.3a Resting Membrane Potential

As soon as the depolarization or excitation of the membrane reaches to its peak i.e. between 60 and 90 milli volt, the permeability of sodium ions decreases and it is followed by repolarization phase. Immediately after this activity the sodium ions are pumped out and potassium ions pumped in again. The membrane returns to its resting state. The difference of potential between the active and resting parts of the nerve causes local electron flow . Electrons travel from a region of high concentration (the cathode/negative electrode) to one of lower concentration (the anode/positive electrode). This sequential depolarization and repolarization of the cell membrane caused by the change of flow of ions across the cell membrane is called action potential(AP)

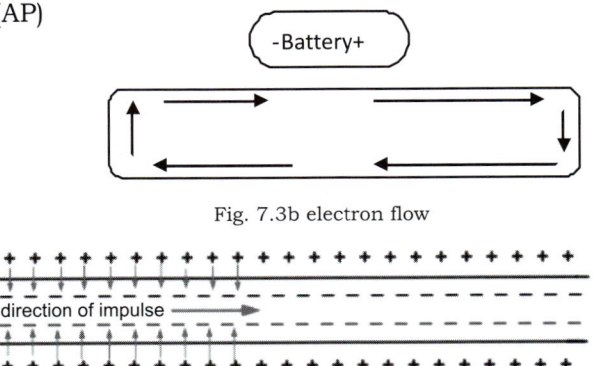

Fig. 7.3b electron flow

direction of impulse ⟶

Fig. 7.3c direction of flow of impulse

When the nerve is at the stage of depolarization and there is no fall in the action potential, nerve cannot be stimulated further. This period is known as absolute refractory and relative refractory period. If the nerve axon fails to respond to the subsequent stimulus this is known as absolute refractory period. Therefore; to get the nerve stimulated a stronger stimulus then the previous stimulus is required, which is known as refractory period. After depolarization just before returning to the resting potential, there is a brief period of membrane hyperpolarization.

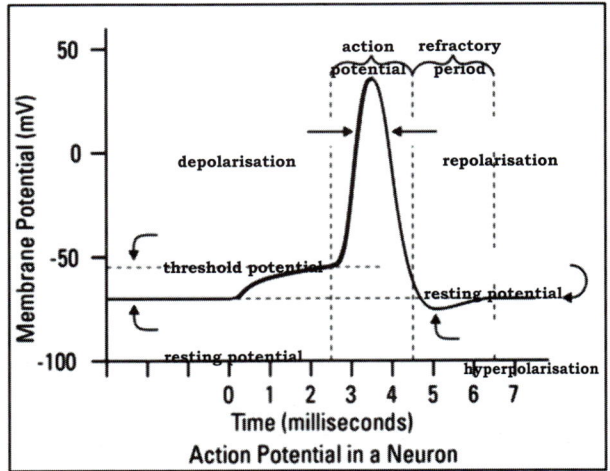

Fig. 7.3d Nerve depolarization, action potential and refractory period

Sensory Nerve Stimulation – The flow of current to the superficial structures on the skin is perceived by the superficial nerve ending, which leads to prickling sensation. The sensory stimulation causes a reflex vasodilatation of the superficial blood vesels which produces slight erythma on the skin (local area).

Motor Nerve Stimulation – A stimulus of sufficient strength (intensity) can stimulate the motor nerve which in turn can cause tetanic contraction of the muscles. Tetanic is the surge which includes series of contractions or pulses of short period. Approximately 50-100 contractions or pulses are produced in .1-1milisecond.

Increase Metabolism – The tetanic like contraction of the muscles or group of muscles increases metabolic rate, with consequent increase in the demand for oxygen, and foodstuff. There is increased output of the waste products including metabolites.

Increase Vasodilatation – Increase metabolism and demand for oxygen increases dilatation of the blood vessels (arterioles and capillaries). A tetanic contraction followed by relaxation exerts a pumping action within and around the vessels. The pumping action helps in increasing venous and lymphatic return.

Denervated Muscle Contraction – Faradic has limited use in the stimulation of the denervated muscles as the current is of short duration. The denervated muscles require more time to get stimulated therefore, galvanic, a long duration current can stimulate the denervated muscles , prevent disuse atrophy, and helps in regeneration of the nerve.

Polarity

Under normal physiological conditions, less current is required from a cathodal stimulus to evoke a muscle contraction of given strength than from an anode stimulus. Therefore the negative electrode is used to evoke the muscle contraction and is termed the active electrode, because depolarization of the biologically excitable tissue is most easily accomplished at the cathode. Excitable tissue under the positive electrode is less prone to depolarization and thus, the anode is often termed the inactive, reference, or dispersive electrode[6]. The strength of a muscle contraction produced by the inactive electrode(anode) is about 70 percent of the contraction produced by the active electrode (cathode) at a given current amplitude[7].

Direct current can induce chemical reactions in body tissues. There is oxidation of the anions at the anode that results in acidic reactions, whereas, at the cathode, reduction of the cations results in alkaline reactions. These electrochemical reactions under the cathode and anode electrodes are referred to a polar reactions. The polar reaction under the anode electrode can cause formation of hydrochloride (HCL), solidification of protein, hardening of the tissues, hyperpolarization and increased nerve excitability. The polar reaction under cathode electrode include formation of sodium hydroxide (NaOH), liquification of protein, softening of tissues, hyperpolarization and increased excitability. To avoid such chemical reactions under the electrodes, their positions are changed intermittently.

Alternating current is a biphasic current, which flows in two direction or bidirection. The electrodes used to deliver the current to the tissues change their polarity as the current changes its direction. Therefore, the chemical reactions formed under the electrodes during one half cycle of phase of the output is neutralized by the next half cycle of the output which is opposite in direction and similar in magnitude. The change of direction in every half cycle changes the polarity of the electrodes and thus avoids formation of any chemical reactions under the electrodes.

Therapeutic Uses

Electrical therapeutic currents have been used for many years to successfully stimulate and contract paralyzed muscles[8, 9]. It has received increasing attention in the last few years because of its potential to serve as a strength training tool for healthy subjects and athletes, a rehabilitation and preventive tool for partially or totally immobilized patients, a testing tool for evaluating the neural and/or muscular function in vivo., and a post-exercise recovery tool for athletes.[10]

Disuse Atrophy-Prevention and Reduction – Disuse atrophy refers to the decrease in muscle cross sectional area or reduction of muscle mass (there is no change in the number of muscle fibers, but rather a decrease in the mean fiber cross sectional area). It may occur as a result of prolonged immobilization of the joint (after fracture), or as a result of central nerve system trauma (stroke or spinal cord injury). Both the type I and type II muscle fibers show atrophy following immobilization. The atrophy of the type I (slow-twitch muscle fibers) begins soon after the immobilization whereas; atrophy in the type II (fast-twitch) muscle fibers begins after months of the immobilization. Therefore, atrophy of the type II muscle fibers is a more gradual process and only observed after months of immobilization.

Electrical stimulation promotes early active range of motion in post surgical and cast immobilized limbs[11].Use of electrical stimulation in preventing the muscle atrophy or decrease the effect of the atrophy is a common practice in the physiotherapy, however; its effectiveness depends upon the parameters of current. The atrophy of the muscle may range from minimal to the severe. To treat the muscles with severe atrophy, the frequency and contraction time (on time) should be as low as possible usually 3-10pps (pulses per second), and 5 seconds respectively. The relaxation period between the two contractions should be at least 25-50 seconds. To treat the muscles with minimal atrophy, the frequency of the pulses per second and contraction period (on time) can be increased to 30-50pps, and 10-15 seconds. The session length should be 15 minutes irrespective of the severity of the atrophy. 3-4 treatment sessions may be repeated daily. If patient achieves voluntary contraction, electrical stimulation can be discontinued, and should be encouraged to the resisted exercises. However, if endurance is the concerned, the electrical stimulation may be continued until the functional goal previously established are achieved or modified.

Pain Control – A stimulus of sufficient strength can stimulate sensory as well as motor nerve. The impulses are carried out by the large-diameter afferent neurons to the spinal cord, where they may travel to higher centers in the central nervous system and eventually be perceived as a pain sensation. While travelling to the higher centers, the large diameter afferent neurons block the small diameter nociceptive impulses at the level of spinal canal, resulting in analgesia.

Increase, Maintain and Restore Range of Motion – Loss of Range of motion following prolong immobilization, injuries, surgery, pain, stroke and spinal cord insult is a common problem. Maintenance and restoration of the range of motion is one of the challenges in the clinical practice. For example, (a) pain in the knee joint due to chronic osteoarthritis limits range of motion of the joint. Stimulation of the quadriceps muscles with low level of intensity for long periods can increase range of motion of the knee joint.[12] (b.) Spasticity in the flexor group of the wrist limits extension range. In a study reported by Baker et al and expanded by Waters and Bowman, a nerve and muscle electrical stimulation program was effective in maintaining wrist and finger range of motion into extension in nearly 80 patients with spastic hemiparesis without joint limitations.[13,14] Munsat et al, reported first time that stimulation of the femoral nerve provided activation of the quadriceps femoris muscle group which improved range of motion of the knee joint.[15] To maintain range of motion of the joint between 50 to 100 cyclic repetitions of range through full joint excursion per treatment session are required. However, to gain range of motion of the joint more aggressive treatment is administered, especially in the presence of spasticity; the number of repetitions must increase to 200 or more pre treatment session.[16] To be optimal, stimulation programs should be done daily, which is often most effectively managed at home.[17]

Decrease Spasticity – Spasticity resulting from trauma, lesion or dysfunction of the central nervous system is a major concern for the physical therapist. The spastic muscles inhibit the weak agonist, prohibiting the patient from using the extremity appropriately. Moderate to severe spasticity not only interferes with the functions but also disturbs the posture, making coordinated movements impossible. Electric stimulation of the antagonists to a spastic muscle, followed by vigorous range of motion exercises can, dramatically decrease the muscle tone. When spasticity impedes volitional control, addition of the electrical stimulation provides significant increase in the management of abnormal muscle tone[18]. The neurophysiologic rationale for the effectiveness of electrical stimulation to the antagonist of the spastic muscle deems to rest on the principle of reciprocal inhibition. However; the effect of the reciprocal inhibition is very short, measurable in milliseconds. The phenomenon known as posttetanic potentiation (PTT) may account for some of the therapeutic effects that exceed the length of the treatment program[19].

Electrical stimulation of the spastic muscles to reduce spasticity and increase voluntary contraction has also been reported in many literatures[37] However, some authors believe that the electrical stimulation of the spastic muscles may result in no effect or slight increase in spasticity.[20] There are two possible rationale for the decrease in tone fatigue following the barrage of electrical stimulation of same motor neurons and antidromic activation of the axon of an alpha motor neuron. The antidromic stimulation of the alpha motor neuron activates the motor unit and, through recurrent collaterals, excites a pool of Renshaw cells. In turn, the Renshaw cells inhibit the alpha motor neuron of the activated pool and the motor neurons of the synergistic muscles.

Improve Inadequate Voluntary Control – The inability to contract the muscles adequately as per demand of the activities of daily living may be due to (a.) peripheral inhibition of the central nervous system such as pain in the knee joint, or (b.) due to decreased descending activation from the cortical and subcortical centers onto the alpha motoneuron pool such as immediately following stroke. Inadequate contraction of the muscle is mainly due to inadequate motoneuron drive on voluntary command. Peripheral inhibition of the motoneuron pool, that decreases voluntary contraction of the muscles can be enhanced by decreasing the patients pain and increasing the sensory drive, by applying the electrical stimulation to the nerve which will excite the motoneuron of the targeted muscles.

Control or decrease Edema - Voluntary contraction of the muscles producers pumping action which aids in venous return. Loss of pumping action of the muscles does not adequately help in venous return that may lead to accumulation of the fluid in the local area or in the limb. Congestion of the body fluid may also occur due to compromised peripheral vascular function such as venous insufficiency. Loss of pumping action of the muscles may occur as a result of injury, prolong bed rest, weakness due to pain, or dysfunction of the central or peripheral nervous system. Application of the electrical stimulation to the weak muscles can cause contraction that improves the pumping action and thus improve circulation to the area. Bipolar electrodes of one or more channels are placed over the agonist and antagonists muscles for reciprocal contraction and relaxation. The ratio of contraction and relaxation of the muscles should be 1:2 respectively to allow weak muscles to relax. Treatment session should be approximately 20-30 minutes, however;

time may be increased or decreased as per the patient's tolerance. The technique used to reduce edema is known as faradism under pressure which is described later in this chapter.

Muscle Re education and Facilitation Prolonged immobilization following fracture or injury, weakness due to dysfunction of central nervous system or peripheral nervous system, un-ables the patients to contract the muscles by voluntary demand. In other words, simply the muscle forgets its own action. For example, (a,) in patients with long standing flat foot the intrinsic muscles become unaware of their own action, (b,) spasticity in the flexor group of the muscles due to dysfunction of central nervous system does not allow active extension of the wrist in response to voluntary demand, (c,) paralysis of one side of the face muscles due to dysfunction of the peripheral nervous system (Bell's palsy) remain stretched to the sound side and (d,) following tendon transfer muscle does not contract voluntarily as it is not aware of the new action. Electrical stimulation not only helps in reeducating the muscle action but also facilitates the action of the muscles by providing proprioceptive, kinesthetic, and sensory input. The electrical stimulation facilitates muscle action during functional training involving gait training.[21]

Tissue Repair – The human body has a mechanism that is engaged in the repairing of the damaged tissues due to injury or trauma. Electrical stimulation at a wound site has been claimed to accelerate and enhance healing by retarding bacterial growth, increasing local circulation, or enhancing the natural process of tissue repair[22]. The electrical stimulation around the wound site can increase the permeability to macromolecules, and marked extravasation of white blood cells occurred from the capillaries. There is migration of epidural cells, fibroblasts, leukocytes, and macrophases by electrical fields. Lateral fields at the edge of wound conceivably could directly promote the inflammatory response, epithelialization, and fibrogenesis associated with wound healing.[23]

Contraindications

i.   Cardiac Pace Maker – Electrical stimulation should not be given over the pace maker directly as this can interfere the function of the pace maker

ii. Over the carotid sinus – Application of electrical stimulation on the carotid sinus may reduce the blood pressure of the patient.

iii. Areas of the venous or arterial thrmbosis or thrombophlebitis - Application of electrical stimulation on the area of venous or arterial thrombosis or thrombophlebitis may increase circulation, and the risk of releasing emboli.

iv. Pregnancy- over the abdomen – The application of electrical stimulation directly or nearby to the fetus area can cause current to pass to the fetus.

v. Impaired sensation – Areas of sensory deficit should well be avoided for electircal stimulation. Application of electrical current directly over the area of impaired sensation can cause electrical burn.

vi. Malignant Tumor - Application of electrical stimulation on the tumor can enhance the growth of the tissues as the current increases blood circulation and metabolism rate necessary for tissue growth.

vii. Open Wounds – Electrical stimulation is used to enhance the healing and growth of the tissues, but the sensation of the areas (peripheral to the open area) should be tested and the intensity may be kept low to avoid any adverse effects.

Motor Point

A motor point can physiologically be identified as a specific location on the skin that requires the lowest amplitude of electrical stimulation to produce excitation of an underlying innervated muscle. Anatomically, this area of skin has been found to transversely overlie a muscle's neurovascular hilus, which contain sensory, motor, and autonomic axons, and the zone of innervations, where branches of motor axons terminate on individual muscle fibers.[24,25] This is the point where maximum muscle contraction is achieved than any other area of the muscle with the same amplitude of the current.

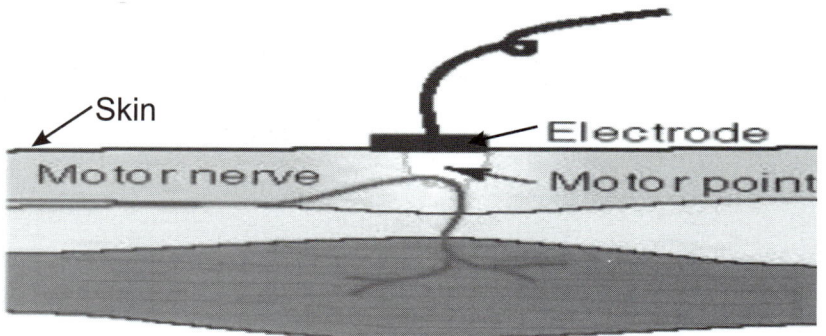

Fig.7.4 Motor Point

Motor points are frequently located at the junctions of the upper and middle one thirds of the fleshy belly of the muscle. There are some exceptions

i.   The motor points of the vastus medialis, whose nerve enters at the lower part of the muscle, is situated a short distance above the knee joint[26].

ii.   The motor point of the extensor hallucis longus can only be elicited at the distal anterior part of the ankle joint as the upper and middle one third of the muscle is deep to the peroneii muscles.

iii. In denervated muscles normal motor point is no longer present as these muscles are deprived of the nerve supply. The contraction is present due to stimulation of the muscle itself, rather than the motor nerve. Hence, the motor point is usually found distal to the normal motor point. However; no contraction is achieved with the short pulse durations.

Technique – Determination of the motor point is essential either to strengthen the weak muscle or to draw strength duration curve for the diagnosis. The individual or specific muscles can be strengthened by stimulating the muscles at the motor points.

Preparation of equipment – The equipment electronic muscle and nerve stimulator and diagnostic should be free from any electric shock. It should have faradic, surge faradic, plane galvanic and interrupted galvanic currents. The parameters of the currents such as frequency, wave forms, and contraction and relaxation periods should be designed very well on the equipment.

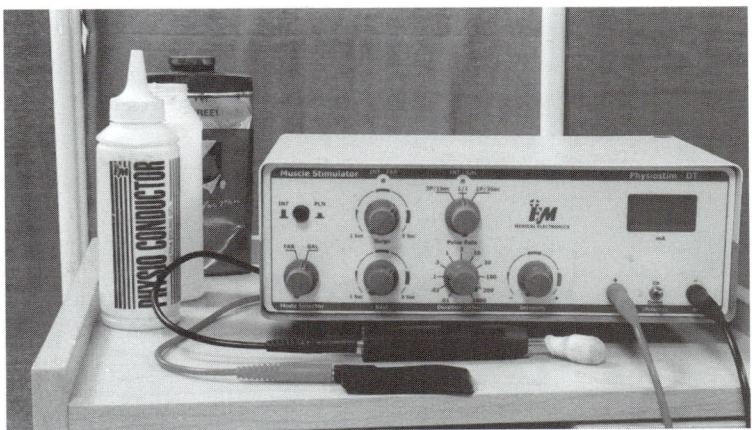

Fig. 7.5 Electrical muscle and nerve stimulator

The equipment should have black and red colored marked points for active and passive electrodes. The electrodes may be made up of carbon and stainless steel (plate). If plate electrodes are used to stimulate nerve and muscles these should be covered with the lint (cloth). The lint is of cotton cloth, which is folded in such a way that eight layers can be made. The plate electrode is inserted into the folded lint that seven layers out of eight remain on one side of it. The seven layer part of the electrode is placed over the skin, whereas' last layer of the lint remain out. However, many therapist cover the plate electrodes with the lint as per the convenience of patient and therapist. The carbon electrodes do not require lint and placed on the patient surface with the gel.

Selection of Parameters – Select the current, pulse duration, and frequency. To elicit the motor points interrupted (galvanic) direct current should be selected, this is because, it is a long duration current and can stimulate both the innervated and denervated muscles. On the other hand faradic current is a short duration current which cannot stimulate the denervated muscles, therefore, if surge faradic current is selected it would not elicit the motor points of the denervated or partially denervated muscles.

Self Testing of the equipment – If all the parameters are set and electrodes are prepared for eliciting the motor points, it is important to test the equipment before applying the current to the patient to know whether the equipment is working satisfactorily or not. For self testing the therapist places both the electrodes under the palmer aspect of hand and the intensity is increased gradually. A fine visible contraction with comfortable current can be elicited. If the examiner feels discomfort with the current with increasing intensity and the current unables to elicit the visible contraction it may probably be due to the malfunctioning of the equipment. It should not be tried on the patient.

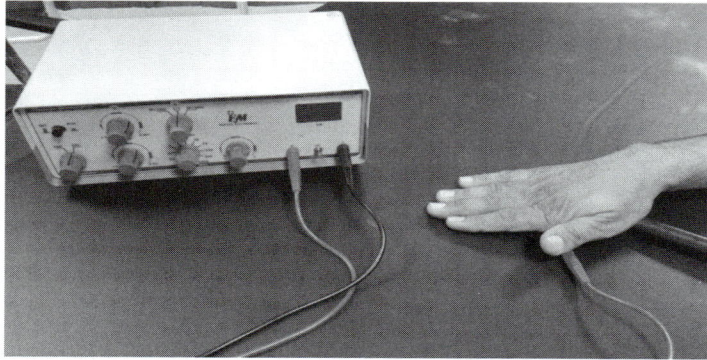

Fig. 7.6 self testing of the equipment.

Preparation of patient – The patient is placed in a comfortable position. Muscle which is being stimulated must be exposed adequately from origin to the insertion. The skin must be cleaned with the warm water and soap or alcohol to remove any dirt to decrease the skin resistance. If the muscles of the extremity are to be stimulated, place joint at neutral position to see the visible contraction (for motor points) or place the extremity with appropriate support in a semi flexed position for the desired movement (for strengthening).

Placement of the electrodes – To elicit the motor points of the muscles two electrodes- Pencil and plate or pad (carbon) are used. The pencil and pad electrodes are called active and passive electrode respectively. The knob of the active electrode is a metal peace which is placed over the muscle belly. The metal knob of the electrode must completely be covered by a lint or cloth. The knob of the electrode with lint or cloth is soaked repeatedly into the water to conduct the current to the tissues through the lint. An active electrode is placed directly on the muscle belly to find out the motor point.

There are three criteria for placement of the passive electrode (i.) on the origin of the muscle, (ii.) on the respective nerve trunk, and (iii.) on the spinal cord (spine). Efforts should be made to place the electrode over the origin of the muscle, but if it is difficult especially when the motor points of the small muscles (facial) are elicited or there is difficulty in exposing the origin of the muscles for privacy such as quadriceps and hamstrings. For these reasons the passive electrode is placed over the trunk or spinal cord. The advantage of the placement of the electrode over the nerve trunk is that all the muscles supplied by the respective nerve can be stimulated without changing the passive electrode.

Elicitation of motor point – After preparing the patient and selecting the parameters of the current, explain the procedure to the patient. The passive electrode is placed over the desired position as mentioned above and active electrode is placed randomly on the upper and middle one thirds of the fleshy belly of the muscle. Ensure that the intensity knob is at the zero before switching the equipment on. The intensity is increased gradually. The examiner must keep the eyes on the muscle which is being stimulated to see the visible contraction. As soon as a visible contraction is observed the intensity is stopped increasing further. The examiner now moves the active electrode over the upper and middle one thirds of the fleshy belly of the muscle to find out maximum contraction. The point where maximum contraction is achieved is termed the motor point of the said muscle. The examiner must ensure that the electrode is kept perpendicular to the muscle and pressure should also be same throughout the procedure. The electrode must not be lifted off the muscle belly while searching the motor point and intensity if on.

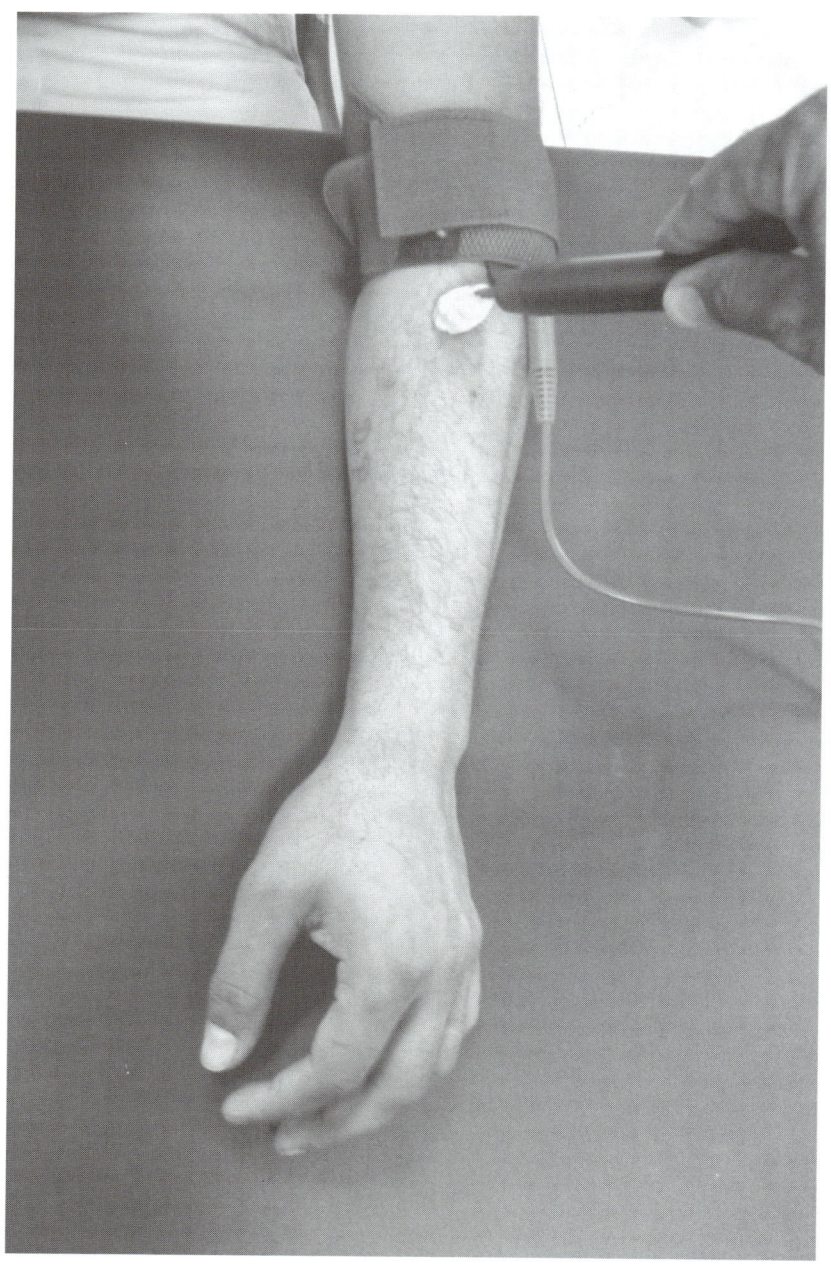

Fig. 7.7a Elicitation of Motor Point

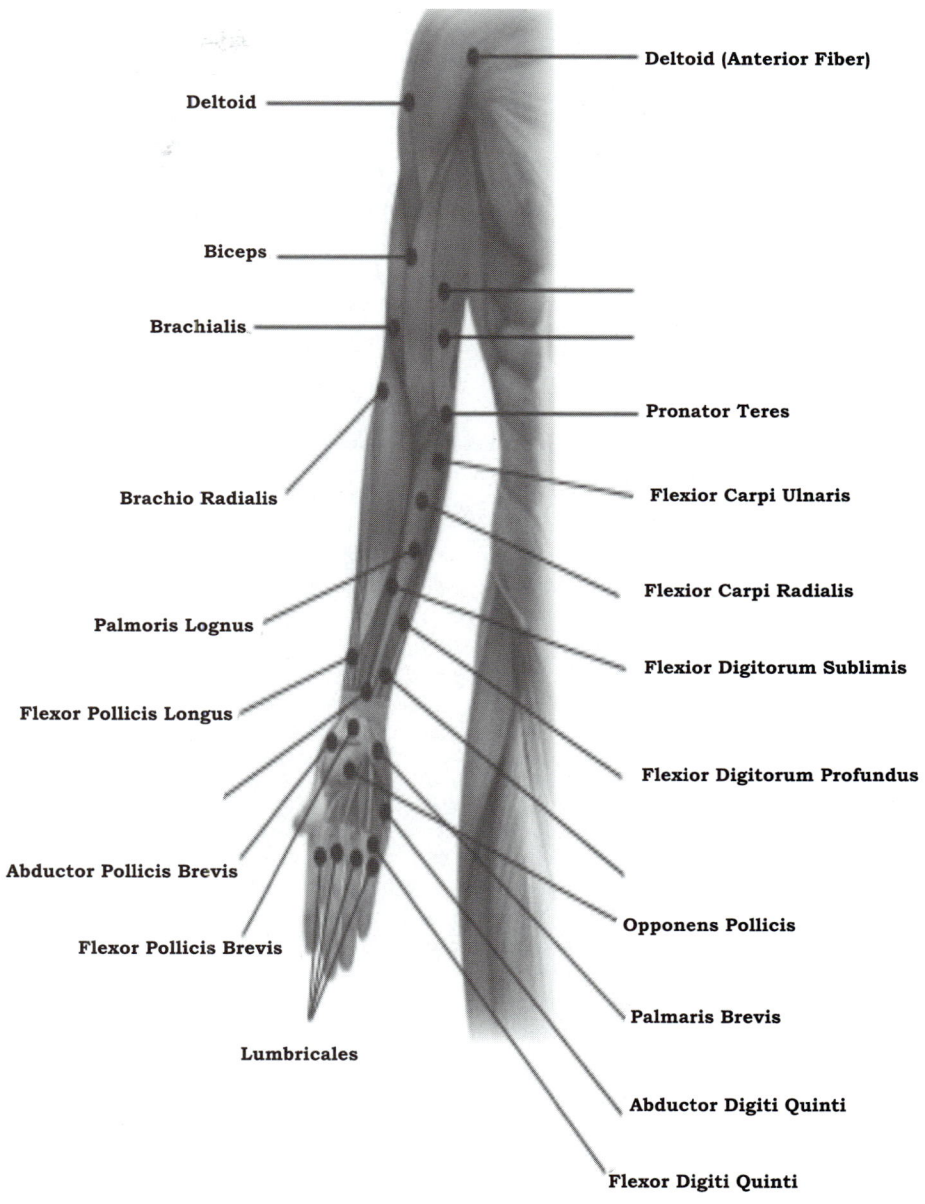

Deltoid (Anterior Fiber)

Deltoid

Biceps

Brachialis

Pronator Teres

Brachio Radialis

Flexor Carpi Ulnaris

Flexor Carpi Radialis

Palmoris Lognus

Flexor Digitorum Sublimis

Flexor Pollicis Longus

Flexor Digitorum Profundus

Abductor Pollicis Brevis

Flexor Pollicis Brevis

Opponens Pollicis

Lumbricales

Palmaris Brevis

Abductor Digiti Quinti

Flexor Digiti Quinti

Fig. 7.7b Illustration of Motor points of upper extremity (palmer view)

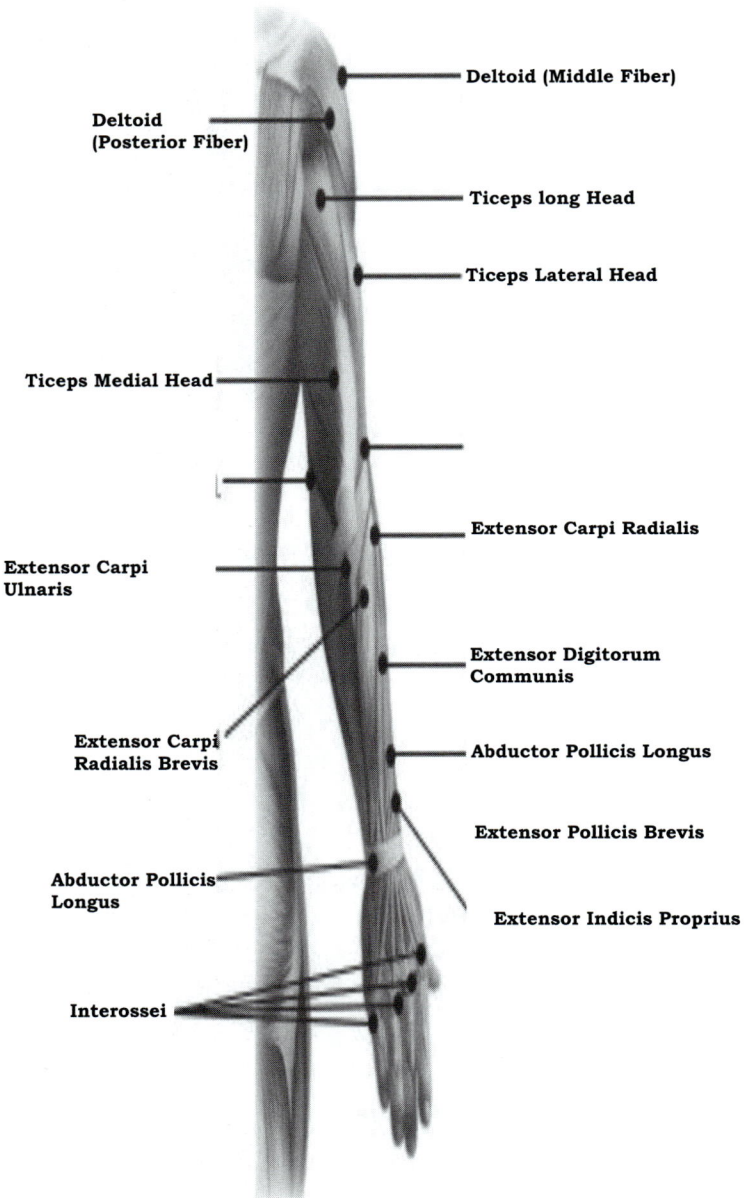

Deltoid (Middle Fiber)

Deltoid
(Posterior Fiber)

Ticeps long Head

Ticeps Lateral Head

Ticeps Medial Head

Extensor Carpi Radialis

Extensor Carpi
Ulnaris

Extensor Digitorum
Communis

Extensor Carpi
Radialis Brevis

Abductor Pollicis Longus

Extensor Pollicis Brevis

Abductor Pollicis
Longus

Extensor Indicis Proprius

Interossei

Fig. 7.7c Illustration of Motor points of upper extremity (dorsal view)

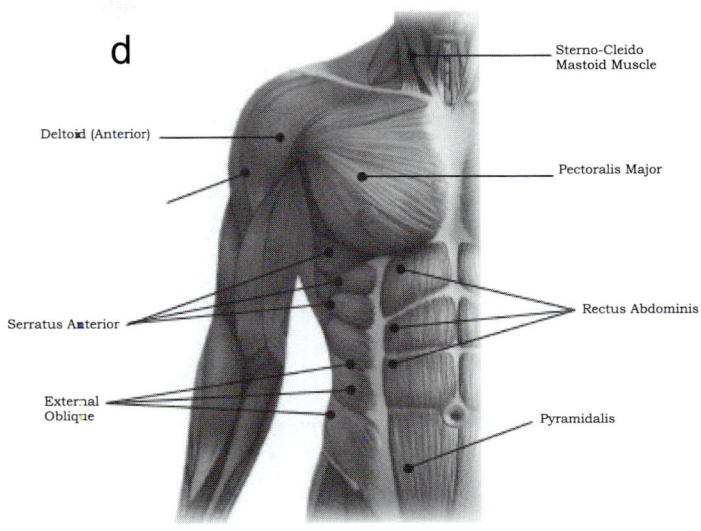

d

Sterno-Cleido Mastoid Muscle

Deltoid (Anterior)

Pectoralis Major

Serratus Anterior

Rectus Abdominis

External Oblique

Pyramidalis

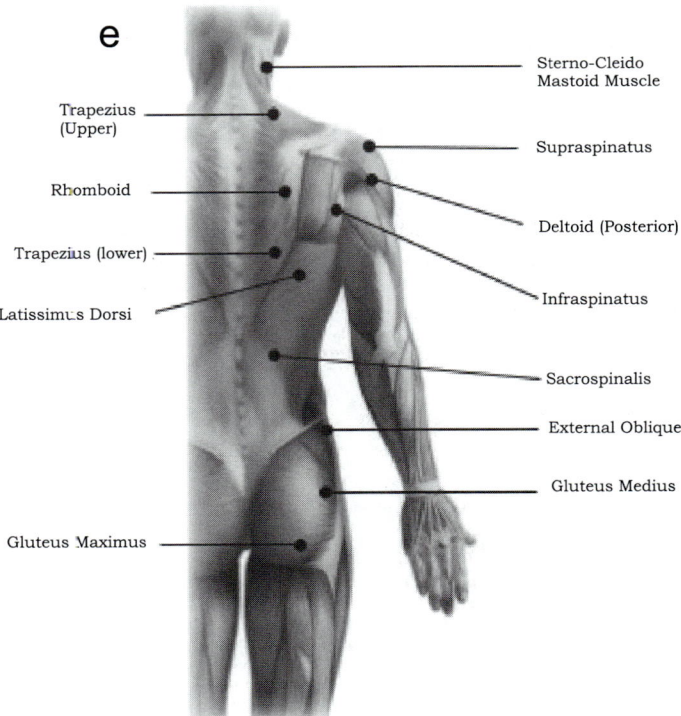

e

Sterno-Cleido Mastoid Muscle

Trapezius (Upper)

Supraspinatus

Rhomboid

Deltoid (Posterior)

Trapezius (lower)

Infraspinatus

Latissimus Dorsi

Sacrospinalis

External Oblique

Gluteus Medius

Gluteus Maximus

Fig. 7.7d&e Illustration of Motor points of chest and back

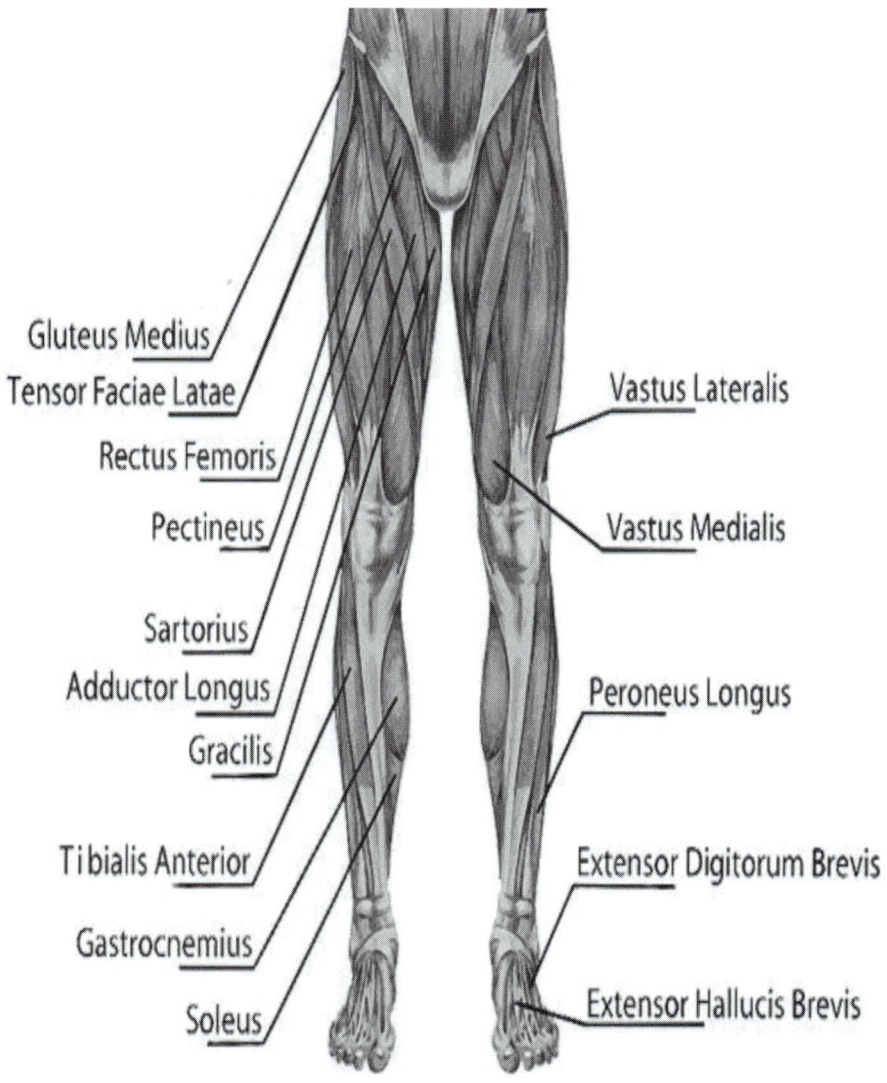

Gluteus Medius

Tensor Faciae Latae

Rectus Femoris

Pectineus

Sartorius

Adductor Longus

Gracilis

Tibialis Anterior

Gastrocnemius

Soleus

Vastus Lateralis

Vastus Medialis

Peroneus Longus

Extensor Digitorum Brevis

Extensor Hallucis Brevis

Fig. 7.7f Illustration of Motor points of lower extremity (anterior view)

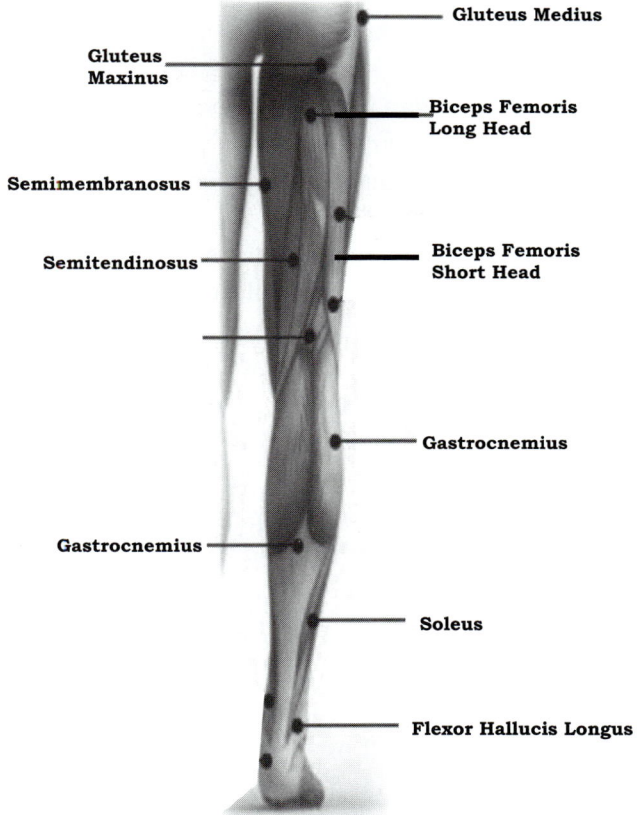

Gluteus Medius

Gluteus Maxinus

Biceps Femoris Long Head

Semimembranosus

Biceps Femoris Short Head

Semitendinosus

Gastrocnemius

Gastrocnemius

Soleus

Flexor Hallucis Longus

Fig. 7.7g Illustration of Motor points of lower extremity (posterior view)

Motor Points of Facial Muscles

The facial muscles are supplied by the seventh cranial nerve. Bell's palsy and upper motor neuron lesion can affect the contraction of the facial muscles. Bell's palsy is a lower motor neuron lesion in which paralysis of same side of facial muscles occurs following pain in the ear (Herpes Zoster infection) whereas; in upper motor neuron lesion paralysis of the muscles of opposite side of the face occurs, the later may affect both the sides of muscles.

The facial nerve divides into three nerve trunk – upper, middle and lower. To stimulate the facial muscles the passive electrode (pad/plate) can either be placed over the nerve trunk of the seventh cranial nerve or over the cervical spine as it is difficult to place over the origin of the muscles because they are very short. An active electrode is placed directly over the muscle belly which is being stimulated. The intensity is increased gradually till a visible contraction is achieved. After achieving the visible contraction the intensity is stopped to increase further and active electrode is moved over the muscle to find out the maximum contraction (motor point). The active electrode is kept perpendicular to the muscle. The point where maximum muscle contraction is achieved is the motor point of that particular muscle. The motor points of all the muscles can be elicited by using this procedure. The examiner must ensure that the intensity is at zero before moving to the next muscle.

Accommodation

When adequate amplitude of current is transmitted in to the nerve it can cause potential difference which results in excitation of the nerve. The rise and fall of the current produce the nerve excitation. The accommodation is described as a phenomenon in which the threshold of membrane excitability automatically rises or ceases which the membrane is stimulated with a stimulus of slowly increasing intensity. If the variation of the current is gradual there is time for accommodation to take place, and the muscle (s) fails to respond to the stimulus, therefore; a greater current is needed to be effective than if the variation is sudden. A current that changes very slowly does not initiate a nerve impulse at all. It is, therefore, to avoid accommodation to take place in the nerve, a current of square wave form pulse, which rises or falls suddenly is used as it is more effective in initiating an impulse than one which changes slowly.

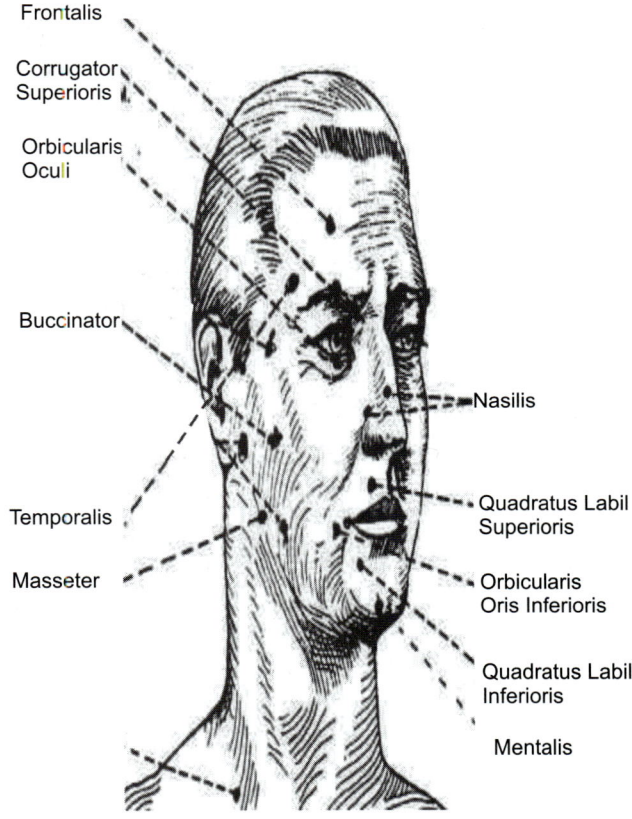

Frontalis

Corrugator
Superioris

Orbicularis
Oculi

Buccinator

Nasilis

Temporalis

Quadratus Labil
Superioris

Masseter

Orbicularis
Oris Inferioris

Quadratus Labil
Inferioris

Mentalis

fig.7.8 Motor points of facial muscles.

Faradic Foot Bath

Faradic foot bath is the technique of application of faradic current to stimulate and strengthen muscles of foot in the water. The foot ailments such as flat foot, Hallux valgus,and metatarsalgia can be treated with the faradic currents. It is difficult to stimulate the foot muscles by using the motor points technique as there are four layers of the muscles in the foot. The water makes perfect contact with the foot tissues and also reduces skin resistance. Position the patient in high sitting with back support. Place the foot in the bath. The level of water should be at the web of toes as shown in the image. If the water level is above the web of toes, this would unnecessoraly stimulate the dorsal muscles (foot). For Lumbrical Muscles: - Place each pad electrode under the heel and metatarsal heads transversely. For Planter Interossei Muscles: - Place one electrode on each side of the foot at the level of the metatarsal shafts. For Abductor Hallucis: -Place the pad electrode under the heel and pencil (active) electrode on the muscle belly of the abductor hallucis. Select the surge faradic current with an appropriate contraction and relaxation periods. The relaxation period should be larger than the contraction period to allow the muscles to relax and to avoid fatigue. Increase the intensity gradually till a strong contraction is achieved. Several contractions for 3-5minutes are repeated for improving the strength. The patient is encouraged to contract the muscles voluntarily with the electrical stimulation. Once the patient achieves voluntary contraction, the stimulation is discontinued.

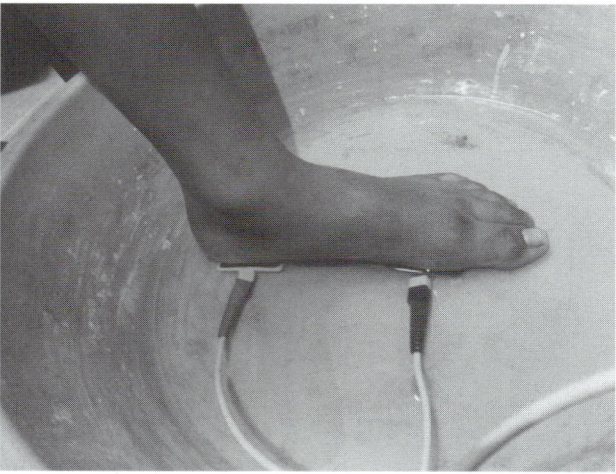

Fig. 7.9 faradic foot bath

Therapeutic Currents

Faradism Under Pressure

Faradism under pressure is the application of surge faradic current combined with the elastic crepe bandage to reduce swelling and edema of the distal part of the extremities. The elastic crepe bandage increases the pressure on the vessels when the muscles contract in response to electric stimulation and exerts a further pumping effect as the muscle relaxes during the relaxation phase of the current.

For Upper Extremity- Place the patient in supine position with the arm elevated above the heart level to enhance venous return. Remove all the jewellary and clothing to expose the extremity. Privacy of the patient must be the concerned. Clean the flexor aspect of the arm and forearm with the soap and warm water to reduce skin resistance. Place pad electrodes each over the flexor aspect of the arm and forearm. Apply an elastic crepe bandage from distal to proximal (hand to the proximal arm). The bandage is applied with maximum pressure at the hand and decreasing gradually towards the arm. There should not be any gaps between the turns of the bandage.

For Lower Extremity - Place the patient in supine position with the concerned leg elevated above the heart level to enhance venous return. Remove all the jewellary and clothing to expose the extremity. Privacy of the patient must be the concerned. Clean the posterior leg and the plantar surface with the soap and warm water to reduce the skin resistance. Place one pad electrode over the mid calf muscles and other pad electrode over the plantar aspect of the foot. Apply elastic crepe bandage with maximum pressure at the toes of the foot and decreasing gradually towards the proximal calf muscles. There should not be any gaps between the turns of the bandage.

Select the surge faradic current with appropriate pulse contraction and relaxation periods. Test the equipment whether it is working satisfactorily or not by placing each electrodes on the thenar and hypothenar surface of the hand. The rate of contraction must be slow, to allow maximum contraction of the muscle. The relaxation period should also be adequate preferably double of the contraction period to allow the vessels to refill. Ensure that the intensity knob is at zero before turning the stimulator on. Increase the intensity gradually till a strong contraction but tolerable is achieved. Total treatment time for reducing edema should be thirty minutes.

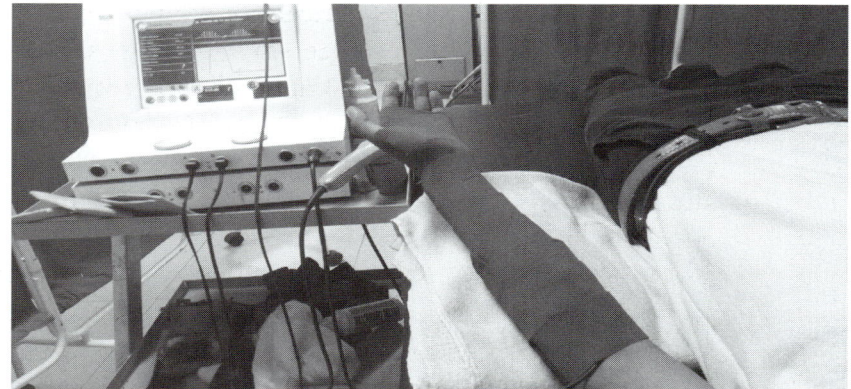

Fig. 7.10. Faradism Under Pressure.

Strength Duration Curve

The strength-duration curve is a technique of plotting of the threshold current (I) versus pulse duration (d) required to stimulate excitable tissue.[36] Plotting Strength duration curve is one of the techniques of testing of electrical reaction in peripheral lesions. It was the technique most widely used in the clinics till 1960s, and after that declined sharply with the development of nerve conduction velocity test and electromyography. The muscle is contracted to see the strength of impulses of various durations. Normal muscle responds to the electrical stimulation of pulse duration of ranged from .01 millisecond to the 600 millisecond. The longer the duration, the lesser the strength (in intensity) required to stimulate the muscle; and vice versa. The muscle deprived of nerve innervations do not respond to the electrical current of short pulse duration usually .01, .03, .1, .3 and 1 millisecond, but may respond to the longer pulse duration usually 100ms and above.

Application of electrical stimulation with appropriate parameters and proper positioning of the electrodes on motor points can provide reliable and accurate information on the status of the peripheral nerve innervations and dennervation to the muscles. The results of the strength curve can be as objective as nerve conduction testing and electromyography. The disadvantage of the technique is that in large muscles only a proportion of the fibers of the muscle respond to the current, so that the full picture is not clearly shown and also an SD curve does not indicate the site of the lesion. These limitations can only be overcome by testing several muscles, innervated by that particular nerve.

To plot an SD curve, a electrical stimulator capable of producing square-wave monophasic pulse stimuli of at various precise pulse duration range from .1 to 300millisecond is required. The stimulus must have a meter preferably digital for an accurate reading of intensity (strength) at various precise pulse durations. Most of stimulators are designed with the constant voltage and constant current. Wynn Parr's discussed the strength curve properties using a constant voltage stimulator rather than constant current stimulator and related that although the output of the constant current is more stable (because it compensates for changes in tissue impedence), both types of stimulators give equally accurate results and the constant voltage is more preferred in interest of the patient comfort and tolerance[27].

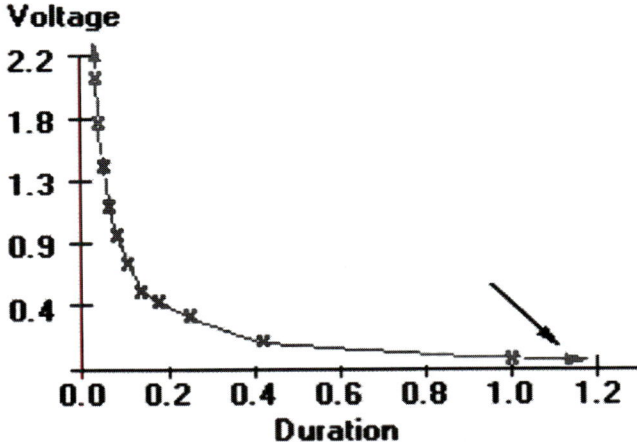

Fig.7.11a Strength Duration (S.D.) Curve for normal muscle (Constant Voltage)

The part which is being tested for strength duration curve is exposed adequately and the skin is cleaned with the warm water and soap. Passive electrode (pad) is either placed on the nerve trunk or origin of the muscle which is being tested, if both locations are not convenient the third choice of placement of passive electrode is on the lumbar spine for the lower extremities, and cervical spine for the upper extremity and facial muscles. Active (pencil) electrode is placed directly on the muscle belly. Interrupted direct galvanic current with constant voltage or constant current is selected. The frequency of the pulses should ideally be thirty pulses per minute. Strength duration curve plotting should be started from the longer durations for example 300millisecond pulse duration is selected first and the intensity is increased till a visible or palpable contraction is achieved.

The point where muscle starts showing visible contraction is the strength of the stimulus at the 300millisecond pulse duration. This amplitude (intensity) shown by the meter is recorded. The intensity is reduced to zero and next shorter pulse duration is selected i.e. 100millisecond. The intensity is increased gradually till a visible contraction is achieved. The point where muscle starts showing visible contraction is the strength of the stimulus at the 100millisecond pulse duration. This same procedure is repeated for each length of the stimulus. The minimum visible contraction should be same for all the pulse durations to get the accurate results. The examiner should ensure that the location of the active electrode must be in the same position with the same pressure throughout the session. Change in the location of electrodes and pressure can distort the findings.

Significance of strength duration curve- The strength duration curve helps in detecting whether the concerned muscle is deprived of the nerve innervation partially or completely. The special characteristic features can identify the innervation of the nerve to the muscle.

Complete Denervation – The muscles with complete nerve denervation do not respond to the short pulse duration impulses. As the pulse duration is decreased the stimulus strength is increased rapidly to elicit the muscle contraction, therefore, curve rises steeply. Muscles do not respond to the stimulus strength to shorter impulses usually less than 1millisecond.

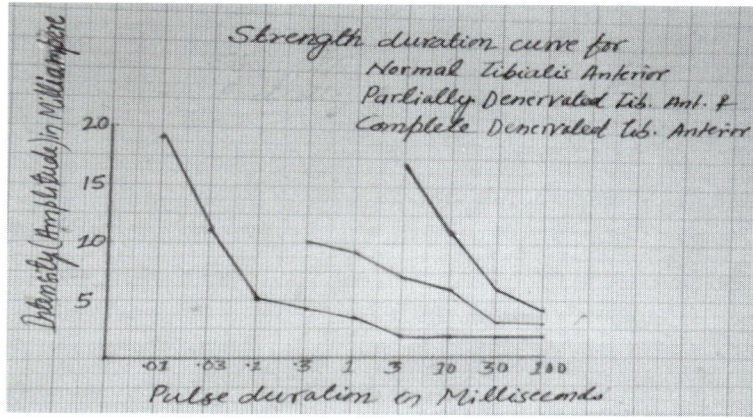

Fig. 7.11b Strength duration curve, A- Normal Muscle, B- Partially Denervated Muscle, and C- Complete Denervated Muscle.

Partial Denervation- The nerve innervations to the muscle is not completely cut, nerve fibers are still intact to supply the muscle. There are some muscle fibers, deprived of the nerve supply whereas, remaining muscle fibers are innervated. Initially, the stimulus strength (intensity) stimulates the innervated and denervated muscle fibers. But the curve rises steeply as the denervated muscles respond less readily to the shorter impulses. With decreasing the pulse duration, the innervated muscle fibers start contracting with the less amplitude, therefore, the curve falls steeply and forms an angle which is known as kink. Kink is actually a point between the stimulating of denervated and innervated muscle fibers. It is a feature of partially denervated muscles.

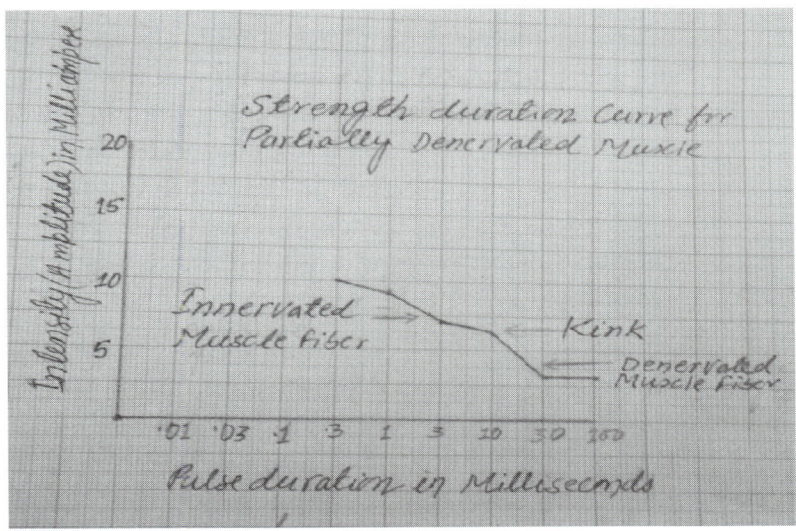

Fig. 7.11c Strength duration curve, for partial denervated muscle

Note: - In wallerian degeneration, alterations in the myelin sheath and axon distal to the lesion occurs in 2-3 weeks; therefore; a strength duration curve test will not reveal an accurate picture of denervation if it is performed earlier than fourteen days after an injury. The follow up of the strength duration curve should not be scheduled so frequently as an average axonal regeneration is one millimeter per day. To see the prognosis several strength duration curve must be plotted over several weeks. The two important points on the curve are rheobase (b) and chronaxie (c), which correlates to twice the reheobase (2b).

Rheobase

Rheobase is the minimal amplitude or intensity of a current that is required to elicit a minimal visually perceptible muscle contraction.[31] at infinite pulse duration, usually 100ms for the clinical practice[26] It is represented as "b". In neuroscience, rheobase is the minimal current amplitude of infinite duration (in a practical sense, about 300 milliseconds) that results in the depolarization threshold of the cell membranes being reached, such as an action potential or the contraction of a muscle.[35] When the strength duration curve is plotted the contraction of the muscle depends on the two variables: the strength of the stimulus and the duration of the stimulus.[36] The strength and duration of the stimulus are inversely related to each other. As the strength of the stimulus is increased to contract the muscle, the duration of the stimulus required to stimulate the muscle is decreased. The two important points on the curve are rheobase (b) and chronaxie (c), which correlates to twice the rheobase (b). Strength-duration curves are useful in studies where the current required is changed when the pulse duration is changed. The rheobase of same muscle of different patients varies due to skin resistance.

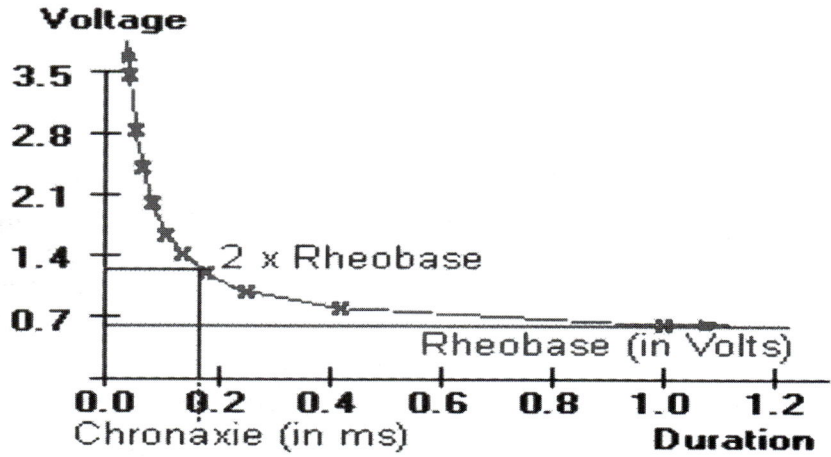

Fig.7.12 Rheobase (constant voltage)

Chronaxie

Chronaxie refers to the minimal pulse duration of the stimulus required to stimulate the muscle for minimally visible contraction. It is the double of the rheobase. The chronaxie value for the normal muscle is found less than 1 millisecond, usually a pulse duration of .1

millisecond, while the chronaxie for the fully denervated muscle is detected much longer, usually 20 to 50 millisecond. It is, therefore, that the muscles deprived of their nerve supply require higher rheobase (amplitude), whereas, muscles with intact nerve supply require less rheobase (amplitude) at the same pulse duration. This is the reason that the muscles deprived of their nerve supply do not respond to the current at the lower pulse duration usually less than 1 millisecond.

Pulse duration in millisecond	Amplitude of Right Tibialis anterior in m.A.	Amplitude of right Anterior (denervated Tibialis) in m.A.	Amplitude of right tibialis anterior (partially denervated) in m.A.
100	2	4	3
30	2	6	3
10	2	11	6
3	2	17	7
1	3	No response	9
.3	4		10
.1	5		No response
.03	11		
.01	19		

Table 7.1 Determination of Rheobase and Chronaxie in the strength duration curve

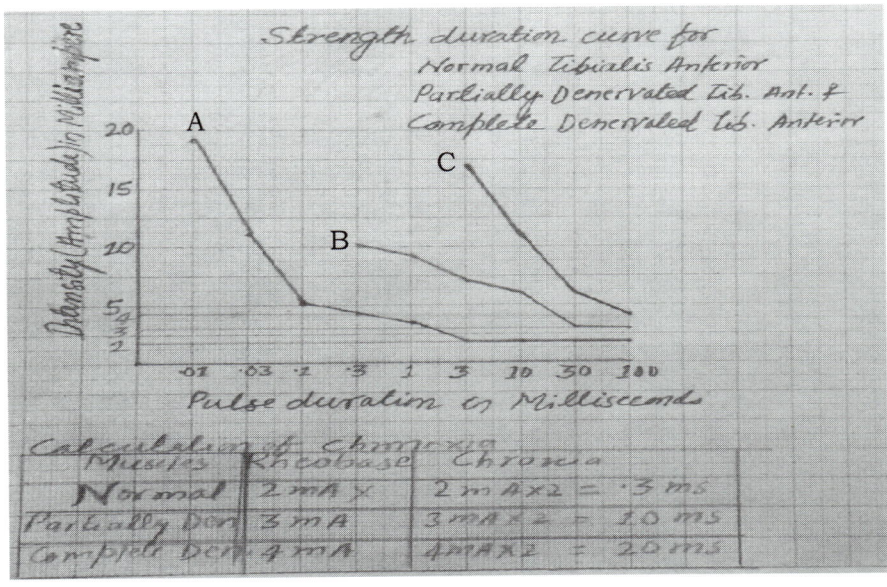

Fig. 7.13 Determination of Rheobase and Chronaxie in the strength duration curve

Therapeutic Currents

The Rheobase (b) and chronaxie(c), can be determined from the SD Curve as under:- (Fig 7.13)

i.   For the right normal tibialis anterior (curve A) rheobase (b) is 2miliampere, whereas, the chronaxie (double of the rheobase) is .3milisecond.

ii.   For the left complete denervated tibialis anterior the rheobase is 4miliampere, whereas, the chronaxie is 20 milisecond.

iii. For the left partially denervated peroneus longus the rheobase is 3miliampere and chronaxie is 10milisecond.

From the curve A,B, and C, it can be inferred that the normal muscle has chronaxie less than 1 millisecond, whereas, the partially denervated and complete denervated muscles have chronaxie 10 ms and 20 millisecond respectively.

Reaction of Degeneration Test

It is the screening procedure for assessment of paralytic muscles following lower motor neuron injuries. It is used as a quick screening test for differentiating a muscle with normal peripheral innervations from a muscle with peripheral denervation. The reaction of degeneration test is also referred as faradic and galvanic test as both the currents are used in the procedure. A motor point is searched with the help of small, hand held electrode or pencil electrode.

First, faradic current of more than 20Hz repetitions at less than 1 millisecond pulse duration is applied to he motor point. This would produce a tetanic or sustained contraction of the muscle of interest. It is called no reaction of degeneration. If no response or sluggish response is seen, peripheral deneravation is likely occur. Now, the muscle of interest is stimulated with the galvanic, a long pulse duration current (monophasic), at 100 millisecond pulse duration or longer. A slow, or sluggish response to the current is due to either partially or completely denervation of the nerve.

Disadvantage – The reaction of degeneration test is very inaccurate. The sluggish response of the innervated muscles may also be recorded if their temperature is below normal or in certain conditions such as myxoedema, on the other hand, the contraction of denervated may be brisk if as their temperature rises.

Iontophoresis

Iontophoresis is the noninvasive, sterile and relatively painless technique of transferring medically useful ions into the tissues through the skin by using direct current[28]. Iontophoresis, based on the principle that an electrically charged electrode will repel similarly charged ions, was described by Le Duc in 1903. The negative ions are placed under the cathode. This electrode would be known as the active electrode. Application of direct current would propel the ions into the skin and tissues.

There is a wide use of iontophoresis such as in the treatment of edema, ischemic skin ulcers, hyperhidrosis, fungal infection, gouty arthritis, calcific tendinitis, and other conditions. Technique of iontophoresis to transfer the ions into the tissues is primarily used by the physiotherapist for musculoskeletal inflammatory conditions, edema, producing local and topical anesthesia of the skin. Harris[30] has reported significant improvement in the symptoms of bursitis and tendonitis following application of dexamethasone sodium phosphate with xylocaine by using iontophoresis technique for twenty minutes. The intensity was increased gradually at the rate of 1mA per minute till five minute and then kept constant at 5mA for next fifteen minutes. Magistro[31] used hyaluronidase in the study of 100 patients with edema and found significant improvement in the reduction of edema. Most studies have demonstrated penetration of the drugs to a depth of 3mm to 20mm.[32] Lai PM and et al. demonstrated that sodium ethanolamine and lidocaine could be detected up to 2cm laterally away from the iontophoresis treatment electrode in the intact skin of rats.[33]

Application

Determine appropriate medication or solution for the condition. The area which is being treated should be cleaned with the soap and warm water to reduce skin resistance. There are two electrodes, one is used for the transfer of the ions which is also known as delivering electrode, whereas, other is placed at least three inches away from the first electrode. Place medication under the delivering electrode and place other electrode distal or proximal to the delivery electrode. The therapist must ensure same polarity of the ions and delivery electrode. Secure both the electrode with the Velcro or bandage. Explain the procedure to the patient. Select the direct current and set the treatment for twenty minutes. Increase the intensity gradually. Observe the patients response to the treatment and discontinue if there is any discomfort. Remove the delivery electrode at the end of the treatment time and inspect the area for any adverse effects of the procedure. The other electrode is of opposite ion which attracts the ions from the delivery electrode.

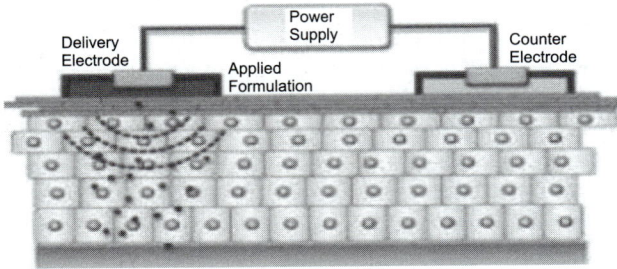

Fig.7.14a Iontophoresis. Placement of drugs under the electrode of same polarity which propel the ions away from the electrode.

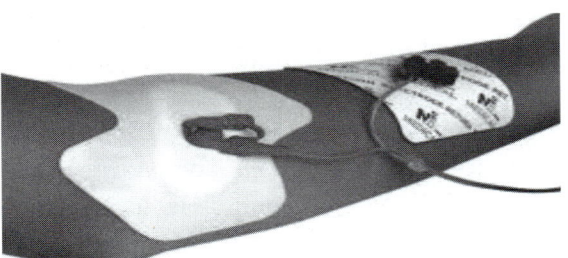

Fig.7.14b Iontophoresis, the placement of electrodes

Ion	Polarity	Indications
Dexamethasone	-	Musculoskeletal inflammatory conditions
Acetate	-	Calcium deposits
Lidocaine	+	Analgesic agent
Hyaluronidase	+	Edema reduction
Zinc	+	Ischemic ulcer
Copper	+	Fungal infection

Table 7.2 Commonly used ions with the Iontophoresis method[34].

Russian Currents

It was first investigated by Dr. Y M Kots in the Russian literature. Russian current is actually a medium frequency current which produces low frequency current to elicit muscle contraction. From a strict electronic perspective, Russian current can be defined as "time modulated alternating current". In 1970 claims were published that this 2500 Hz medium frequency interrupted current (Russian current) could produce greater muscle force (contraction) than a maximal voluntary contraction. Russian current with frequency of 2500Hz is applied as a series of separate bursts having pulse duration of 0.2ms (200microseconds) which is interspersed (interrupted) with 10 ms (100microseconds) that produces low frequency faradic type of current. Each burst is actually a polyphasic pulse waveform.

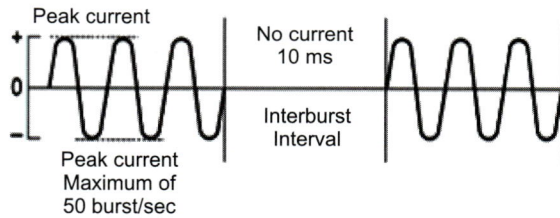

Fig. 7.15 Russian currents

Parameters

Channels: single or two channel

Mode: continuous or interrupted

Waveform: time modulated alternating current

Phase duration: 50-200microseconds

Pulse rate: 1-100Hz

Indications: Russian current is indicated to improve muscle strength and reduce the muscle spasm. To improve muscle strength the parameters of the current should be frequency- 50-70Hz, with pulse duration of 150-200microseconds, and amplitude should be tetanic type to produce comfortable contraction. The patient is asked to contract the muscles isometrically, or slow isokinetically in short arc during the current to achieve good results. For reduction of muscle spasm the therapist can select frequency- 50-70Hz, with pulse duration of 50-175 and amplitude- tetanic type to produce comfortable contraction within the tolerance.

Contraindications: All the contraindication of low frequency currents are applied here, some of them are as under:-

    i.   Cardiac pacemakers and Arrhythmias
    ii.   Hemorrhagic condition
    iii.   Thrombosis and thrombophlebitis (inflammation of wall of vein)
    iv.   Early tendon transfer and repair
    v.   Pregnancy: On pelvic, low back and abdomen
    vi.   Unconscious patient
    vii.   Recent radiotherapy
    viii. Carotid sinus
    ix.   Child with mental disturbance
    x.   Malignancy
    xi.   Infected wound and skin lesion

Diadynamic Current

It is a monophasic pulsed current that was developed in the 1950's, and attributed to Bernard (a French Dentist). Diadynamic current uses usually a sine wave at a carrier frequency of 100Hz, which either has half-wave or full-wave rectified. The resulting monophasic pulses have a duration of 10 msec (milliseconds). Half wave rectification yields a pulse rate of 50pps with 5 msec interpulse interval it is known as MF current, whereas, the full wave rectification yields 100 pps with no interpulse duration it is known as DF current.

Diadynamic current can be modified into courtes periods (CP) and longer periods (LP). In courtes periods MF and DF are exchanged every 1 sec. whereas, longer periods (LP) involve ramps up and down every other pulse over a period of 5 to 7 seconds.

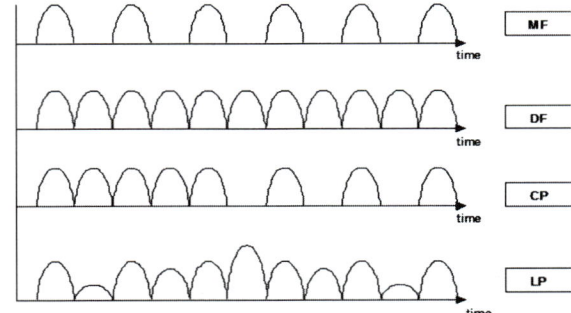

Fig. 7.16 Diadynamic Current

Diadynamic current due to its long pulse duration, and relatively short (or absent) interpulse interval is very uncomfortable.

Therapeutic Currents

References

1. Ranvier, Louis-Antoine (1874). "De quelques faits relatifs à l'histologie et à la physiologie des muscles striés". Archives de physiologie normale et pathologique (in French) 6: 1–15.

2. Denny-Brown, D. (1929). "On the Nature of Postural Reflexes". Proceedings of the Royal Society B 104 (730): 252–301.

3. Buller, AJ; Eccles, JC; Eccles, RM (1960). "Interactions between motoneurones and muscles in respect of the characteristic speeds of their responses". The Journal of physiology 150: 417–39.

4. Pette, Dirk; Smith, Margaret E.; Staudte, Hans W.; Vrbová, Gerta (1973). "Effects of long-term electrical stimulation on some contractile and metabolic characteristics of fast rabbit muscles". Pflügers Archiv European Journal of Physiology 338(3): 257.

5. Angela Forster, Nigel Palastanga. Clayton's Electrotherapy, theory and practice ninth edition,pp80..

6. Pfleuger, EFW: Uberdie tetanisierende Wirkungdes constantent Stromes und dass Allgemeingeesetz der Reizung. Virchow's Arch 3:13, 1858.

7. McNeal, DR and Baker, LL : Effects of joint angle, electrodes and waveform on electrical stimulation of the quadriceps and hamstrings. Ann Biomed Engg16:299, 1998.)

8. Geddes LA. A short history of the electrical stimulation of excitable tissue including electrotherapeutic applications. Physiotherapist 27 (suppl): S-2, 1984,

9. Speilholz NI. Electrical stimulation of denervated muscles. In clinical electrotherapy; 3rd ed. Stamford, CT: Appleton and Lange, 1999, 411-446..

10. Maffiuletti, Nicola A.; Minetto, Marco A.; Farina, Dario; Bottinelli, Roberto (2011). "Electrical stimulation for neuromuscular testing and training: State-of-the art and unresolved issues". European Journal of Applied Physiology111 (10): 2391–7.

11. Knight KL: Electrical stimulation during immobilization. Phys Sport ed. 1980;8:147 Eriksson E, Haggmark T:Comparison of isometric training in the recovery after major knee ligament surgery. Am J Sports Med. 1979;7:169-171)

12. Zizic TM, Hoffman KC, Holt Pa et al. the treatment of osteoarthritis of the knee with pulsed electrical stimulation. J

Rheum 22:1757-1761, 1995).

13. Baker LL, Yeh C, Wilson D, Waters RL,. Electrical stimulation of wrist and fingers for hemiparesis patients. Phys Therapy Association 1979.

14. Waters RL, BowmanBR, Multicenter functional electrical stimulation evaluation for contracture prevention and correction. Final report to veteran Administration, No. V790, p1441, Washington DC, 1981.

15. Munsat TL, McNeal D, Waters R: effects of nerve stimulation on human muscle, Arch Neurol, 33:608-617, 1976).

16. Baker LL, McNEAL dr, Benton LA, Bowman BR, Waters RL,. Neuromuscular electrical stimulation – Apractical Guide (third edition) Downey, CA, Los Amigos Research and education institute, 1993.

17. Roger M. Nelson, Karen W. Hayes, Dean P Currier,Clinical Electrotherapy third edition, p361).

18. Levine MG, Knott M, Kabat H. Relaxation of spasticity by electrical stimulation of antagonist muscles. Arch Phys Med, 33:668-673, 1952).

19. Roger M. Nelson, Karen W. Hayes, Dean P Currier Clinical Electrotherapy, third edition, pp382).

20. Bowmam BBajd T. influence of electrical stimulation on skeletal muscle spasticity. Proc Intern Symp External ControlHuman Extremities. Belgrade, Yugoslavia, committee for electronics and Automation, pp561-576, 1981).

21. Uros Bogatal, Nusa Gros, et al: restoration of gait during two to three weeks of therapy with multi-channel electrical stimulation. Phys Ther. 1989;69:319-327).

22. Bernadette Hecox, Tesega Andemicael Mehreteab and Joseph Weisberg Physical agents, a comprehensive textbook for physical therapists, page 290.

23. Roger M. Nelson, Karen W. Hayes, Dean P Currier, Clinical Electrotherapy third edition, p209).

24. Roger M. Nelson, Karen W. Hayes, Dean P Currier, Clinical Electrotherapy third edition, p313. Gunn CC, Motor points and motor lines. Am J A cupunct, 6:55-58, 1978.

25. Walthard KM, Tchicaloff M. Motor points. In Licht S(ed), electrodiagnosis and electromyography, vol 3. Baltimore, MD, Waverly Press, pp153-170, 1971).

26. Clayton's Electrotherapy, theory and practice ninth edition p68. Angela Forster, Nigel Palastanga).

27. Wynn Parry, CB; Strength duration curves. In Licht, S(ed): electrodiagnosis and electrophysiology , ed 3, Elizabeth Licht, New Havens, 1971, pp141 .

28. Meryl Roth Gersh, Electrotherapy in Rehabilitation, first Indian edition, pp338.

29. Le Duc in 1903. Le Duc, S.: Electric ions and their use in medicine. Rebman, Liverpool, 1903.

30. Harris, PR: Iontophorsis: Clinical research in musculoskeletal inflammatory conditions. J Orthop SportsPhys Ther 4:109,1982.

31. Electrotherapy in Rehabilitation, FA Davis Company Philadelphia, pp106

32. Glass JM, Stephen RL, Jscobsen SC : The quality and distribution of radiolabeled dexamethasone delivered to tissue by iontophoresis, Int J D Eermatol19:519-525, 1980).

33. Lai PM, Anissimov YJ,   Roberts MS: Lateral iontophoresis solute transport in skin, J Pharm Res 16 (1): 46-54, 1999).

34. Kamala Shanar, Kenneth D. Randall, therapeutic physical modalities, , first edition, pp40.)

35. Ashley, et al. "Determination of the Chronaxie and Rheobase of Denervated Limb Muscles in Conscious Rabbits". Artificial Organs, Volume 29 Issue 3 Page 212 - March 2005.

36. Geddes, L. A. (2004). "Accuracy limitations of chronaxie values". IEEE Transactions on Biomedical Engineering, 51(1).

37. Lee WJ, McGovern JP, Duvall EN. Cutaneous tetanizing (low voltage) current for relief of spasm. Arch Phys Med Rehabil, 31;766-771, 1950).

Chapter 08

Transcutaneous Electrical Nerve Stimulation (TENS)

Transcutaneous electrical nerve stimulation (TENS) is a non-invasive analgesic technique that is used to relieve nociceptive, neuropathic, and musculoskeletal pain.[1] TENS is the use of electric current produced by a device to stimulate the nerves for therapeutic purposes. TENS, by definition, covers the complete range of transcutaneously applied currents used for nerve excitation although the term is often used with a more restrictive intent, namely to describe the kind of pulses produced by portable stimulators used to treat pain.[2] In the clinical context, it is most commonly assumed to refer to the use of electrical stimulation with the specific intention of providing symptomatic pain relief

Over 77% of pain specialists use transcutaneous electrical nerve stimulation (TENS) to manage chronic pain, and over half of chronic pain patients have given TENS report that they find it beneficial and wish to continue using it.[3] Transcutaneous electrical nerve stimulation (TENS) is used clinically by a variety of health care professionals for the reduction of pain.[4] Long before the invention of the TENS unit – thousands of years earlier, in fact – the ancient Egyptians discovered that the shocks administered by electric eels offered relief from pain. Heiroglyphs dating as far back as 2500BC show an electric fish, or eel, being used as a form of treatment. The first recorded use of electricity for pain relief appeared in compositions Medicae, written in 46A.D. by Scribonis Largus, a Roman physician. A live torpedo fish (also called the electric ray) was used for the treatment of gout and headache, its electrical discharge being used to shock the affected body part into numbness.[5]

By the 19th Century, scientists had invented a number of machines that administered static electricity specifically to relieve pain. Interest was re-awakened in 1965 by Melzack and Wall, who provided a physiological rationale for electro-analgesic effects. They proposed that the transmission of noxious information could be inhibited by activity in large diameter peripheral afferents or by activity in pain inhibitory pathways descending from the brain.

These inventions, somewhat larger and far less sophisticated than the modern TENS machine, proved very popular until the emergence of medical painkillers, when interest waned. The American Neurosurgeon and pain relief pioneer, Clyde Norman Shealy, had designed the first modern TENS unit patented in 1974.[6]

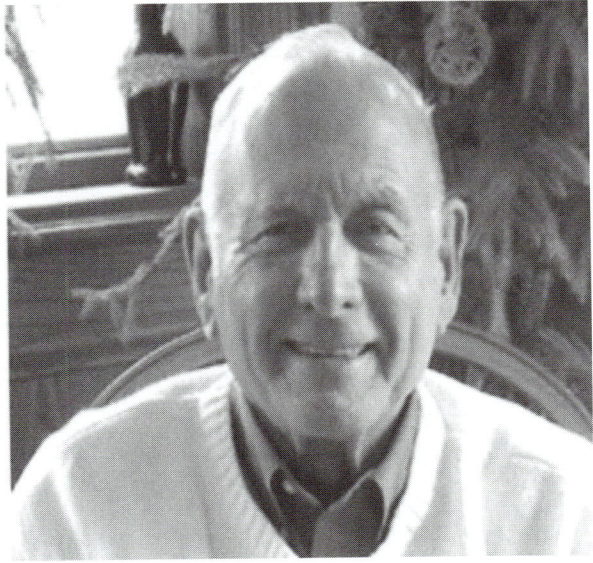

Fig. 8.1 Clyde Norman Shealy is credited with the invention of transcutaneous electrical nerve stimulator.

Mechanism of Use of TENS

The use of conventional (high-frequency) TENS was originally based on the gate-control theory of pain,[7] which suggested that counter stimulation of the nervous system could modify the perception of pain. Later studies suggested that with low-frequency, high-amplitude ("acupuncture-like") stimulation, TENS could also raise endorphin levels in the spinal fluid.[8]

Gate Theory

In 1965 Melzack and Wall proposed the gate theory of pain which they subsequently reviewed in 1978. They originally postulated that interneurons in the substantia gelatinosa in the dorsal horn of the spinal cord acted as a gate to modulate sensory input.[10] This theory has been credited with rekindling interest in electrical control of pain and inspiring research with important scientific and clinical ramification.[11] The essence of this theory is that small diameter myelinated A-delta neurons and small diameter, un-myelinated C fiber also known as pain carrying nociceptives project to the spinal cord where they synapse directly or via interneurons with the transmission cells (T cells) in the dorsal horn of the grey matter. The T cells relay the small diameter pain carrying sensation to the higher centers.

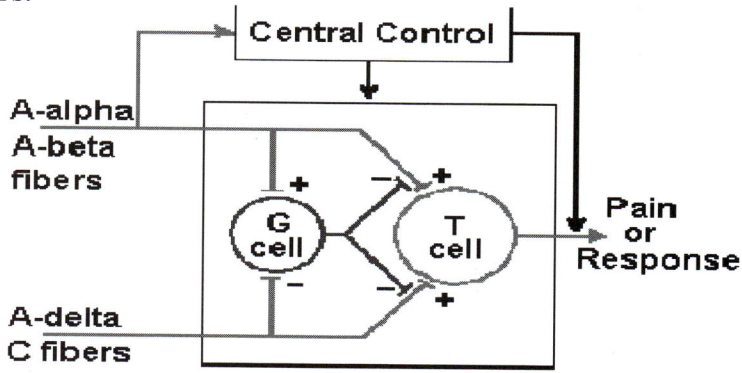

Fig. 8.2 Schematic Diagram. Pain gate Control

Large diameter myelinated A beta and alpha fibers also known as pain inhibiting fibers arise from the peripheral part and terminate on T cells through substantia gelatinosa of the spinal cord. The stimulation of the mechanoceptors large diameter fibers (A beta and alpha) inhibit the nociceptors at the T cells and prevent transmission to the higher centers. The inhibitory input caused by activation of the large diameter, mechanosensitive afferent is said to close the gate to nociceptor transmission. This is also known as "Pain Gate Control Theory".[19]

Opiod activation

Another mechanism proposed is activation of descending inhibitory pathway, through release of endogenous opioids.[9] The areas involved in descending inhibition include nucleus raphe magnus in rostral ventral medulla (RVM) and the periaqueductal gray (PAG). The PAG sends projections to the RVM, which in turn send projections to the spinal dorsal horn. The stimulation of PAG or the RVM produces inhibition of dorsal horn nucleus including spinothalamic tract cells. Specific and different opioid receptors are activated through release of endogenous opioids by different frequencies of TENS. Application of low frequency TENS causes activation of δ-opioid receptors and high

Transcutaneous Electrical Nerve Stimulation (TENS)

frequency TENS activates μ-opioid receptors. These opioid receptors in turn activate the PAG-RVM pathway

Parameters of TENS

Clinical trials suggests that adequate doing, particularly intensity, is critical to obtaining pain relief with TENS.[10] Most of TENS units produce an electric output having one characteristic waveform, usually of symmetric or balanced asymmetric biphasic type with zero net current to minimize skin irritation.[11] The judicial selection of various parameters such as waveform, frequency, pulse width, amplitude and frequency modulation can have great role in effectively management of pain.

Amplitude: The Tens units have amplitude control switch range from 1mA to 100mA. Intensity from 1mA to 100mA is sufficient because the primary target is the sensory nerves, in addition to that it is sufficient to depolarize the sensory nerves. The intensity of amplitude depends on the condition and severity of pain. The use of high-intensity (9- to 12-mA) stimulation was significantly more effective in decreasing the postoperative analgesic requirements than a low intensity (4–5 mA) of stimulation when used as an adjunct to PCA (patient controlled analgesia).[12] Furthermore, intermittent electrical stimulation for short intervals (30 min) has been found to be more effective than prolonged or continuous stimulation.[13]

Frequency: The selection of frequency of TENS is one of the important parameters which may alter the results if selected wrongly. The frequency may range from 1 Hz to 120 Hz. The frequency is one of the criteria of classification of the TENS. High-frequency TENS reduces primary hyperalgesia to heat and mechanical stimuli for up to 1 day after treatment. In contrast, low-frequency TENS is ineffective in reducing primary hyperalgesia.[14,15] Hansson P et al. reported that the use of high-frequency stimulation produced greater analgesic effects.[16] They reported comparable analgesic effects at both low and high frequencies of stimulation; however, the patients "preferred" high-frequency stimulation. It has also been reported that low-frequency stimulation requires a higher intensity to produce pain relief equivalent to high-frequency stimulation.[17]

Pulse Width: Pulse width is actually a length of time the current acts on the nerve. It ranges from 40 microseconds to 250 microseconds. A microsecond is a millionth of a second and such short duration pulses are used to achieve analgesic effects as the target is the sensory nerve which tends to have relatively low thresholds. Long duration impulses are not required in order to force a sensory nerve to depolarize, therefore, stimulation for less than a millisecond is sufficient. The 200 microsecond pulse duration in clinical practice is commonly used by the clinicians; however, pulse width can be modified accordingly.

Waveform: Presently the waveform used in the physiotherapy practice in the TENS is biphasic which has positive and negative phases. The biphasic nature of the pulse means that there is usually no net DC component (often described in the manufacturers as 'zero net DC'), thus minimising any skin reactions due to the build up of electrolytes under the electrodes.

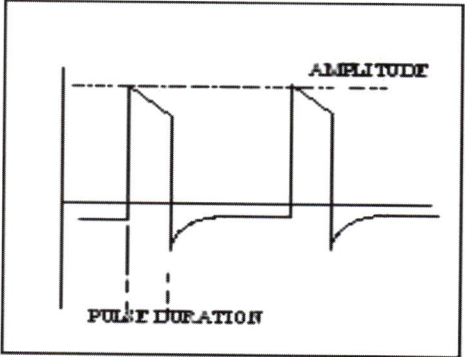

Fig. 8.3 Biphasic Wave Form, which has negative and positive waves..

The waveforms can be modified into square, triangular, rectangular, and sine waves.

Modulation: The pulses of different frequency, intensity, and pulse duration are modulated in such a way that leads to less irregular pulses. This modulation helps in minimizing the effects of accommodation which are often occurred with electrical stimulation of nerve and muscles.

Duration: Transcutaneous electrical nerve stimulation currents are used for longer period of time. Many authors suggest that analgesic effect of the TENS does not remain for longer period of time, therefore; these can be used for hours to days especially in post operative acute cases. However; it is not feasible in the clinical set ups to use TENS for more than 30 minutes. Yannick Tousignant-Laflamme and et al. studied the comparison between 15 minute and 30 minute duration of acupuncture like TENS. They observed that a longer application of

AL-TENS (30 minutes versus 15 minutes) induced neither longer duration of analgesia nor greater magnitude (greater analgesic effect).[31] However, many other authors recommended TENS for many hours to days.

TENS Modes

Six types of TENSs have been discussed with regularly in the literature.[18] The classification of transcutaneous electrical stimulation is based on the frequency and amplitude.

Conventional: Conventional TENS is also known as high TENS as it is characterized by high frequency and low amplitude. Conventional mode has the frequency ranged from 10Hz to 100Hz and the amplitude that produces comfortable cutaneous stimulation without muscle contraction.[19] The studies have shown that the frequencies approximating 60Hz are optimal for relieving pain[20] on the other hand frequencies above 80 to 200 Hz may worsen pain of some patients[21] A short pulse duration 50 to 100 microseconds favors preferential stimulation of large diameter myelinated afferent neurons, the target of this mode of TENS.[22] This mode is mostly used by the clinicians. The conventional TENS stimulates selectively large diameter A beta fibers, without stimulating the pain nociceptor A delta and C fibers. The A beta fibers block the pain carrying A delta C fibers to reach to the higher centers at the spinal cord. This mode of TENS elicits segmental analgesia. To prevent accommodation the current must be periodically increased in order to maintain adequate perception of electrical paresthesia.

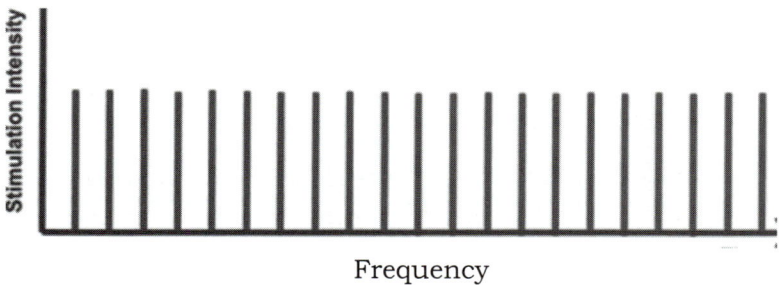

Fig 8.4a Conventional TENS with high frequency and low amplitude

Acupuncture Like TENS: Acupuncture mode of Tens is also known as strong low-rate mode TENS. This mode of TENS has the frequency below 10 Hz, and the most commonly used frequency is 1 to 4 Hz with pulse duration ranged from 100 to 300 microseconds. The amplitude is usually high (above 30mA) than the conventional TENS to produce visible strong and rhythmical muscle contraction. Acupuncture like TENS selectively stimulates the A delta and C fibers that releases endogenous opiod like substances at cord level. The substance like enkephalins and beta endorphins block the transmission of pain stimuli and elicits extrasegmental analgesia. This type of TENS is effective in chronic and deep situated pain.

Brief-Intense Mode TENS: It is a high amplitude and high frequency TENS. This type of mode of TENS has the frequency ranged from 60Hz to 150Hz, pulse duration 50-250 microseconds and amplitude is adjusted to produce either uncomfortable tetanic muscle contraction (high setting) or nonrhythmic muscle fasciculation (low setting). The aim of such type of TENS is to produce significant muscle fatigue with continuous stimulation. The brief intense mode of TENS activates small diameter afferents to elicit peripheral nerve blockade and extrasegmental analgesia

Pulse Burst Mode: This type of TENS is also called burst or pulse train[18] and even acupuncture-like TENS. It consists both high setting (high amplitude) and low setting (low amplitude). The patient experiences either uncomfortable tetanic muscle contraction (high setting) or nonrhythmic muscle fasciculation (low setting). This type of TENS is characterized by a high carrier frequency 50-100 Hz which is modulated by a low burst frequency 1 to 4Hz. The 1-4Hz frequency is a series of pulses (train) with the pulse duration of 50 to 100 microseconds.

Fig. 8.4b Pulse Burst Mode

Modulated Mode: This type of TENS is designed to prevent accommodation to occur and to improve patient tolerance. The modulated mode allows one of the parameters of the TENS such as pulse duration, or amplitude, or frequency to change (modulate) automatically by a given percentage from an initial set level.

Transcutaneous Electrical Nerve Stimulation (TENS)

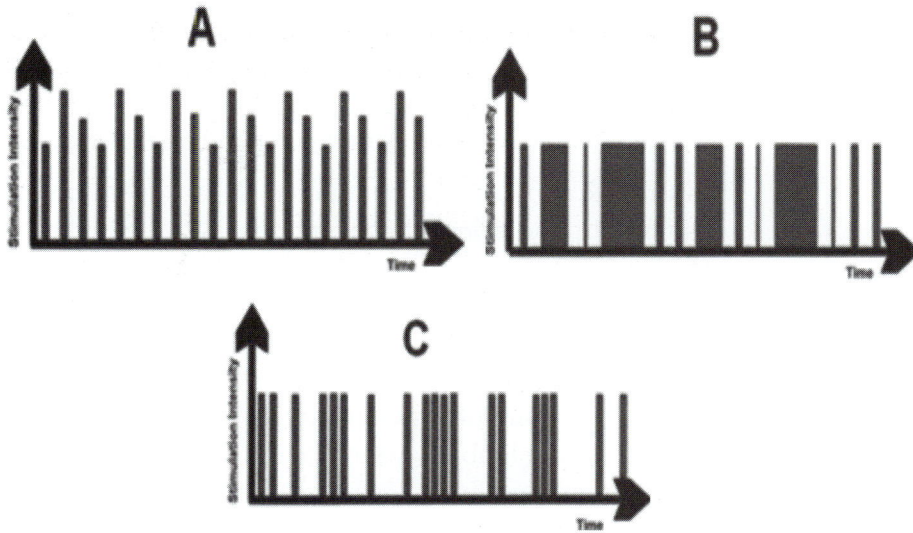

Fig. 8.4c Modulated Mode TENS in which the parameters of TENS are modulated. A-Intensity, B- Pulse Duration, C-Frequency

Hyperstimulation Mode: This type of TENS is also known as noninvasive electroacupuncture TENS. It is the only mode that regularly utilizes either direct or monophasic pulsed currents. Hyperstimulation mode uses high amplitude that produces very noxious cutaneous stimulation which is sharp and burning in character, without resultant muscle contraction. This type of TENS is applied through a small probe type electrode, with a tip that may be only 1 to 3 mm in diameter. The pulse duration required for such type of TENS is very long i.e. 500msec and the frequency can exceed 100Hz with the amplitude not exceeding higher than 50 mA.

Indications

The primary indication for TENS have been recognized as the symptomatic relief and management of chronic intractable pain and as an adjunctive treatment in the management of postsurgical and post traumatic acute pain.[23]

Phantom and Stump Pain: Phantom pain or sensation is experienced by the individuals after the amputation. The patients feel that they have the intact leg or arm, their finger and toes are still working. These patients often fall in the morning when they try to stand on the amputed leg. The feeling of presence of normal leg can be eliminated with help of TENS. Mulvery MR and et al applied the TENS for 60minutes to generate a strong but comfortable TENS sensation at the site of stump pain or projected into the site of phantom pain.This study has demonstrated that TENS has potential for reducing phantom pain and stump pain at rest and on movement.[24]

Matthew R. Mulvey et al conducted the study on phantom pain and stump pain and selected conventional TENS with the parameters of continuous pulse pattern, pulse duration of 80 microseconds, pulse frequency of 100 Hz, strong but comfortable intensity. Study found that participants tolerated TENS delivered to a painful phantom and/or stump and that TENS may reduce pain both on movement and at rest. The study also found that TENS sensation can be projected into a phantom limb and that the TENS sensation feels as if it arises from a prosthetic limb. This may prove a useful aid for perceptual embodiment of an artificial limb.[25]

Post Surgical Pain: TENS undoubtedly has a place in the postoperative pain treatment, although its effect is not as strong as that of epidural analgesia with local anesthetics. TENS, however, is easy to administer, lacks side effects, and can be administered by the patients themselves.

Inga Arvidsson et al compared the effectiveness of TENS with placebo TENS and epidural analgesia with dilute local anesthetics in 15 patients with open knee surgery. The results showed that placebo-TENS had no significant effect on either pain perception or on IEMG. High frequency TENS given for 15 min to 20 min decreased pain perception by 50% at rest and by 11% after quadriceps contraction. High frequency TENS increased muscle contraction ability by 305%, compared with the initial contraction before treatment. Epidural injection of a dilute local anesthetic decreased pain perception by 90% at rest and by 67% after contraction, and increased muscle contraction ability by 1,846%.[26]

Jan Magnus Bjordal et al. investigated the literature of randomized placebo-controlled trials to find out if transcutaneous electrical nerve stimulation or acupuncture like TENS can reduce analgesic consumption after surgery. The study used adequate treatment pulse frequency 1-8Hz for the ALTENS and 25 -150 Hz for the TENS with intensity above 15mA,to produce strong, definite, subnoxious, maximal tolerable contraction. The electrodes were placed over the incision area. The study found that the TENS, administered with a strong, subnoxious intensity at an adequate frequency in the wound area, can significantly reduce analgesic consumption for postoperative pain.[27]

Gerson Cipriano et al. conducted a prospective and randomized investigation to evaluate the effects of transcutaneous electrical nerve stimulation (TENS) in the postoperative management of pain in patients who were submitted to different cardiac surgeries. The study found that TENS presented with beneficial effects not only in postoperative pain, but also in selected pulmonary-mechanical properties and electrical activity of thoracic and girdle muscles. These data point out for a relevant role of TENS in the postoperative care of cardiac surgery patients.[28]

Neuropathic Pain: G. L. Y. Cheing and M. L. M. Luk have examined the clinical effectiveness of high-frequency transcutaneous electrical nerve stimulation for reducing hypersensitivity of the hand. The authors found significant improvement in the pain and sensitivity after day eleven of the transcutaneous electrical nerve stimulation.[32] Nearly half of those suffering from a spinal cord injury (SCI) are at risk of developing neuropathic pain. Spinal cord injury related neuropathic pain is often difficult to relieve.[33] In patients with spinal cord injury and pain, nonpharmacological treatments conservative management such as physical therapy, relaxation, and acupuncture—were preferred over the opioids.[34] This preference might be associated with the severity of the side effects experienced, the limited pain relief provided by pharmacological treatment, or both. Treatment with transcutaneous electrical nerve stimulation (TENS) is rarely associated with negative side effects and has been reported to be effective in patients with peripheral neuropathic pain,[35] e.g., patients with diabetic neuropathy,[36] and patients with pain of differing origin but less effective in patients with central neuropathic pain.[37]

Dysmenorrhoea: Dysmenorrhoea is a very common complaint that refers to painful menstrual cramps in the uterus. The stimulation of the cutaneous sensory nerves directly over the area through the transcutaneous electrical nerve stimulation (TENS) relives pain. It is thought to alter the body's ability to receive and perceive pain signals rather than by having a direct effect on the uterine contractions. The studies found that high-frequency TENS may help in the relieving the pain pertaining to dysmenorrheal[38]

Labour: TENS is a device that emits low-voltage currents and which has been used for pain relief in labor. A significant number of TENS machine brands have been targeted for use for labor pain. In 1987, it was observed that some mothers were not responding to traditional pain relief methods during labour, causing intense discomfort and possible complications during birth. Ray Kriesler set about creating one with that purpose. First trialed in Melbourne, Australia. TENS application reduced the duration of the first stage of labor and the amount of analgesic drug administered. There were no adverse effects on mother or newborns."

Contraindications and Precautions

Serious adverse effects of TENS on skin and underlying structures are not common like interferential therapy and other low frequency currents. However, occasional superficial electrical burns have been noted by the patients and clinicians may be because of improper placement of electrodes. Some patients experience mild autonomic responses and minor skin irritation beneath electrodes.

Pacemakers and cardiovascular disorders: TENS has been shown to interfere with pacemaker function. Therefore, it should not be applied directly over the pace maker, however; some clinicians advise the TENS on the chest away from the site of pacemaker. To be in the safer side the application of the TENS even away from the pace maker should be done with consultation to concerned cardiologist. TENS is often used over the chest for angina with much success; again, the situation should be discussed with a cardiologist. The application of TENS on anterior and posterior areas of the chest should never be advised as this may compromise pulmonary ventilation due to excessive stimulation of the intercostal muscles.

Haemorrhage: The contraction of muscles during application of high or burst TENS increases the blood circulation in the local area that may lead to further increase in the size of haematoma. Therefore, electrodes should not be placed over areas where there has been recent haemorrhage as the currents may cause further haemorrhage.

Thrombosis: The application of TENS is absolutely contraindicated on the calf muscles and other potential area for thrombosis especially with post surgical patients because of the potential for embolism.

Pregnancy: There are many studies which state that the use of TENS during labor and delivery[29] is beneficial and reduces the duration of the first stage of labour and the amount of analgesic drug administered However, TENS should not be administered over the abdomen or pelvis during pregnancy because the effects of TENS on fetal development are still unknown and currents could inadvertently cause uterine contractions and induce premature labour.[30]

Carotid Sinus: Application of TENS overt the carotid sinus, may reflexly induce slowing of the heart a fall in blood pressure, or fainting, should also be recognized to be hazardous.

Epilepsy: TENS is not absolutely contraindicated on the patients with epilepsy. The clinicians should be cautious when applying TENS to patients with epilepsy and should not apply electrodes on the neck or head.

Undiagnosed pain: TENS should be applied with caution to the patients with undiagnosed pain

Application of TENS

Electrodes: Different sizes and shapes of electrodes are available in the market. There are reusable, disposable, nonsterile, and presteriliized electrodes, out of which reusable nonsterile electrodes are more often used in the clinics. The electrodes are basically carbonized rubber and siliconized carbon rubber. The electrodes are cleaned with the mild soap and warm water, thoroughly rinsed, and patted dry with a soft towel. These are the reusable non sterile electrodes which can be used for long period of time, however; cuts and irregular surfaces these should be checked prior application of the electrodes, and use of these electrodes for more than six month is not advisable.

Placement of electrodes: There are four basic options especially for the two electrodes. The first option is the placement of electrode directly over the painful areas or proximal to the site of pain. Second option is the placement of electrodes just outside the proximal and distal margins of the painful region in a manner that 'bracket' this area. For an example, if the site of pain is in the vertebral column, the electrodes should be placed on either side of the column. The third option of placement of electrodes is basically for the radicular or referred pain. One electrode is placed over the painful area (proximal part) while other electrode is placed over the distal area related to the spinal nerve root. The fourth option of electrode placement is crisscross or modified in which four electrodes of two channels are used. For an example, painful knee joint. Two electrode of one channel can be placed directly over the painful site and other two electrodes can be placed adjacent to the painful area. **Nerve-** The electrodes over the course of peripheral nerve especially where located superficially can also be placed. The stimulation of proximal part of the nerve is preferred over the distal, if two electrodes are used. **Trigger points –** The trigger point is a painful area on compression with some referred pain. The electrodes can be placed relative to a trigger point. One electrode can be placed directly over the trigger point and other electrode is place over its relative referred pain. **Motor point –** Motor point is the area of the muscle where nerve enters into the muscle, it is usually situated proximal $1/_3$ of the muscle. Such points would seem well suited to afford input to the central nervous system, permit efficient stimulation of muscle contractions.[18] The electrodes are secured on the body or extremities with the help of surgical tape, or a variety of paper or foam adhesive patches. The Velcro tapes and bandages may also be used to secure the electrodes firmly on the treatment area.

Placemnt of electrodes for Phantom pain: Both the high frequency and low frequency can be used for the phantom pain. High-frequency TENS- the electrodes are placed on each paravertebral region in the same segment as the pain. If sensitivity is normal, then both the electrodes are placed on the contralateral side, such as the foot. Low-frequency TENS: Both the electrodes are placed on the contralateral side in the same myotome as the pain.

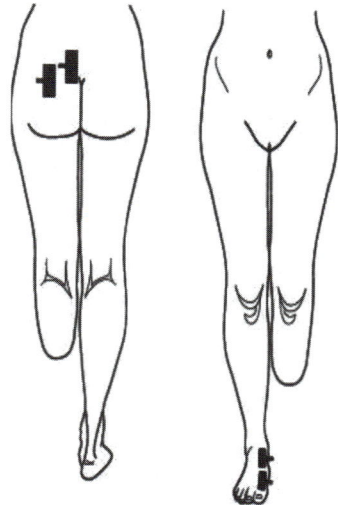

Fig. 8.5a Placement of electrodes for Phantom Pain.

Placement of electrodes for Low Back Pain: To relieve pain localized in the lower back area single channel (two electrodes) or two channel (four electrodes can be used). In case of single channel the electrodes are placed on either side on the paravertebral region of the site of pain. If two channel or four electrodes are used-two electrodes of one channel are placed on the right paravertebral region and two electrodes of second channel are placed on left paravertebral region of the painful area.

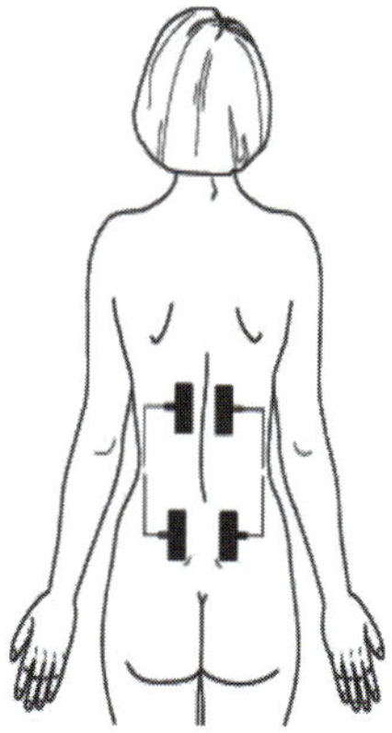

Fig. 8.5b Placement of electrodes for Back Pain.

Placement of electrodes for sciatica: Two channels are used for the sciatic pain. Two electrodes of one channels are placed on either side on the paravertebral region of the nerve roots. The electrodes are not placed directly over the nerve roots. The electrodes of other channel are placed on the sciatic notch and distal posterior thigh. If pain distribution is in the whole course of the sciatic nerve then one electrode is placed on the paravertebral region of the same side, second electrode of the first channel is placed on the sciatic notch. The third electrode is placed on the mid posterior thigh and the fourth electrode is placed on the mid posterior calf muscles.

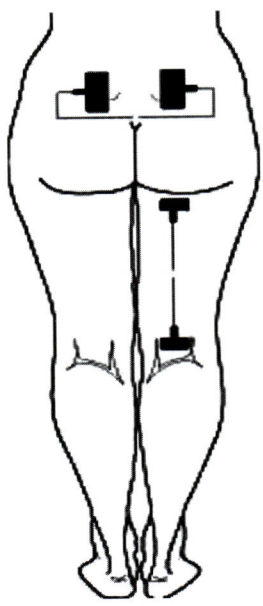

Fig. 8.5c Placement of electrodes for Sciatic Nerve Pain (Sciatica).

Electrode placement for Labor: Single channel or two channels can be used for the labor. To use single channel electrodes are placed over the painful area, usually the sacral region. To use four electrodes (two channel) the electrodes of first channel remains in the same position, while the electrodes of second channel are placed on the hips down towards the groin. Method II - one pair of electrodes is placed paravertebrally at the level of T10-L1 and another pair of electrodes at the level of S2 to S4 (Fig. 8.5d). The woman controls the intensity of the current by turning an intensity knob and varies the stimulation pattern with a thumb switch or by adjusting knob on her TENS unit. Note: Electrodes shall not be placed directly on the uterus.

Electrode placement for Menstrual Pain or Cramp – Single channel is used. The electrodes are placed directly over the painful area. High frequency with high amplitude is preferred for the acute ischemic pain.

Transcutaneous Electrical Nerve Stimulation (TENS)

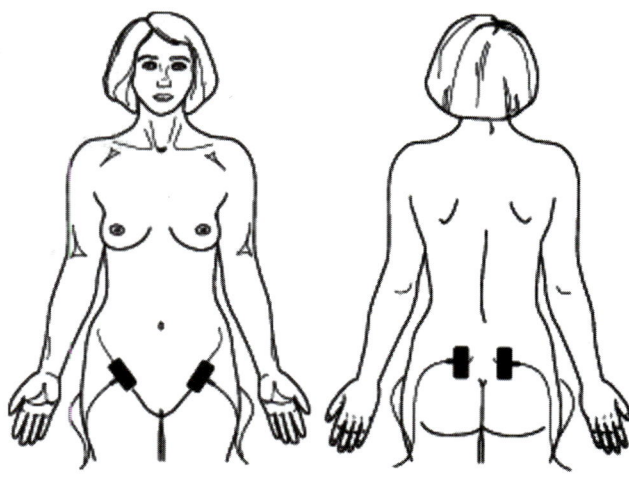

Fig. 8.5d Placement of electrodes for Menstrual Pain or Cramp.

Placement of electrodes for Knee joint: Single channel or two channel electrodes can be used depending on the area of pain. The electrodes of single channel are placed directly over the painful area. When using four electrodes these are arranged in a crisscross manner on each side of the knee joint which allow functional movements (flexion and extension) also.

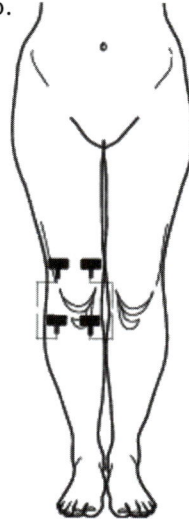

Fig. 8.5e Placement of electrodes for Knee Joint.

Placement of electrodes for the Shoulder Joint – Similar to the knee joint single or two channel electrodes can be used for the shoulder joint. If the area of the pain is small one electrode is placed directly over the joint line or painful site and other electrode is placed on the insertion of the deltoid lateral fibers.

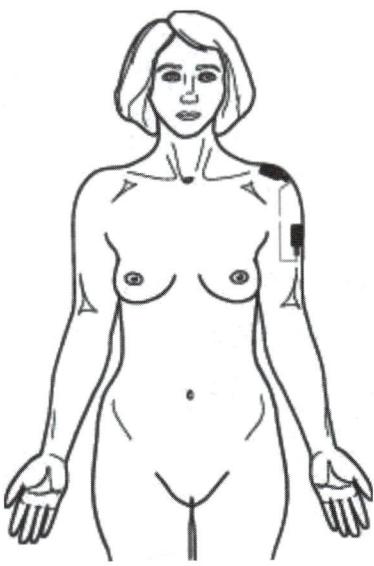

Fig. 8.5f Placement of electrodes for Left Shoulder.

Procedure

The patient is screened for the contraindication to the TENS. There should be thorough check of the skin for cut and abrasions. The electrodes should also not being used for long period of time. The area of treatment is also inspected after the treatment for skin allergy to the electrode or gels. After securing electrodes firmly on the treatment area the patient is explained about the sensation of current he or she is going to experience. The intensity of the current is increased gradually till a desired muscle contraction or sensation is achieved.

References

1. Johnson M. Watson T. Transcutaneous electrical nerve stimulation, Electrotherapy: Evidence-based Practice. , 2008 Edinburgh Churchill Livingstone (pg. 253-96)

2. Robertson, Valma J.; Alex Ward; John Low; Ann Reed (2006). Electrotherapy Explained: Principles and Practice (4th ed.). Butterworth-Heinemann (Elsevier). ISBN 978-0-7506-8843-7.

3. Berman BM, Bausell RB. The use of non-pharmacological therapies by pain specialists. Pain. 2000;85:313–315. .

4. Kathleen A. Sluka,Transcutaneous electrical nerve stimulation: Basic science mechanisms and clinical effectivenessThe Journal of Pain Volume 4, Issue 3, April 2003, Pages 109-121

5. Kellaway P. The William Osler medal essay: The part played by electrical fish in the early history of bioelectricity and electrotherapy. Bull His Med, 20:112-137, 1949. On Roger M. Nelson, Karen W. Hayes, Dean P. Currier: Clinical Electrotherapy, Appleton & Lange, Stamford, Connecticut, third editionpp292.

6. Top TENS, tens.net

7. Melzack R, Wall PD. Pain mechanisms: a new theory . Science 1965; 150:971–9.

8. Sjolund BH, Eriksson MBE. . Endorphins and analgesia produced by peripheral conditioning stimulation . Adv Pain Res Ther 1979; 3:587–90.

9. Sluka KA, Walsh D. Transcutaneous electrical nerve stimulation: Basic science mechanisms and clinical effectiveness. J Pain. 2003;4:109–21 [PubMed]

10. Josimari M. DeSantanaEmail author, Deirdre M. Walsh, Carol Vance, Barbara A. Rakel, Kathleen A. Sluka: Effectiveness of transcutaneous electrical nerve stimulation for treatment of hyperalgesia and pain, Current Rheumatology Reports, December 2008.

11. Roger M. Nelson, Karen W. Hayes, Dean P. Currier: Clinical Electrotherapy, Appleton & Lange, Stamford, Connecticut, third editionpp293.

12. Wang B, Tang J, White PF, Naurse R, Sloninsky A, Kariger R, Gold J, Wender RH: Effect of the intensity of

transcutaneous acupoint electrical stimulation on the postoperative analgesic requirement. Anesth Analg 1997; 85:406–13.

13. Romita VV, Sul A, Henry JL: Parametric studies on electroacupuncture-like stimulation in a rat model: Effect of intensity, frequency, and duration of stimulation on evoked antinociception. Brain Res Bul 1997; 42:289–96.

14. Priya Gopalkrishnan, MS, Kathleen A. Sluka, PhD: Effect of varying frequency, intensity, and pulse duration of transcutaneous electrical nerve stimulation on primary hyperalgesia in inflamed rats Archives of Physical Medicine and Rehabilitation, Volume 81, Issue 7, July 2000, Pages 984–990

15. Johnson MI, Ashton CH, Bousfield DR, Thompson JW: Analgesic effects of different frequencies of transcutaneous electrical nerve stimulation on cold-induced pain in normal subjects. Pain 1989; 39:231–6

16. Hansson P, Ekblom A: Afferent stimulation induced pain relief in acute orofacial pain and its failure to induce sufficient pain reduction in dental and oral surgery. Pain 1983; 15:157–65

17. Andersson SA, Hahsson G, Holmgren E: Evaluation of the pain suppressant effect of different frequencies of peripheral electrical stimulation in chronic pain condition. Acta Orthopaed Scand 1976; 47:149–57

18. Mannheimer C, Lampe GN, clinical transcutaneous Electrical Nerve Stimulation (TENS) Philadelphia, PA, FA Davis,1984 on Roger M. Nelson, Karen W. Hayes, Dean P. Currier: Clinical Electrotherapy, Appleton & Lange, Stamford, Connecticut, third editionpp293.

19. Erikson MBE, Sjolund BH, Nielzen S. Long term results of peripheral conditioning stimulation as an analgesic measure in chronic pain. Pain, 6:335-347, 1979.

20. Barr JO, Nielsen DH, Soderberg GL. Transcutaneous electrical nerve stimulation characteristics for altering pain perception. Phys Ther, 66:1515-1521,1986

21. Picaza JA, Cannon BW, Hunter SE, et al. Pain suppression by peripheral nerve stimulation, Part I: Observation with

22. Howson DC, Peripheral neural excitability: Implication for transcutaneous electrical nerve stimulation. Phys Ther, 58:1467-1473, 1978.

23. American National Standards for Transcutaneous Electrical Nerve Stimulation. ANSI/AAMI NS4-1985. Arinlington, VA, Association for the Advancement of Medical Instrumentation, 1986 Roger M. Nelson, Karen W. Hayes, Dean P. Currier: Clinical Electrotherapy, Appleton & Lange, Stamford, Connecticut, third editionpp29.

24. Mulvey MR, Radford HE, Fawkner HJ, Hirst L, Neumann V, Johnson MI. Transcutaneous electrical nerve stimulation for phantom pain and stump pain in adult amputees. Pain Pract. 2013 Apr;13(4):289-96.

25. Matthew R. Mulvey, PhD, Helen E. Radford, BSc, Helen J. Fawkner, PhD; Lynn Hirst, BSc; Vera Neumann, MD; Mark I. Johnson, PhD. Transcutaneous Electrical Nerve Stimulation for Phantom Pain and Stump Pain in Adult Amputees*Faculty of Health and Social Sciences, Leeds Metropolitan University, Leeds, U.K.; † Leeds Pallium Research Group; ‡ Leeds Teaching Hospitals NHS Trust

26. Inga Arvidsson, Dr MedSc, RPT; Ejnar Eriksson, MD Postoperative TENS Pain Relief After Knee Surgery: Objective Evaluation: Orthopedics, October 1986 - Volume 9 · Issue 10: 1346-1351.

27. Jan Magnus Bjordal, Mark I. Johnson, Anne Elisabeth Ljunggreen, Transcutaneous electrical nerve stimulation (TENS) can reduce postoperative analgesic consumption. A meta-analysis with assessment of optimal treatment parameters for postoperative pain. Europeun Journal of pain Volume 7, Issue 2, April 2003   Pages 181–188

28. Gerson Cipriano, Jr. Antonio Carlosde Camargo Carvalho Graziella França Bernardelli Paulo Alberto Tayar Peres. Short-term transcutaneous electrical nerve stimulation after cardiac surgery: effect on pain, pulmonary function and electrical muscle activity. Interact CardioVasc Thorac Surg (2008) 7 (4): 539-543.

29. Angustinsson LF, Bohlin P, Carlosson CA et al. Pain relief during delivery by transcuraneous electrical nerve stimulation. Pain, 4:59-65,1977 Roger M. Nelson, Karen W. Hayes, Dean P. Currier: Clinical Electrotherapy, Appleton & Lange, Stamford, Connecticut, third editionpp293.

30. Iain Jones MB ChB FRCA Mark I Johnson PhD Transcutaneous electrical nerve stimulation Continuing Education in Anaesthesia, Critical Care & Pain j Volume 9 Number 4 2009.

31. Yannick Tousignant-Laflamme, Marilyne Brochu, Cynthia Dupuis Michaud, Catherine Page, Draga Popovic, and Marie-Eve Simard. Duration of Analgesia Induced by Acupuncture-Like TENS on Experimental Heat Pai.n International Scholarly Research Notices Pain Volume 2013 (2013).

32. G. L. Y. Cheing, M. L. M. Luk, Transcutaneous Electrical Nerve Stimulation for Neuropathic Pain. Journal of Hand Surgery (European Volume), First Published February 1, 2005.

33. Cecilia Norrbrink, RPT, PhDTranscutaneous electrical nerve stimulation for treatment of spinal cord injury neuropathic pain. Journal of Rehabilitation Research & Development, Volume 46 Number 1, 2009, Pages 85 — 94.

34. Haythornthwaite JA, Wegener S, Benrud-Larson L, Fisher B, Clark M, Dillingham T, Cheng L, DeLateur B. Factors associated with willingness to try different pain treatments for pain after a spinal cord injury. Clin J Pain. 2003;19(1): 31–38. [PMID]

35. Cruccu G, Aziz TZ, Garcia-Larrea L, Hansson P, Jensen TS, Lefaucheur JP, Simpson BA, Taylor RS. EFNS guidelines on neurostimulation therapy for neuropathic pain. Eur J Neurol. 2007;14(9):952–70. [PMID]

36. Carroll D, Moore RA, McQuay HJ, Fairman F, Tramer M, Leijon G. Transcutaneous electrical nerve stimulation (TENS) for chronic pain. Cochrane Database Syst Rev. 2001; 3:CD003222. [PMID]

37. Meyler WJ, De Jongste MJ, Rolf CA. Clinical evaluation of pain treatment with electrostimulation: A study on TENS in patients with different pain syndromes. Clin J Pain. 1994;10(1):22–27. [PMID]

38. Proctor M, Farquhar C, Stones W, He L, Zhu X, Brown J. Transcutaneous electrical nerve stimulation for primary dysmenorrhoea. Cochrane Database of Systematic Reviews 2002

Chapter 09

Interferential Currents

Interferential therapy is a form of transcutaneous application of two alternating medium frequency currents to generate a low frequency current in the deep structures. It is a noninvasive, safe and effective alternative treatment to manage chronic intractable, post-surgical and post-traumatic pain. Interferential therapy was developed in 1950s by Dr. Hans Namec in Vienna, and became increasingly popular in the United Kingdom during the 1970s.[1] Interferential Therapy has been widely used in therapy for many years.[2,3] Popularity of interferential current in the United States has become evident in the last 35 to 40 years, following a vigorous advertising campaigns.[4]

Interferential current therapy is used widely to stimulate tissues that lie deep within the body. The effects can be local or more general depending upon the configuration of the current applied to the skin. Unlike other methods of low frequency electrical stimulation, these currents encounter a low electrical resistance and can thus penetrate deeply without causing undue discomfort.[5] It is difficult to produce low frequency currents directly to the deeper structures because of considerable skin resistance. This is due to the impedance of the skin being inversely proportional to the frequency of the stimulation. In other words, lower the stimulation frequency, greater the impedance to the passage of the current & so, more discomfort is experienced as the current is 'pushed' into the deeper tissues against this barrier. On the other hand, skin resistance to the medium frequency currents is very low, that allows conduction of the current easily at any depth of the tissues. It is therefore; the lower frequency current can be produced at any dept of the tissues without considerable skin resistance by using the medium frequency currents.

Surveys consistently reported that interferential therapy is the most commonly used electrotherapeutic modality in Britain and Ireland for the physiotherapeutic management of patients with low back pain.[16,17] Foster at el[16] observed that interferential therapy was preferred by 44.1% of 813 physiotherapist. This modality has widespread ownership, popularity, and usage among physiotherapist in Australia and Canada.[20]

Production

The transformer in the equipment boosts up the common house electricity frequency to the desired medium frequency currents. Two alternating medium frequency currents are applied simultaneously to the body through the skin. These currents are applied in such a way that they must cross each other in the tissues. The sites of the tissues where the two alternating medium frequency currents cross each other cause interference.

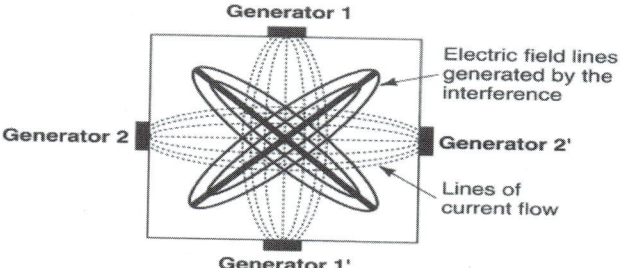

Fig 9.1 production of medium frequency currents

The interference of these two medium frequency currents produces a low frequency current which is known as "beat frequency. Each beat (or envelop) seems to cause excitation of peripheral nerves much like a single of a monophasic or a biphasic pulse and therefore, can also be termed as polyphasic pulses. The beat frequency is equal to the number of times each second the current amplitude increases to its maximum value and then decreases to its minimum value, or the simply the difference between the frequencies in circuit 1 and 2.[6] The resultant low frequency current (beat frequency) is actually a difference of the two medium frequency currents. For an example, two medium frequency currents are 4000Hz and 4050Hz respectively.

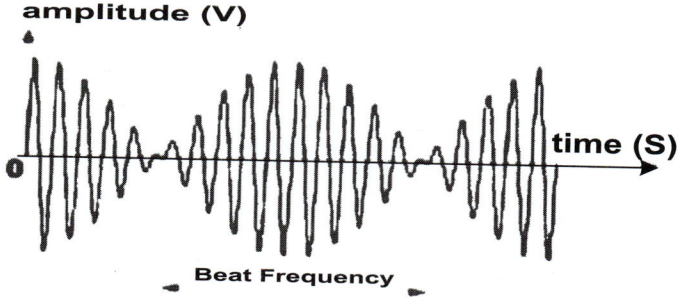

Fig 9. 2 production of resultant beat frequency current in the tissues.

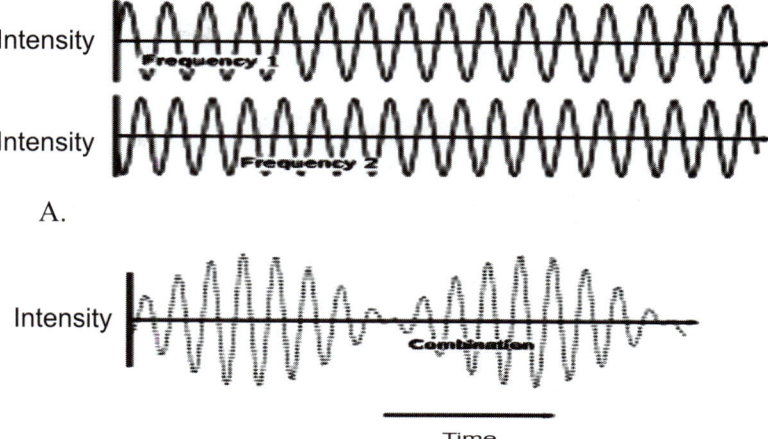

A.

Fig 9.3 The production of resultant amplitude modulated interferential current by the two medium frequency currents. A. two medium frequency currents, B resultant amplitude modulated interferential current.

Therefore, the resultant low frequency current would be 50Hz.

Amplitude modulations are variations in the peak amplitude in a series of pulses or cycles. **Frequency modulations** are variations in frequency in a series of pulses. **Phase or pulse duration modulations** are also variations in phase or pulse duration in a series of pulses.[8]

Similar, to the Conventional TENS, most of interferential currents apparatus allow modulation of the pulse rate, amplitude, and pulse duration. If the beat frequency remains constant the cycle duration of each cycle within a beat would also remain constant. However, if there is any variation in the beat over the time, the cycle duration within the beat would also vary. For example, an interferential apparatus, generating the carrier frequency of 4000Hz and the beat frequency is 100Hz. A constant beat frequency of 100beats per second, each beat would have duration of 10 millisecond with the 40 cycles or pulses, each of which has duration of 250microseconds. However, if the beat frequency is reduced to 10beats per seconds, then the beat duration (100ms), as well as the number of cycles per beat (400) and the duration of the cycles within each beat (25), would also vary.

Physiological Effects

The literatures suggest that the interferential currents simply represents a different electronic approach to achieve the same basic physiologic and clinical response achieved by other TENS devices. J. Gareth Noble et al conducted the study and found some evidence of a putative vasodilatory effect caused by interferential current therapy when applied through suction electrodes at a modulated frequency of 10–20 Hz.[9] An adequate intensity and other parameters of the interferential currents is capable of contracting the muscles involuntarily that increases localized blood flow. The optimal frequency for stimulation of most of voluntary muscle appears to be 40-80 Hz[10,11] whilst visceral muscle, supplied by the autonomic nervous system, is stimulated optimally at 10-50Hz[12] The increased local blood circulation helps in improving healing and reducing swelling. This also helps in removing damaged tissue and brings nutrients necessary for healing to the injured area. The interferential current stimulates A beta large diameter fibers which block the transmission of the pain sensitive fibers at the pain gate. There is stimulation of the sensory nerves also which is experienced by the patient as tingling or prickling sensation.

Indications

i. **Relief of Pain** – Interferential current is used for the reduction of pain and muscle guarding. The muscles guard the joint to prevent pain. The frequency between 80-100Hz of analgesic effect helps in relieving pain and spasm. Interferential therapy current is more effective in the chronic musculoskeletal pain and spasm rather than the acute and post surgical pain.

ii. **Reduction of Swelling** – Interferential current claimed to be effective as a treatment to promote the reabsorption of edema in the tissues. The evidence is very limited in this respect and the physiological mechanism by which it could be achieved as a direct effect of the current remains to be unestablished. The preferable clinical option in the light of the available evidence is to use the current to bring about local muscle contraction which combined with the local vascular changes that will result could be effective in encouraging the reabsorption of tissue fluid. The use of suction electrodes may be beneficial, but also remains unproven in this respect.

Following soft tissue injury there is rupture of the muscle fibers or vessels on the skin or underlying structures. The organization of the exudates leads to the formation of adhesions (hematoma) that results in impairment of functions. Frequency between 1-30Hz causes muscle contraction (increased permeability of the cell membrane, which helps in movement to and from cells) venous and lymphatic flow, and tone of tissues and vessels which aid in the relief of edema progress. The frequency between 1-10Hz produces muscle contraction and vasodilatation, and has a vigorous pumping effect which will have physiologic mechanisms for the absorption of the exudates.

iii. **Stress Incontinence –** The incontinence is more commoner in the females than the males may be due to the anatomy of the female created for child bearing which alters the control mechanisms to prevent incontinency. The stress incontinence is a situation where a patient cannot maintain normal passive continence of the bladder when subjected to stress such as coughing and sneezing. It appears due to the internal sphincter being very well identified in the male and not easily identified in the female. With males the sphincter is strong enough to exert a closure effect due to a muscular ring which does not exist with a female. This is probably due to the fact the female's absence of the muscular ring is for reproductive purposes and not uro-dynamic.

The use of interferential therapy with the frequency of 0-10 Hz stimulates and activates the external striated sphincter, smooth muscle surrounding the urethra, and periurethral muscles of the pelvic floor. Due to the physical ability of small diameter autonomic fibers to polarize and repolarize the suggested rate, frequency is 1- 10 Hz. This is because the affected fibers lack the ability to repolarize in shorter time intervals, unlike faster large diameter fibers. To get good results the patient is asked to contract the muscles voluntarily with the current.

Contraindication

I.   Arterial disease - The stimulatory effect of the current could produce emboli

ii. Deep Vein Thrombosis - In the acute phase, it is possible to dislodge the thrombi or increase the inflammation of the phlebitis

iii. Infective conditions – Contraction of muscles by interferential current could spread the infection or exacerbate the condition. Hence, interferential current directly over the infective site should be avoided.

iv. Malignant tumors - Direct stimulation of the muscles over the tumor is contraindicated, but referred pain from cancer or metastasis can be treated

v.   Pregnant Uterus - Not safe for fetus - may however be used on other areas such as hip joint and sacroiliac joint strain during pregnancy.

vi. Danger of hemorrhage – The strong contraction of the muscle or group of the muscles can cause increase in blood circulation in the local area or may rupture tiny blood vessels which may produce haematoma in the area.

vii. Artificial pacemakers – A demand unit senses the electrical activity of the heart, thus avoid an electric device that may interfere with it

viii. Large open wounds - These will cause concentration of the current and distortion of the interferential field.

ix. Dermatological conditions – The current may exacerbate the dermatological conditions in the area being treated.

Application Parameters

The parameters of the interferential therapy are the set of guidelines for the safe and effective use of the modality. Many textbooks and literature have explained the parameters of interferential therapy such as carrier frequency, beat frequency, amplitude modulated frequency, swing frequency, pulse duration, two pole, four pole, treatment time, and electrode placement. Most of the therapists are inconsistent with these parameters and they administer interferential treatment on a trial and error basis[18] and are solely based on the anecdotal evidence.[19] However the parameters of the modality such as placement of the electrodes are at the discretion of the individual therapist. The following parameter should be used for safe and effective treatment.

Frequency Sweep:- There is a tendency of the nerves to get accommodated with the constant current. To overcome the accommodation the frequency of a current is set in a manner which allows that to change repeatedly. A range of frequency as per the required physiological effects is set from base to the top which changes from the base to the top usually over the six seconds, however some of the equipments may offer 1 or 3 second options. For an example, base frequency is set at the 90Hz and the top frequency is set at the 130Hz for over a period of 6 seconds. It means the frequency would sweep from 90Hz (base) to the 130Hz (top) over a period of 6 seconds. The important part of this is also that the frequency may also sweep in the patterns over the given time. The patterns are usually, triangular, rectangular and trapezoidal. In triangular pattern the frequency would sweep gradually from the base (90Hz) to the top (130) over the period of six seconds, and then sweep gradually from the top to the base.

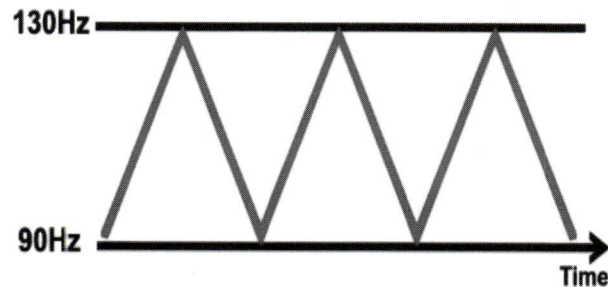

Fig 9.4a: Frequency Sweep Triangular.

In rectangular pattern the frequency would sweep from the base to the top and remain constant for a while and then sweeps from the top to the base. Hence, in this pattern, the frequency switches' between these two specific frequencies rather than gradually changing from one to the other

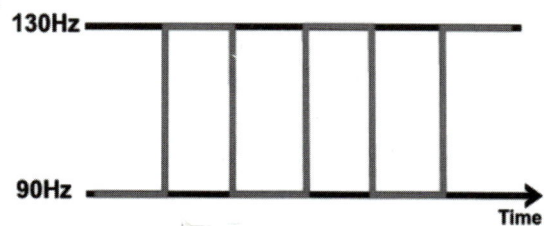

Fig 9.4b: Frequency Sweep Rectangular

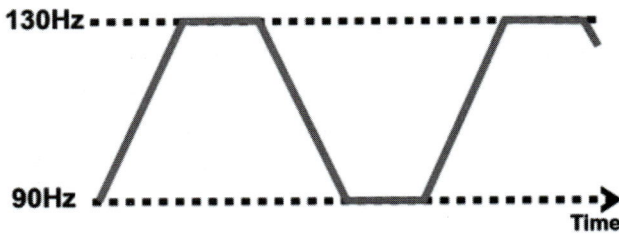

Fig: 9.4c. Frequency Sweep Trapezoidal.

The trapezoidal pattern of the frequency is the combination of both the triangular and rectangular patterns

Amplitude Modulated Frequency: - Amplitude modulated frequency is actually an equal to the mean of two medium frequency currents.[7] For an example, one medium frequency current is normally of fixed frequency, say about 4000Hz, and the other medium frequency current adjustable is of 4100Hz. These two medium frequency currents (4000Hz and 4100Hz) summate or cancel each other out in a predictable manner, and produce a resultant amplitude modulate interferential current of 4050 Hz which is known as **"Amplitude Modulated Frequency".** Theoritically, the medium frequency currents summate or cancel each other out in a predictable manner, producing the resultant "amplitude modulated interferentid current" . It is difficult to show categorically that this is the case in the tissues but it is reasonable to suggest that the resultant current (AMF) will be stronger than either of the 2 input currents.

The addition of an amplitude-modulated frequency parameter to interferential therapy did not influence mechanical pain sensitivity in healthy subjects. Amplitude-modulated frequency is therefore unlikely to have a physiological hypoalgesic effect.[13]

2 Pole and 4 Pole Mode: - The application of the interferential currents may either be bipolar or four polar. However; the physiological effects produced by the 2 pole and 4 pole interferential currents are more or less similar. The use of 2 pole (bipolar) interferential stimulation is made possible by electronic manipulation of the currents - the interference occurs within the machine instead of in the tissues, hence the current is 'pre modulated'. The patient experiences more intensity under the electrodes. The wide dispersal of the area of interference with the bipolar technique may reduce the effectiveness of the treatment.[14] The application of four pole interferential current produces amplitude modulated current in the center of the four electrodes. Therefore, the electrodes should not be placed directly on the targeted treatment area. The treatment area should be in the center of the four electrodes to achieve effective results. The four pole application of interferential therapy produces current in the deeper structures than the bipolar application.

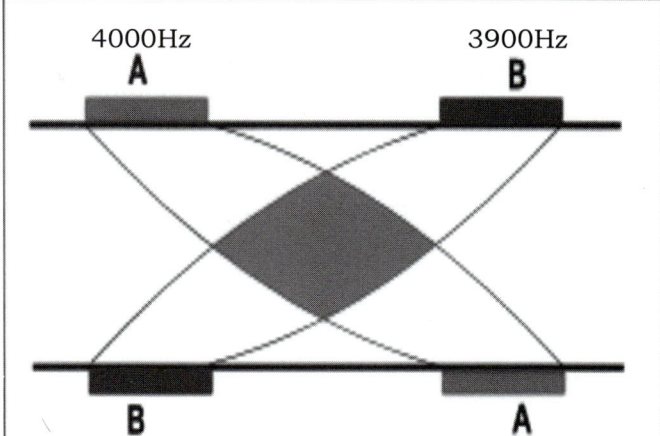

Fig 9.5. Two medium frequency currents A and B of 4000Hz and 3900Hz produce a low frequency current of 100Hz and an amplitude modulated frequency current of 4050Hz in the tissues.

Vector – Many of the interferential current equipments show vector mode on the display board. The application of vector mode is to scan the treatment area. Normally, the low frequency current is produced in the specific area between the electrodes; therefore; some treatment area remain untreated. The vector mode allows scanning movement of the interferential field from deeper to the superficial so that the whole part between the electrodes subjected to the maximum interferential effect.

Electrodes – Interferential currents can be applied to the body through the plate, carbon electrodes or suction electrodes. The plate electrodes require adequate covering with the wet lint. The whole electrode must be covered with the lint; leaving any part of the lint can cause burn or electric shock. The carbon electrodes are applied with adequate gel for good conduction. Suction electrodes are also being used to transfer the interferential current to the body. The advantage of the suction electrode is that these can be applied easily to the patient. These do not require any gel, clothing and straps. The suction electrodes are also good option for the less accessible anatomical areas.

Interferential Currents

Treatment Duration – The treatment duration depends on the conditions of the patients; however' no longer than the twenty minutes and shorter than 10 minutes is suggested by many authors. The most of painful conditions require ten minutes of interferential therapy.[15]

Intensity – The gradual increase in the intensity causes prickling and tingling sensation to the treatment area. The intensity is increased till a strong sensation is produced within the comfortable zone of the patient. The tolerance to the current varies from patient to patient therefore; therapist must ensure that the intensity is not out of the comfort zone of the patient, otherwise this can cause burn. Lower beat frequency can produce strong visible contraction of the muscles.

Application Procedure -

Equipment Preparation– Prepare the equipment for the treatment. Self testing – test the equipment whether it is working or not. Place the electrodes under the hand and increase the intensity gradually to see the prickling and tingling sensation. If equipment is working satisfactorily, select the parameters according to the condition or requirement of the patient. **Patient Preparation**– Screen the patient for contraindications to the interferential current. Explain the type of current to the patient that he or she would experience. Explain that the prickling, tingling and involuntary contractions are considered as normal; however; any other discomfort symptoms during the treatment need to report immediately. **Electrode Placement** – It is explained already that the interferential current can either be applied through bipolar or quadripolar electrodes. The bipolar is the pre modulated current whereas, the quadripolar produces amplitude modulated current in the tissues. In quadripolar method the four electrodes, two black and two red are used and placed around the treatment area, whereas in the bipolar mode both the electrodes of same color either of red or black are placed directly over the treatment area.

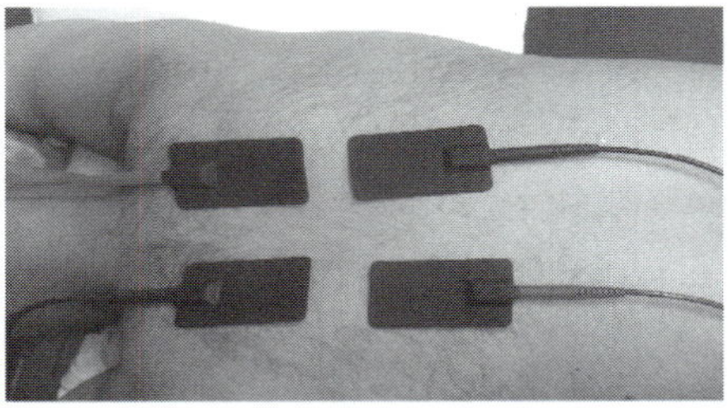

Fig 9.6a. Application of IFT upper dorsal region.

Interferential Currents

b 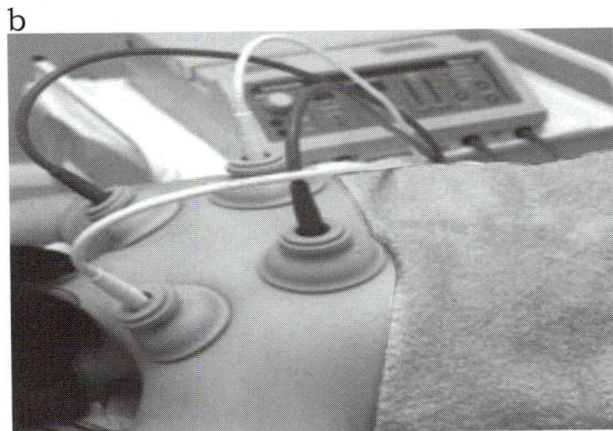 c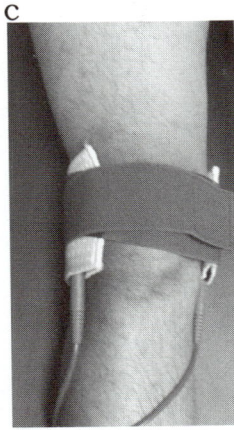

Fig 9.6 b. Application of the four pole vacuum electrodes interferential current on the dorsal region.

Fig 9.6 c. Application of IFT on knee joint mediolateral .

In quadripolar, the four electrodes are placed in such a way that the two channels cross each other in the treatment area. The treatment area should be in the center of the four electrodes. When the current pathways intersect, they will either be in phase, or out of phase. This means that they will either summate (add to each other) or neutralize (cancel each other out). To treat the knee pain situated in the deep area, two channels can be applied so that they cross each other in the deep area of the knee joint and mimic the low frequency current. **Intensity –** The intensity is increased gradually until the patient feels a tingling or pins and needle sensation at the contact area of the electrodes and also in the deep situated area. The intensity should be increased within the patients comfort level. Stronger intensity is preferred for more beneficial effects but it should not be turned up so high as to cause it to be uncomfortable. The patient should be asked for any discomfort during the treatment. **Duration –** Treatment may be advocated between 10 to 20 minutes per session as per the condition of the patient. The intensity is turned to zero after completion of the treatment session. The electrodes are removed and skin is cleaned at the end of the treatment.

Suggested Frequencies for various conditions

Pain gate sensory fiber stimulation   1-100Hz (Wadsworth and
                                        Chanmugam, 1980
                                        80-100Hz De Domenico, 1982
                                        0-100 Savage, 1984

	100 Hz Goats, 1990
Increase circulation Sympathetic fibers stimulation	0-100Hz Wille, 1969
	100 Hz Ganne, 1976, Nikolova, 1987
	100 Hz, 90-100Hz, 1-10Hz Wadworthand Chanmugam, 1980
	Less than 80 Hz De Domenico1982
	0-5Hz Savage 1984
Descending pain Suppression/ nociceptive fiber stimulation	10-25 Hz De Domenico,1982
	130 Hz Savage, 1984
	15Hz Goals, 1990
Physiological block of nociceptive C fibers	less than 50 Hz; A delta fibers less than 40Hz (De Domenic 1982) 40Hz larger diameter (Goals, 1990)
Placebo Response	None specifically implicated

Stress incontinence – To produce an adequate stimulation the position of the electrodes should be an appropriate. For females one posterior electrode is placed under the ischial tuberosities, and the second electrode is placed over either side of the gluteal cleft, anterior to the anus. Disposable gamagee pads are recommended to prevent cross infection. A variety of electrodes, some internal, some external have been used with varying degrees of success. For males, one electrode is placed over the coccyx and other electrode is placed over the pubic symphasis. The aim of treatment is to strengthen the pelvic floor muscles and to prevent incontinence.

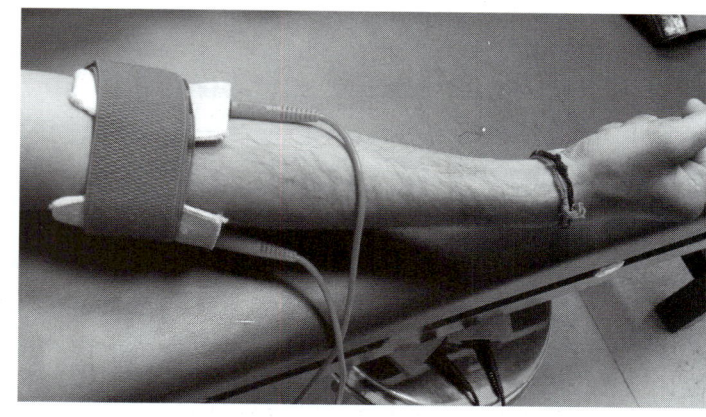

Fig 9.6 d. Application of 2 pole IFT Elbow Joint

Interferential Currents

Reference

1. Shiela Kitchen, Electrotherapy Evidence Based Practice, Eleventh edition, Churchil Livingstone, pp 287.

2. Pope, G. D. et al. (1995). "A survey of electrotherapeutic modalities: ownership and use in the NHS in England." Physiotherapy 81(2): 82-91.

3. Shah, S. and A. Farrow (2012). "Trends in the availability and usage of electrophysical agents in physiotherapy practices from 1990 to 2010: a review." Physical Therapy Reviews 17(4): 207-226

4. Roger M. Nelson, Karen W. Hayes, and Dean P. Currier: clinical electrotherapy, third edition, Appleton and Lange, Stamford, Connecticut, pp82

5. C.G. Goats, Interferential current therapy, Br. J. Sports Med. , Vol 24, No. 2, 91.

6. Meryl Roth Gersh, Electrotherapy in Rehabilitation, contemporary Perspective in Rehabilitation, Japee Brothers Medical Publishers (P) Ltd. New Delhi, India, pp203.

7. Shiela Kitchen,Electrotherapy Evidence Based Practice, Eleventh edition, Churchil Livingstone, pp288.

8. Roger M. Nelson, Karen W. Hayes, and Dean P. Currier: clinical electrotherapy, third edition, Appleton and Lange, Stamford, Connecticut, pp28.

9. J. Gareth Noble, Gail Henderson, A. Fiona L. Cramp, Deirdre M. Walsh and, Andrea S. Lowe. The effect of interferential therapy upon cutaneous blood flow in humans. Article first published online: 28 JUN 200. DOI: 10.1046/j.1365-2281.2000.00207.

10. De Domenico, G. New Dimension in interferential Therapy: A Theoritical and Clinical Guide. Ist Edn Reid Medical Books, 1987, Lindfield, NSW, Australia.

11. De Domenico, G. and Strauss, G.R. Motor stimulation with interferential current Aust J Phsiother 1985, 31 (6), 225-230.

12. Laycock, J. and Green, R.J. Interferential therapy in the treatment of incontinence Physiotherapy 1988, 74 (40161-168.

13. Fuentes C J[1], Armijo-Olivo S, Magee DJ, Gross D. Physiotherapy. 2010 Mar;96(1):22-9. doi: 10.1016/j.physio.2009.06.009. Epub 2009 Sep 4. Does amplitude-modulated frequency have a role in the hypoalgesic response of interferential current on pressure pain sensitivity in healthy subjects? A randomised crossover study.

14. Basant Nanda, Electrotherapy Simplified, 2nd edition, Jaypee the health science publisher, new Delhi, pp245.

15. Wadsworth and Chanmugam,APP 1980 Electrophysicla agents in physiotherapy. Therapeutic and diagnostic Use. Science Press, Marrickville, NSW, Electrotherapy evidence based practice Shiela Kitchen, 11th edition pp 292.

16. Foster NE, Thompson KA, Baxter GD, AllenJM, Management of non specific low back pain by physiotherapist I Britan and Ireland: a descriptive questnaire of current clinical practice Spine 1999, 24;1332-42.

17. Gracey JH, Mcdonough SM, Baxter GD, Chartered physiotherapist of low back pain in Northern Ireland, Kinesither Sci 1998; 383;10-1.

18. Johnson M, Tubasam G, A questnaire survey on the clinical use of interferential currents by physiotherapist. Proceedings of the pain. Society of Great Britain Annual Conference; Leicester (England): 1998 MM DD

19. Watson T, Shrewsbury Mesical interferential guidelines. Archam, Shapshire (UK): Shrewsbury Medical; 1987.

20. Lindsay DM, Dearness J, McGinley CC. Electrotherapy usage trends in private physiotherapy practice in Alberta.Physiol Can, 1995,47:30-4.

Chapter 10

Cryotherapy

Cold, in the form of cryotherapy, has been used since the time of the ancient Greeks, as an analgesic modality to reduce inflammation after acute musculoskeletal injury or trauma.[1] Cryotherapy consists of the lowering of tissue temperature by withdrawing heat from the body to achieve an analgesic effect.[3] The withdrawing of the heat from the body occurs through the conduction as the cold surface extracts energy or heat from the warmer surface. The general rule is, larger the temperature difference between the two surfaces, the greater the drop in the tissue temperature.[8,9] The application of ice on the skin can decrease the tissue temperature through conduction deep to the area of application, including intra-articular area.[10]

The application of cold not only increases the pain threshold but also prepares the athletes for readiness for physical activity, and general recovery from fatigue and stressful bouts of sports training.[4] The investigators, however, have also suggested that nerve conduction velocity decreases in a linear fashion with tissue cooling[5] and not skin cooling[6] and the rate of decrease in muscle tissue temperature depends on the cooling temperature.[7]

Cryotherapy is commonly used to reduce tissue temperature, metabolism, inflammation, pain, circulation, tissue stiffness, muscle spasm, and symptoms of delayed-onset muscle soreness.[2] Contemporary sports activities impose extremely high physical demands on athletes. Many of them are subjected to treatments that involve local changes in body temperature to obtain therapeutic effects.

Hemodynamic Effects

Initial Vasoconstriction - When cold is applied over the skin the immediate response is vasoconstriction of the cutaneous blood vessels that results in reduction in blood flow. The vasoconstriction of arterioles and venules occurs through direct and indirect mechanisms. The direct mechanism involves activation of the cutaneous cold receptors that stimulates the smooth muscles of the blood vessel walls to contract. The increased tone of the smooth muscles of the blood vessels wall following application of the cold will reduce the diameter of the vessels. Any influence that will cause vascular smooth muscles to contract will reduce vessel diameter. The reduced diameter of the vessels would reduce the blood flow. Decrease tissue temperature also decreases the production and release of the vasodilator mediators, such as Histamine and Prostaglandins which further contributes to the vasoconstriction.

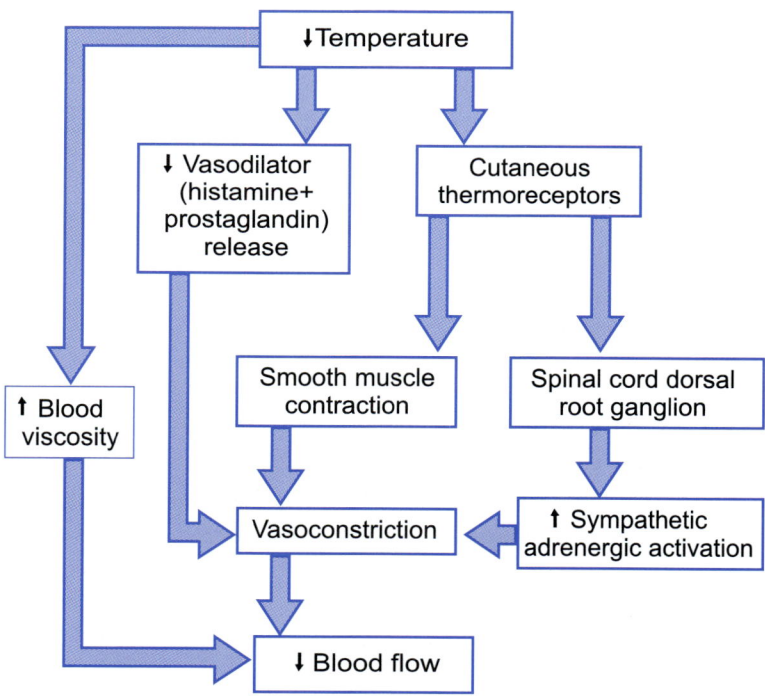

Fig 10.1a schematic diagram of physiological effects of ice on tissue

Further in the process decrease tissue temperature stimulates cold thermal receptors situated in the skin which in turn causes a reflex activation of sympathetic adrenergic neurons or fibers, resulting in cutaneous vasoconstriction. This reflex vasoconstriction produces generalized cutaneous vasoconstriction. The blood flow decreases following cold application also increases the blood viscosity and thereby, increasing the resistance to blood flow. Increase viscosity of the blood reduces the circulation rate. Reducing circulation results in a greater decrease in the tissue temperature in the area that is directly cooled and lesser extent in the area distant from the site of cold application. Contralateral changes resulting form generalized cutaneous vasoconstriction were less pronounced.

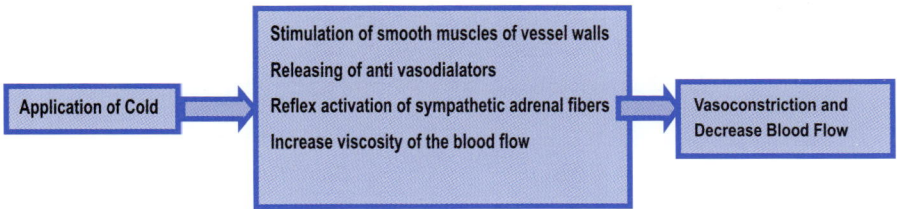

Fig: 10.1. B. schematic diagram of initial vasoconstriction

Therefore, stimulation of smooth muscles of the vessel walls, releasing of anti vasodilators, reflex activation of sympathetic adrenergic fibers and increase viscosity of the blood all help in vasoconstriction and reducing significant blood flow following application of cold.

Later Cold Induced Vasodilatation and Lewis Hunting Response - When tissue temperature is reduced below 10^0 C, or ice application is allowed for a long time usually for more than 11 minutes, a cold induces vasodilatation can follow the initial period of vasoconstriction. However, vasodilatation has not been found to be consistent response to prolonged cold application[11]. This phenomenon was first recognized and reported by Lewis[12] in 1930. He found that when fingers were immersed in an ice bath, skin temperature decreased during the first 15 minutes. This reduction in temperature was followed by cyclic periods of increasing and decreasing temperature, which he correlated this with the vasodilatation and vasoconstriction, respectively. This reaction of "hunting" for a mean point of circulation is called "Lewis's Hunting Reaction". Lewis felt that the hunting response was mediated by activity within an axon reflex. As skin was cooled to less than 10^0 C, pain would result, causing afferent sensory impulses to be carried antidromically towards skin arterioles. An unidentified neurotransmitter, termed "H" similar in action to histamine, was hypothesized to be released, resulting in arteriolar vasodilatation. The vasodilatation would increase the temperature of the area as the increased blood flow will provide more warm blood in the area. As the temperature rises above 10^0 C the, ice bath was again effective in causing vasoconstriction. However, during cyclic periods, temperature never returned to near-pre-immersion values. The hunting response appears to occur predominantly in apical areas, where, arteriovenous (AV) anastomoses are located in the skin.[13, 14]

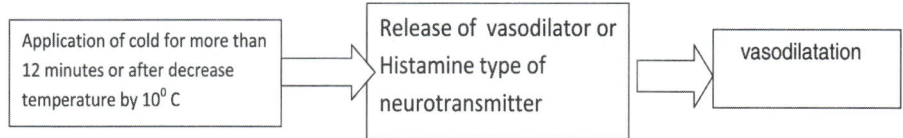

Fig: 10.1. C schematic diagram of cold induced Vasodilatation

As cooled blood returns to the general circulation, it stimulates the heat conservation area in the preoptic region of the anterior hypothalamus. Stimulation of the area will result in further reflex cutaneous vasoconstriction. If the area being cooled is smaller, the Lewis hunting response would occur and thermal injury to the tissues be prevented by cyclic vasoconstriction and vasodilatation. However, if the area being cooled is larger, shivering would occur as a heat retaining mechanism.

Neuromuscular Effects

Application of cold can alter the neuromuscular functions such as decrease nerve conduction velocity, elevate pain threshold, altering muscle force generation, decreasing spasticity, and facilitating contraction.

Effects on Peripheral Nerves – Application of ice on the nerves can significantly decrease the motor as well as sensory nerve conduction velocity. The quantity of change in the nerve conduction velocity depends upon the duration of the ice application and degree of the temperature alteration. Following application of ice, A delta fibers which are small diameter, myelinated, pain transmitting fibers, demonstrate the greatest decrease in conduction velocity in response to cooling. The large diameter A alpha fibers are affected last. The fibers least sensitive to cold were small diameter unmyelinated fibers. Ice packs over the ulnar nerve for 20 minutes resulted in an average decrease in motor conduction velocity of 29.4% from precooling values.[16] Zankel[17] conducted study on the ulnar nerve and found that after thirty minutes of the ice application, the conduction velocity was still 8.3 lower than before ice application, suggesting a long lasting effect when ice is given for a longer duration. Synaptic transmission can also be impeded or blocked. Li[18] demonstrated in the rate that neuromuscular synaptic transmission was impeded when the temperature dropped to 15^0 C, and that it was blocked at 5^0C. the peripheral nerve stopped conducting impulses at 4^0C.

Effects on Muscle Strength – The tension generated in the muscle can significantly be increased or decreased by application of the cold. McGown has found that the application of ice for a short period of time for five minutes can increase the isometric strength of the muscle.[18] The possible explanation for the observed increased strength could have been the effect of short duration cold on motor nerve excitability.[19] Clendenin[20] noted that facilitation of a single motor unit was seen after one to two minutes of icing over the biceps brachii muscle of healthy human subjects. In addition, those received ice could have been psychologically motivated to perform better post test.

On the other hand the increase in duration of cold application can decrease the strength of the muscles. Oliver and associates[21] found that the muscle strength of planter flexors was decreased following cold immersion for 30 minutes of normal legs at 10^0 C to 12^0 C. Over 45 minutes of the post immersion, planter flexion strength began to increase over pretreatment values and continued to do so for the next three hours.[21, 22, 23] The proposed mechanism for the reduced muscle strength after prolonged cooling include reduction of blood flow to the muscles, slowed motor nerve conduction, increased muscle viscosity , and increase joint or soft tissue stiffness.

Metabolic Effects

The immediate effect of the cold on tissues is vasoconstriction that decreases the blood flow of the local area. Application of cold also increases viscosity of the blood which offers resistance to the blood flow, therefore, increase viscosity of the blood further contribute to decrease blood flow and lowers the local tissue temperature. Consequently, decrease cell growth, cell reproduction (cellular metabolism), increase cellular survival, decrease local metabolism, and enzymatic activity and decrease oxygen demand. When using cold at extreme temperature, it destroys the cells by crystallizing the cytosol (intracellular fluid).

Indications

Cryotherapy is commonly used to reduce tissue temperature, metabolism, inflammation, pain, circulation, muscle spasm, and symptoms of delayed-onset muscle soreness.2 Contemporary sports activities impose extremely high physical demands on athletes. Many of them are subjected to treatments that involve local changes in body temperature to obtain therapeutic effects. The following are the indications of the cryotherapy.

Edema Control – Cold is the first choice of modality used most widely by the clinicians for treating acute injuries. Cooling can reduce swelling.[24] Following acute injuries there is microtear or rupture of the vennules, capillaries, vessels, and fibers of the muscles; resulting blood comes out of these structures into the interstitial tissues or extracellular tissues, and forms a *"haematoma"*, also known as blood clot. This process is continued for first 24 hours to 48 hours of the acute injury. However, it may be shortened if the injury is mild. The hematoma prevents normal functions of the tissues.

Vasoconstriction, following application of cold, not only decreases blood flow in the tissues but also allows less fluid infiltration into the interstitial tissues and prevents dramatic increase in microvascular permeability.[25] The cold also controls increase in capillary permeability by reducing the release of vasoactive substance such as "histamine". The second effect of cold on tissues which helps in preventing edema formation is increasing viscosity of the blood. Increase viscosity of the blood itself offers resistance to the flow of blood; therefore, it decreases the blood circulation into the injured tissues. The third effect of cold on tissues is decreased metabolism rate. Knight hypothesized that efficacy of cold for the care of acute injuries is due to the reduction in metabolism rate thus a decrease in secondary hypoxic injury.[26]

As far as prevention of edema formation after acute injuries is concerned, the most important part which needs to be taken into account is - *duration of the application of cold and intensity of cold application.* Exposure of the tissues to cold beyond the length of time of vasoconstriction does not help in reducing the edema formation, but increases the swelling in the tissues. Therefore, to prevent and control edema the duration of cold application should not be more than 10 to 12 minutes, however, it may repeated every hour. In addition to that if the clinician adds elevation of the part which is being immersed with compression by the elastic crepe bandages to the ice aplication, it further helps in achieving better results. Use of cold, at temperatures ranging from 5^0C to 15^0C for 24 hours had more swelling than the patients treated without application of cold.[26] The increase in swelling after application of the cold could have been caused by cold induced vasodilatation and thermal damage as a result of prolonged and intense cold exposures. Therefore, to treat acute injuries the clinician should not apply cold at intense temperatures for more than 12 minutes.

Pain Control and Reduction – Elevation of the pain threshold has been demonstrated in patients with rheumatoid arthritis[27] immediately following treatment but declines within thirty minutes. A relief of pain in patients with arthritis may be due to the adverse effects of cold on the activity of destructive enzymes within the joints.[28, 29] A delta fibers which are small diameter, myelinated, pain transmitting fibers, demonstrate the greatest decrease in conduction velocity in response to cooling. Application of ice for 10-15 minutes or longer can control pain for one or more hours. This prolonged effect is thought to be the result of blocking conduction of A delta fibers and by gating of pain transmission by the cutaneous thermal receptors.[16] The part may be treated with the ice pack at the less intense cold for an hour to relieve pain for a long period of time. Hence, the mechanism by which cryotherapy elevates pain threshold and decrease pain include antinociceptive effect on the gate control system, a decrease in nerve conduction, reduction in muscle spasm, and prevention of edema after injury.

Spasticity Reduction - Spasticity is the pathological state of increased muscle tone resulting from lesion to the upper motor neurons. There is increased tone in the extrafusal muscle fibers, when the hypertonic spastic state appears. Spastic patients suffer from muscle contracture, muscle cramp with pain, and involuntary movement of the limbs. Spasticity interferes with the gait, exercise, and range of motion of joints.

Local application of cold is used clinically to diminish the resistance of spastic muscle to rapid stretching and to decrease or abolish clonus.[30] Cold therapy in conjunction with exercises significantly reduced spasticity temporarily, increased range of motion and improved hand function in children with spastic cerebral palsy.[31] Suppression of clonus by cold highlights the importance of peripheral input in relation to central mechanisms.[32]

Decrease spasticity after application of cold is thought to be caused by a decrease in gamma motor neuron activity and, later, a decrease in afferent spindle and Golgi tendon organ activity.[33] Passive movements are performed to reduce further spasticity. Once the spasticity is reduced, active and active assisted movements of the contra-lateral group of muscles are initiated in order to achieve functional and voluntary movements. The functional activities such as sitting, standing, and gait training are also incorporated with the voluntary contraction of the muscles or group of the muscles.

Spasticity can be reduced by using two methods of cryotherapy. **Ice massage –** It Involves rubbing plastic or foam cup (with edges peeled back) of ice over the belly of spastic muscles. It is used mostly for small areas or over group of muscles to the parallel direction for 10-15 minutes until there is significant amount of spasticity reduced. The second method of reducing spasticity is **ice taping.** This method involves taping of ice cubes over the muscles antagonistic to the spastic muscles. Application of ice taping helps in facilitating the contraction of the muscles.

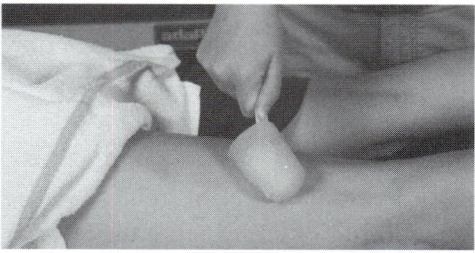

Figure 10. 2. ice massage

Cryotherapy

When cold is applied in an appropriate way on the skin, this can increase the excitatory bias around the anterior horn cell. Combined with other forms of excitation (brushing, tapping) and with the patients' volitation, this can often produce contraction of an inhibited muscle (only with intact peripheral nerve supply). This effect can also be used when muscle are inhibited postoperatively or in the later stages of regeneration of a mixed peripheral nerve

Contraindications

 Application of cold sometimes can cause damage to the tissues and alter the recovery of the patients. The following conditions such as cardiac, psychological, peripheral nerve injuries, vasospastic disease, peripheral vascular disease and cold sensitivity should be ruled out before application of cold.

1.   **Cold Hypersensitivity (Cod Induced Urticaria)** – Cold induced urticaria is the condition in which some individual develop slightly elevated patches, which are redder or more pale than the surrounding skin are often produce severe itching in response to cold. The systemic response may include – facial flushing, a drop in blood pressure, an increase in pulse rate & syncope.

2.   **Raynaud's Phenomena and Disease:- Raynaud's Phenomenon** is a paroxysmal digital cyanotic condition often associated with connective tissue disorder. It exhibits cycles of pallor, cyanosis, rubor & normal color in the hands & feet in response to cold. Numbness, tingling or burning may also occur. Rayanaud' Phenomena may be associated with thoracic outlet syndrome, carpal tunnel syndrome, or trauma. Raynaud's disease is the primary and idiopathic form of paroxysmal digital cyanosis which is caused by the some regional or systemic disorders. The symptoms of Raynaud's disease are similar to the phenomenon but bilateral and symmetrical even when ice is applied to one part.

3.   **Cryoglobinaemia:-** An abnormal protein present in the blood, can form a precipitate at low temperatures blocking blood vessels & thus causing local ischemia. It is not common, but can be found in association with some of connective tissue disorders such as multiple myeloma, systemic lupus

erythematosus and rheumatoid arthritis. It is characterized by the presence of blood in the urine.

4. **Cod Intolerance:-** Following application of cold some individual's complaints of severe pain, numbness, and color changes. These patients should not be given cold therapy.

5. **Cardiac diseases:-** Coronary thrombosis & anginal pain have sometimes been provoked by cold.

6. **Compromised circulation or sensation:-** Application of cold can cause burn and tissue damage, if the blood supply of the area is compromised as the temperature is not dissipated to the adjacent area.

7. **Peptic Ulcer:-** Cold application to the abdomen causes gastrointestinal motility and gastric acid secretion, therefore; it is contraindicated to those patients with known peptic ulcer disease.

8. Local limb ischemia

9. History of vascular impairment

Precautions and adverse effects

Prolonged joint cooling with topical ice can lead to nerve palsy and extensive axonotmesis. Many studies have found ulnar and peroneal nerve damage following prolong application of ice.[34] Therefore, intense cold with prolonged period should be avoided.

Tissue death, frost bite, nerve damage, freezing of tissues etc are the common adverse effects of the cold application.

Methods of Application

Cold application is a simple and inexpensive therapeutic approach which has been accepted for decades as an effective non-pharmacological intervention for pain management. It increases the pain threshold, decreases the inflammatory reaction and spasm. Cold is administered by a variety of methods such as cold packs, ice packs, ice massage, cold baths, vapocoolant sprays, and controlled compression units.

Cryotherapy

Cold Packs – Cold packs are of various sizes designed to cover different parts and contours of the body. The cold packs contain silica gel or sand-slurry mixture encased in vinyl. These materials hold the heat for more than twenty minutes. The cold packs are placed in a refrigerator unit which has temperature of approximately -5degrees for at least two hours before use; however, thirty minute in the refrigerator is enough if placed between the treatments. The part which is being treated should be exposed adequately, and inspected for any contraindications before the initiation of the treatment. The cold pack is wrapped in a towel preferably in a damp towel and is placed on a part to be treated with an adequate bandaging to ensure good contact with the skin for 10-15minutes.

Prawit Janwantankul found that the application of an ice bag directly to the skin is a more effective cryotherapy technique than that of ice bag over a damp towel barrier. Thus, clinicians should consider using an ice bag directly to an area to achieve greater cooling effects.[10] However, any sign of burn or tissue damage during the treatment should carefully be observed.

Ice packs- Ice Pack is a crushed ice or cubes placed in a plastic bag. The bag with crushed ice is wrapped in a dry towel as ice packs provide more aggressive cooling than cold packs. Cold or ice pack can also be placed directly on the treatment area. To achieve intense cooling effects the ice packs are placed on the treatment area and secured with the elastic bandage this procedure is known as ice pack compression bandaging.

Cold or ice packs are placed on the treatment area for 10-15 minute to reduce pain and spasm. In acute injuries, where prevention of swelling is the goal of treatment, ice application should be limited to the 12 minutes to avoid vasodilatation (thermal effects), however, this can be repeated every two hours. To reduce spasticity the application of ice should be longer, up to 30minutes. The area is inspected at every 10minutes for any adverse effects, especially, if the cold application is intensed. Skin redness and dark pimples during and following application of ice are considered normal.

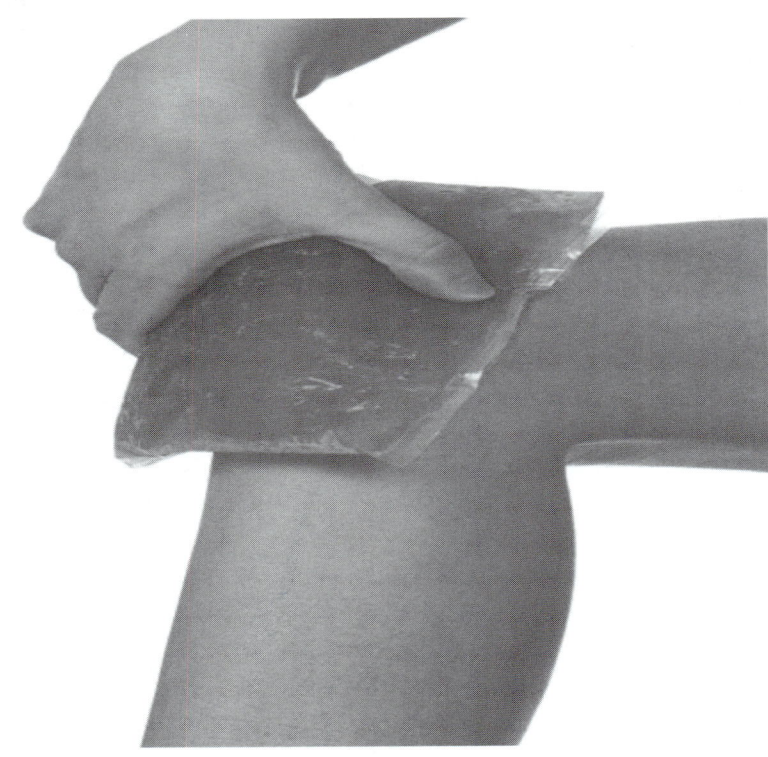

Fig: 10.3a Cold Pack on knee joint

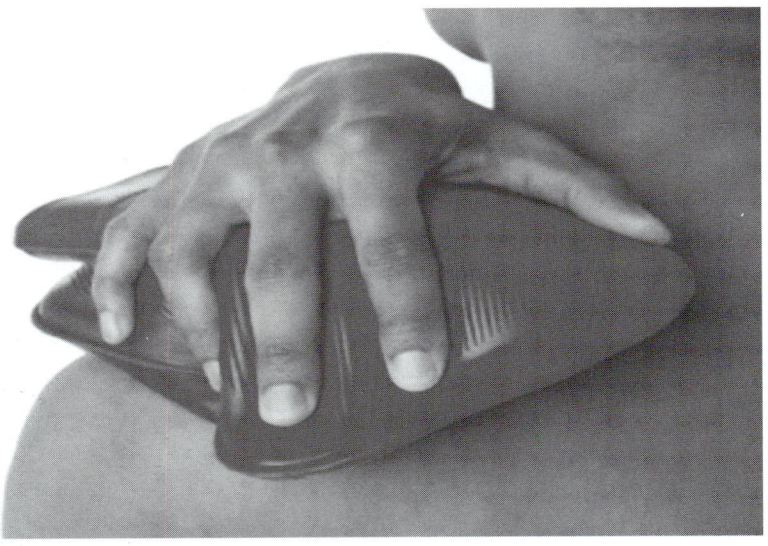

Fig: 10.3b Cold Pack on shoulder joint

Cryotherapy

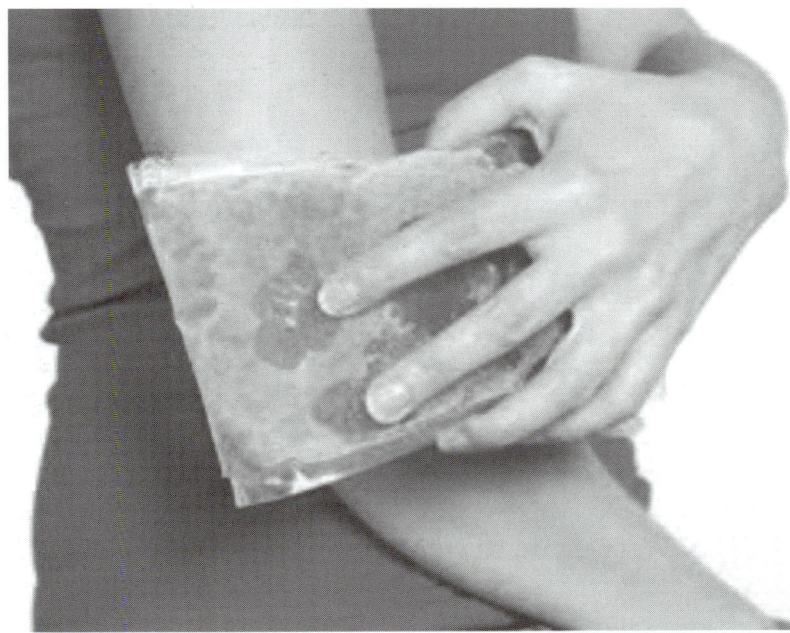

Fig: 10.3c Cold Pack at elbow

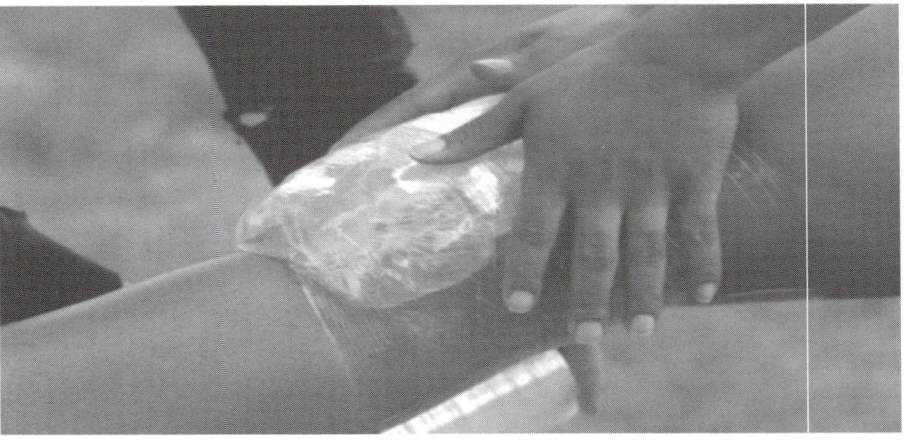

Fig: 10.3d Ice Pack secured with bandage at the leg.

Ice Massage- This is an application of ice cube directly over the treatment area to achieve more intense cooling effects. The small sized Styrofoam or plastic cup is filled with the water with the stick in the center and placed in the refrigerator for at least two hours. The ice is removed from the cup and placed directly over the treatment area. It is moved over the area during the entire treatment session with the help of stick.

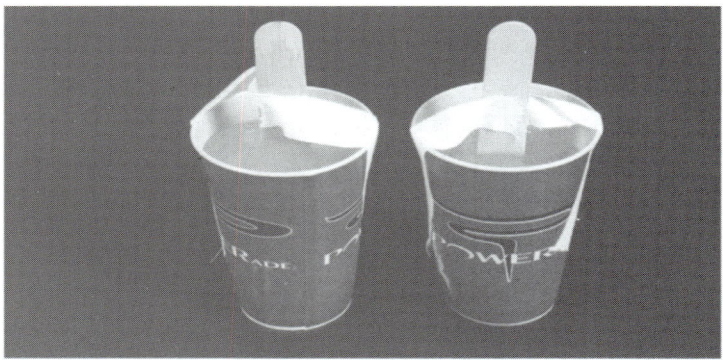

Fig: 10.4 Ice Cup

Cold Water Immersion: Water immersion is increasingly being used by elite athletes seeking to minimize fatigue and accelerate post-exercise recovery. Accelerated short-term (hours to days) recovery may improve competition performance, allow greater training loads or enhance the effect of a given training load. However, the optimal water immersion protocols to assist short-term recovery of performance still remain unclear.

Cold water immersion induces significant physiological and biochemical changes in the body. Much of this evidence is derived from full body immersions using resting healthy participants.[35] Cold water immersion significantly reduced heart rate and core temperature; however, all other metabolic and endocrine markers were not affected by CWI.[36] Cold water immersion is most widely used for the extremities such as feet and hands. A plastic tub with the larger size of the feet is identified and filled with the water and crushed ice. The temperature of the tub is maintained between 15°C and 20°C.[37] Temperature of the tub can be lowered or increased by adding or removing the crushed ice from the tub depending on the condition. Application at lower temperature requires extremity to dip into the bath intermittently to avoid any adverse effects.

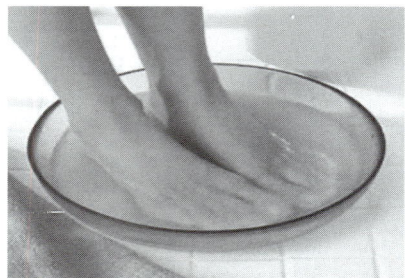

Fig: 10.5. Cold Water Immersion method for feet

Cryotherapy

Controlled Cold Compression Therapy: Controlled cold compression is used frequently following surgeries to prevent postoperative pain, inflammation and edema. This method of compression with cold has proven more significant results than the ice or compression alone. There is an equipment which has two parts the unit and the sleeves. The unit maintains the temperature at desired range which is circulated to the sleeves. The extremity is elevated slightly above the heart and covered with the stockinet before applying sleeves on it. The extremity is wrapped in a sleeve and secured with the Velcro.

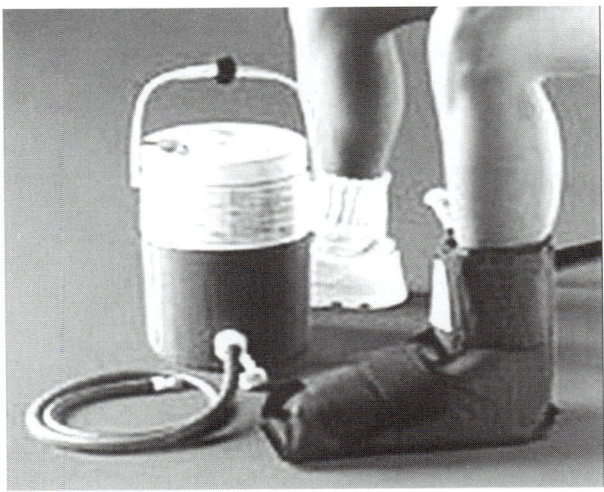

Fig: 10.6 Cold Compression Unit with sleeves at the foot and lower leg.

Vapocoolant sprays

Gebauer's Ethyl Chloride is a vapocoolant (skin refrigerant) intended for topical application to control pain associated with minor sports injuries, injections, starting intravenous. The medium and fine streams are also intended for use as a counterirritant in the management of mayofascial pain, restricted motion, and muscle tension.

A vapocoolant works through evaporation and drops the temperature of the skin to about 8 degrees F instantly. This sends an immediate barriage of signal to the CNS, thus interrupting the pain signal which travels to the CNS on slower conducting nerve fibers. This creates a window of opportunity to move the tissue through normal, pain free range of motion. Travel and Simons said, "stretch is the action, spray is the distraction".

233

Fluorimethane as a vapocoolant spray was formerly used as a common treatment for myofascial trigger points. Now most of the clinicians have replaced fluorimethane with cold spray due to harmful effect of fluorimethane on the environment. However, there is no ban on these sprays and some clinicians still use these vapocoolant sprays. A trigger point in the muscle may result from muscular strain and may be associated with sensitized Nerves, increased metabolism, and decreased circulation. Trigger points are also thought to be present in the skin, ligaments, and fascia. The pioneering work in trigger point localization and therapy was done by Janet Travell, MD. She had designated active and later trigger points.[39] The trigger points usually found in the body area such as cervical spine, shoulder girdle, and lower back are mainly due to the poor body mechanics and faulty posture.

To treat the trigger points with the ice or vapocoolant spray the patient is placed in comfortable position with the skin exposed and the body part supported to permit full relaxation. Before treatment the part is moved through its range of motion so you and the patient can judge changes made by the treatment. With the muscle anchored at one end the ice or vapocoolant is applied in a sweeping motion in a parallel strokes in only one direction over the length of the muscle and then over the referred pain pattern. As the ice or vapocoolant is applied in a rhythmic, unhurried fashion, a slow continual passive stretch is applied progressively to the muscle. Any one area of the skin should receive only two to three strokes of cold before re-warming to achieve optimal results of the ice and stretch technique. The rate at which the ice or vapocoolant is moved over the skin is approximately 4inches (10cm) per second. the stretch force should be light enough that it does not elicit a stretch reflex from the muscle but strong enough to be effective. The application and release of the stretch force should be done smoothly and gradually, not quickly. A cold pack can immediately be applied to further relax the muscle.

It is believed that this technique is effective because of two mechanisms, although they have not been confirmed through research. The gate theory of pain presented by Melzak and the modified gate control theory advanced by Castel postulate that sudden cold and stretch sensations inhibit the pain cycle by blocking pain transmission of pain signals. Ice striking inhibits the pain spasm cycle and allows the muscle to respond to the stretch. The second

Cryotherapy

factor is mechanical: if a muscle is stretched, its sarcomere elongates and releases the actin and myosin elements enough to end the sustained muscle fiber contraction.

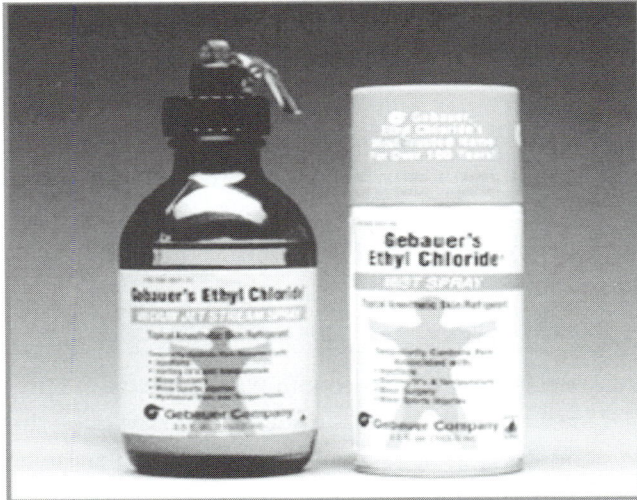

Fig:10.7a. Vapcoolant ethyle chloride

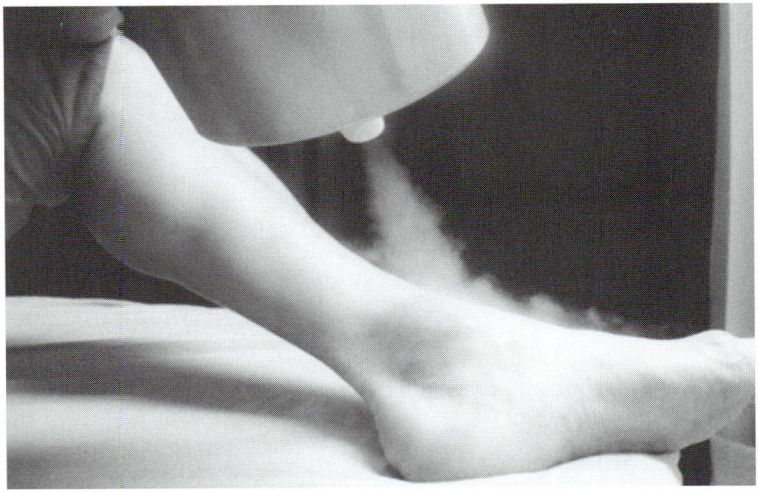

Fig 10.7b. Vapocoolant ethyle chloride spray on the ankle joint.

Cryotherapy

Whole-body cryotherapy: Cold therapy is commonly used as a procedure to relieve pain and symptoms, particularly in inflammatory diseases, injuries and overuse conditions. A peculiar form of cold therapy (or stimulation) was proposed 30 years ago for the treatment of rheumatic diseases. The therapy, called whole-body cryotherapy (WBC), allows exposure to very cold air that is maintained at -110 degrees Centigrade to -140 degrees Centigrade in special temperature-controlled cryochambers, generally for 2 minutes. WBC is used to relieve pain and inflammatory symptoms caused by numerous disorders, particularly those associated with rheumatic conditions, and is recommended for the treatment of arthritis, fibromyalgia and ankylosing spondylitis.

Selection of Cooling Agent

The selection of the cooling agents depend on the size of the treatment area. The therapist must emphasize over the accurate placement of the cooling agent over the treatment area. For small areas such as muscle tendon, bursa, or small muscle belly ice massage effectively produces the desired cooling effects. For joints such as the knee, elbow, shoulder, or a larger muscle mass, such as lumbar or cervical paravertebral muscles a cold pack or ice pack should be the choice of cooling agents. For distal extremity joints such as ankle, leg and hands the cold water immersion should be recommended.

Cryotherapy in acute Ankle Sprains

Acute lateral ankle ligament sprains are common in young athletes between 15 and 35 years of age. Therapies range from cast immobilization or acute surgical repair to functional rehabilitation. There is sufficient evidence to suggest that cryotherapy improves clinical outcome in the management of soft tissue injuries[40]. Cryotherapy is the treatment of choice in the management of acute athletic injuries. The application of heat is not indicated in the immediate treatment of acute athletic injuries. If applied early and injudiciously, heat may adversely affect resolution of the trauma and prolong the rehabilitation of the athlete.[41] There is good evidence that cold application can be useful in certain situation as a therapeutic modality. It seems ideally suited to the acute injury where the reduction in local factors such as hemorrhage and edema can hasten recovery.[42]

Hocutt JE Jr, and et al. conducted the study to assess recovery from ankle sprains. Thirty seven final participants were categorized according to the severity of their injury and they used of cryotherapy versus heat therapy. The study showed that cryotherapy started within 36 hours after the injury was statistically more effective than heat therapy for complete and rapid recovery. Patients received cryotherapy within thiry six hours reached full activity in 13.2 days compared to 30.4 days in a group using cryotherapy initiated 36 hours after injury or to 33.3 days in group using heat therapy.[43]

The lateral ligament comlex includes three capsular ligaments: the anterior talofibular (ATFL), Calcaneofibular (CFL), and posterior talofibular (PTFL). An ATFL is the most common injured in ankle injuries especially when the foot is planter flexed with inversion. Ankle sprains are classified from grade I to III (mild, moderate or severe). Grade I and grade II injuries recover quickly with non operative treatments. A non operative functional treatment includes immediate use of RICE(rest, ice, compression and elevation). Treatment for grade III injuries is more controversial. Functional treatment was complication free, whereas surgery had serious, though infrequent, complications. A comprehensive literature evaluation and meta-analysis showed that early functional treatment provided recovery of ankle mobility and earliest return to work and physical activity without affecting late mechanical stability.[44]

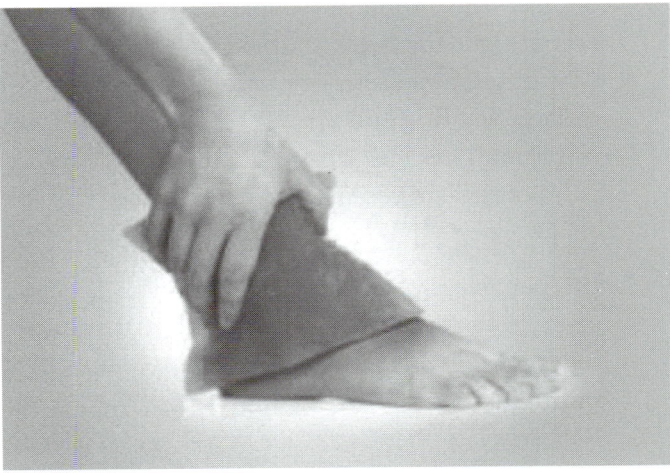

Fig: 10.8. ice pack on ankle in acute injuries ankle in elevated position

Ankle is placed over the pillows to bring it above the level of heart. An ice pack is placed over the ankle covering the dorsum of the foot for 11 minutes. The treatment time must be ensured by the therapist not above 11 minutes as intense cold can cause vasoconstriction and decrease the temperature of the area below 10 degrees. Immediately after reducing the temperature below 10 degrees of the area, an unidentified neurotransmitter, termed "H" similar in action to histamine, was hypothesized to be released, resulting in arteriolar vasodilatation. The vasodilatation would increase the temperature of the area as the increased blood flow will provide more warm blood in the area. The aim of ice packs application immediately after the soft tissue injury should be to achieve vasoconstriction and to avoid vasodilatation to occur. After ten to eleven minutes of treatment a elastic crepe bandage is applied to the ankle joint firmly. The resistance should increase from distal (foot) to proximal ankle joint. The procedure of application of ice may be repeated every two hours or at least thrice daily.

Cryo stretch and cryo kinetic

Cryokinetic- Cryo refers to the ice and kinetic refers to the motion. Cryokinetic is the technique of ice application on the extremities or joints after injuries. The ice is applied for twenty minutes to reduce significant nerve conduction and pain. Immediately after application of ice the joint is allowed to move actively. Cryokinetic is recommended after subsiding the symptoms of acute phase. Cryokinetic exercise re-establishes neuromuscular function and muscle wasting and atrophy of the muscles which is common after the injuries. There is dramatically reduction in swelling through the combination of cooling and exercise.

Cryostretching is a technique of application of ice in combination with the passive stretching exercises. The application of ice and passive stretching reduces muscle spasm and enhances range of motion. The technique involves three phases application of ice for at least twenty minutes, static stretching and PNF technique contract relax. Following application of ice two sets of 65 second stretches are applied with a 20 second rest between sets. Each period of 65 seconds consists mainly of static stretching, with three 5 second isometric contractions interspersed throughout the stretch. There should not be any pain throughout the procedure.

References

1. Swenson C., Sward L., Karlsson J. Cryotherapy in sports medicine. Scand J Med Sci Sport.1996;6(4):193–200. [PubMed]

2. Knight K. L. Cryotherapy in Sport Injury Management. Champaign, IL: Human Kinetics; 1995. pp. 9–11.

3. Knight K. L. Cryotherapy in Sport Injury Management. Champaign, Ill, USA: Human Kinetics; 1995.

4. White G. E., Wells G. D. Cold-water immersion and other forms of cryotherapy: physiological changes potentially affecting recovery from high-intensity exercise. Extreme Physiology & Medicine. 2013;2(26):1–11. PMC [PubMed]

5. Ruiz D. H., Myrer J. W., Durrant E., Fellingham G. W. Cryotherapy and sequential exercise bouts following cryotherapy on concentric and eccentric strength in the quadriceps. J Athl Train. 1993;28(4):320–323. [PMC free article] [PubMed]

6. Todnem K., Knudsen G., Riise T., Nyland H., Aarli J. A. The non-linear relationship between nerve conduction velocity and skin temperature. J Neurol Neurosurg Psychiatry. 1989;52(4):497–501.[PMC free article] [PubMed]

7. Yanagisawa O., Homma T., Okuwaki T., Shimao D., Takahashi H. Effects of cooling on human skin and skeletal muscle. Eur J Appl Physiol. 2007;100(6):737–745. [PubMed]

8. Abramson DI: Physiologic basis for the use of physical agents in peripheral vascular disorders. Arch Phys Med Rehabil 46:2161965.

9. Bocobo C, Fast A, Kingery W, Kaplan M: The effects of ice on intra-srticular temperature in the knee of the dig. Am J Phy Med 70:181-185, 1991.

10. Martin SS, Spindler KP, Tarter JW et al: Cryotherapy : an effective modality for decreasing intraarticular tempetrature after knee arthroplasty, Am J Sports Med May-June; 29(3) : 288-291,2000.

11. Weston M, Taber C, Casagranda L et al: changes I local blood volume during cold gel pack application to traumatized ankle, J Orthop Sport Phy Ther 19 (4): 197-199, 1994.

12. Hartvikksen K: Ice therapy in spasticity, Acto Neurol Scan, 38:79, 1962.

13. Lewis T, Observation upon the reaction of the vessels of th human skin to cold, Heart 15:177, 1930.

14. Fox RH and Wyatt HT: Cold induced vasodilatation I carious areas of the body surfaces in man, J Physiol, 162:289, 1962.

15. Taber C, Countryman K, Fahrenbrunch J et al: measurement of reactive vasodilatation during cold gel pack application to nontraumazed ankle, Phys Ther 72 (4) : 294-299, 1992.

16. Douglas WW and Molcolm JL: The effect of localized cooling on cat nerves, J Physiol 130:53-54,1955.

17. Zankel HT: Effects of physical agents o motor conduction velocity of the ulnar nerve, Arch Phys Med Rehabil 47:787, 1966.

18. McGown HL: Effects of cold application on maximal isometric contraction, Phys Ther 47:185-192, 1967.

19. Knuttesson E, Mattsson E: Effects of local cooling on monosynaptic reflexes I man, Scand J Rehabil Med 52:166-168, 1969.

20. Clendenin MA, Szumski AJ: Influence of cutaneios ice application on single motor units in human, Phys Ther 51:166, 1971.

21. Oliver RA et, Johnson DJ, Wheelsouse WW: Isometric muscle contraction response during recovery from reduced intramuscular temperature, Arch Phys Med Rehabil 60: 126-129, 1979

22. Johnson J, Leider FE: Influence of cold bath on maximum handgrip strength, Percept Mot Skills 44:323-325, 1977.

23. Davies CTM, Young K: Eeffects of temperatre on the contractile properties and muscle power of triceps surae in humans, J Appl Physiol 55:191-195, 1983.

24. Basur R, Shephard E, Mouzos G: a cooling method in the treatment of ankle sprain, Practitioner 216:708, 1976.

25. Dean DN, Tipton J, Rosencrane E et al: Ice reduce edema. J Bone Joint Surg Am, 84 (9) : 1573-1578, 2002.

26. Matson FA, Questd K, Masten AL: The effect of local colling on post fracture swelling. Clin Orthop 109:201, 1975.

27. Curkovic B, Vitulic V, Babic-Naglic D, Durrigle T, The influence off the heat and cold on the pain threshold in rheumatoid arthritis. Schrife Fiir Rheumatology 52: 289-291, 1993

28. Harris ED, McCroskery PA: The influence of temperature and fibril stability on degradation of cartilage collagen by rheumatoid synovial collegenose. New Engalnd Journal of Medicine 290: 1-6, 1974.

29. Peg SMH, Littler TR, Littler EN: A trial of ice therapy and exercise in chronic arthritis. Physiotherapy 55:51-56, 1969.

30. Katz RT. Management of spasticity. Am J Phys Med Rehabil 1988; 67: 108-116.MEDLINE.

31. Gehan M. Abd El-Maksoud[a,] , Moussa A. Sharafb, Soheir S. Rezk-Allah: Efficacy of cold therapy on spasticity and hand function in children with cerebral palsyAm J Phys Med. 1973 Aug;52(4):198-205.

32. Boyraz I, Oktay F, Celik C, Akyuz M, Uysal H.Effect of cold application and tizanidine on clonus: clinical and electrophysiological assessment. J Spinal Cord Med. 2009;32(2):132-9.

33. Wolf SL, Letbetter WD: Effect of cooling on spontaneous EMG, activity in triceps urea of the decerebrate cat, Brain Res 91:151-155, 1975.

34. Collins, K, Storey M, Peterson K: Peroneal nerve palsy after cryotherapy, Phy Sportmed 14:1005-108, 1986.

35. Bleakley CM[1], Davison GW. What is the biochemical and physiological rationale for using cold-water immersion in sports recovery? A systematic review.Br J Sports Med. 2010 Feb;44(3):179-87. doi: 10.1136/bjsm.2009.065565. Epub 2009 Nov 27.

36. Halson SL, Quod MJ, Martin DT, Gardner AS, Ebert TR, Laursen PB. Physiological responses to cold water immersion following cycling in the heat.Int J Sports Physiol Perform. 2008 Sep;3(3):331-46 .

37. Lee JM, Warren MP, Mason SM ,1978, : Effects of ice on nerve conduction velocity. Physiotherapy 64: 2-6.

38. Prawit Janwantankul. Different rate of cooling time and magnitudeof cooling temperature during ice bag treatment with and without damp towel wrap. Physical therapy in Sports. August 2004, volume 5(3):156-161.

39. Susan L. Michlovitz, Thomas P. Noaln, Jr. Modalities for therapeutic intervention, fourth edition, Contemporary Perspective in Rehabilitation, pp53.

40. Collins NC. Is ice right? Does cryotherapy improve outcome for acute soft tissue injury? Emerg Med J. 2008 Feb;25(2):65-8.doi: 10.1136/emj.2007.051664.

41. Kalenak A, Medlar CE, Fleagle SB, Hochberg WJ. Athletic injuries: Heat vs. cold, Am Fam Physician. 1975 Nov;12(5):131-4.

42. McMaster WC. A literary review on ice therapy in injuries, Am J Sports Med. 1977 May-June;5(30: 124-6.

43. Hocutt JE Jr, Jaffer R, Rylander CR, Beebe JK. Cryotherapy in ankle sprains. Am J Sports Med. 1982 Sep-Oct; 10(5): 316-9.

44. Lynch SA, Renstrom PA. treatment of acute lateral ankle ligament rupture in the athlete. Conservative verses surgical treatment. Sports Med 1999 Jan; 27(1):61-71.

Chapter 11

Hydrotherapy

The use of water for various treatments (hydrotherapy) is probably as old as mankind. Hydrotherapy is one of the basic methods of treatment widely used in the system of natural medicine, which is also called as water therapy, aquatic therapy, pool therapy, and balneotherapy.[1] Hydrotherapy is the use of water for accelerating healing, repairing and easing various musculoskeletal and neurological ailments. The benefit of 'water healing' or hydrotherapy have been recognized for thousands of years. In Europe, where hydrotherapy is especially popular, there are numerous health spas and health facilities for all types of 'water cures'.

Ancient civilization recognized the healing power of natural hot and cold springs. Back in the 4th century BC the Greek physician Hippocrates prescribed bathing and deinking spring water for its therapeutic effects. The Greek were the first to appreciate the relationship between physical and mental well being. They developed centers near spring and rivers using them for bathing and recreation. The baths were centers where intellectual, recreational activities, and health and hygiene were pursued. Around AD 339 some baths (built by Greek, and extended by Romans) were used solely for healing purposes and treatment was indicated first of all for symptoms of rheumatic disease, paralysis, and the effects of injuries.

Rationalism of Use of Water as a Physical Agent

Use of water is one of the oldest, cheapest, and safest methods of treating many common ailments. When the body or part of the body in immersed in the water it produces several physiological effects on the body. The buoyancy force generated in the upward direction against the gravity reduces load on the weight bearing joints. The reduction of load on the load on the joints decreases pain and increases the confidence of the patient to exercises in the pool. The hydrostatic pressure exerted by the water on the extremities and body reduces swelling by increasing the venous return.

Biophysical Characteristics of Water

The biophysical characteristics of hydrotherapy rests on the principles and concepts related to the mechanical intrinsic and thermal properties of water.

A. Mechanical Properties

a. **Buoyancy –** There is the upward force in the water which works against the gravity. This fluid force always acts vertically upward. The upward force generated by the water against the gravity is based on Archimedes' Principle, which states that an object or body part, totally or partially immersed in a fluid, experiences an upward, buoyant force equal to the weight of the volume of fluid displaced by that object or body part.[2] The effect of buoyancy reduces the weight and stresses on the weight bearing joints which helps in improving the balance and coordination of patients who find difficulty in standing on ground.

b. **Hydrostatic Pressure –** Hydrostatic pressure is the pressure exerted by the water on the body. According to Pascal's law, when a body part is immersed in the water a pressure is exerted equally at any level in a horizontal direction. This pressure is exerted by the water on all surfaces of the body when it is at rest at a given depth. The hydrostatic pressure increases with the depth and with the density of the fluid (density of the water increases with the depth). Therefore, standing and walking in the water is having greater importance to decrease edema. In standing the distal part of the extremity is the lowest in the water, hence, the pressure gradient between the surface and deeper water favors reduced accumulation of fluid in the distal parts of an extremity. The head out immersion of the body into the water at 35^0C facilitates in increasing venous return and shifting of the fluid from the interstitial space to the capillary.

c. **Hydrodynamic Pressure** – It is the pressure caused by movement of either the object or the water. When the person walks in the water resistance is encountered and demand is made on the walking muscles. The faster one walks, the more demands are made on the walking muscles. This pressure offers resistance against the movements of the limbs; therefore, resistance can be used for strengthening of the muscles.

d. **Turbulence** – It is defined as "the velocity at a given point varies erratically in magnitude and direction". The movements of limbs in the water cause circular patterns of the water and create small whirlpools or eddy currents and turbulence. Movement through turbulent water or against the current than through calm water encounters greater resistance which requires more muscular effort. The circular patterns caused by movement of the legs, arms and body of the patient also known as drag force. The drag force is exerted by water on a submerged and moving objects or body segment.[3] The combined effects of buoyancy and hydrostatic is helpful in balancing the body in the water. The pressure supports the body all around to and equal degree in the horizontal direction while buoyancy maintains the vertical position.

B. **Intrinsic properties – Water exhibits three intrinsic properties such as density, specific gravity and viscosity**

a. **Density** - Different materials usually have different densities, and density may be relevant to buoyancy, purity and packing. The density, or more precisely, the volumetric mass density, of a substance is its mass per unit volume. The symbol most often used for density is ρ Mathematically, density is defined as mass divided by volume $p = m/V$, where p is the density, m is the mass, and V is the volume. the more compactly arranged the molecules, the denser the substance. The density of the material varies with temperature and pressure. Increasing the temperature decreases its density by increasing its volume. Increasing the pressure on an object decreases the volume of the object and thus increases its density.

b. **Specific Gravity** – The specific gravity of the water is unity or 1, because its weight density, as a fluid, equals 9.8 N/L. The object which has the specific gravity greater than 1 would sink in the water. On the other hand the object which has the specific gravity equivalent to the water or less than 1, would float on the water. The specific gravity of human body, which varies depending on the individual's somatotype and residual air volume in the lungs at immersion, is less than 1. Therefore, the human body generally floats on the water when it is totally immersed into the water.

c. **Viscosity** – The viscosity of the water varies from one state to another due to change in the temperature. Viscosity is caused by the chemical binding forces holding the fluid molecules together, such as the forces binding hydrogen to oxygen molecules to form water. The water is more viscous at the lower temperature and its molecules are dispersed at the higher temperatures.

C. Thermal Properties

a. **Specific Heat** – The specific heat value of water is $1 \text{ cal/g}^0\text{C}$ because a heat input of 1 calorie is needed to increase the temperature of 1 g of pure water at 15^0C by 1^0C. Water has the capacity of holding the heat double of the paraffin wax and four times more than the air at any given temperature. A paraffin wax would contain 50% less heat than water at the same temperature. Hence, the patients can tolerate the paraffin wax bath at the 50^0C than the water.

b. **Thermal Conductivity** - Thermal conductivity (often denoted k, λ, or κ) is the property of a material to conduct heat. It is evaluated primarily in terms of Fourier's Law for heat conduction. The higher the thermal conductivity value of the substance the better the substance performs as a heat conductor. The thermal conductivity value of water at 15^0C is

1.42 cal/sec-cm^{0}C. The fat conducts heat 50% slower than the skeletal muscles and 30% slower than the skin. The thermal conductivity of the water is 70 times faster than the air and 2.5 times more rapidly than the paraffin wax.

Physiological Effects

Use of water in various forms and in various temperatures can produce different effects on different system of the body. The temperature is the good conductor of the heat. The temperature of water which is slightly higher than the body temperature produces several physiological changes in the body. The normal temperature of the skin and the subcutaneous tissues is 33^{0}C, whereas, the internal temperature of the body is maintained at 37^{0}C. Superficial cold application may cause physiologic reactions such as decrease in local metabolic function, local edema, nerve conduction velocity (NCV), muscle spasm, and increase in local anesthetic effects.[4] The temperature of the skin varies with cold and hot conditions. The living tissues of the body are affected by temperature in two fundamental ways –

A. The direct effects of the temperature on the body includes increase metabolic rate, increase collagen tissue extensibility and decrease viscosity.

   a. **Metabolic Activity** - Metabolic activities are the series of chemical reactions which increase as temperature increases and decrease with fall of temperature. An appropriate rise in temperature increases all cell activities including cell motility and synthesis and release of chemical mediators. Excessive temperature above 45^{0}C of the body causes so much protein, cell and tissue destruction. If the temperature of body rises by 1^{0}C it increases 13% metabolic activities.

   b. **Decrease Viscosity** – The resistance to flow blood in a vessel depends directly on the viscosity of the fluid and inversely on the fourth power of the radius of the vessel. As the temperature rises, the blood vessels get dilated and the viscosity of fluid also decreases. The resistance to flow to the blood decreases.

B. Systemic Changes - One hour head-out water immersions (WI) in various temperatures (32°C, 20°C, and 14°C) produced various effects. Immersion at 32°C did not change metabolic rate (MR) and rectal temperature, but it lowered the heart rate (HR) by 15%, systolic blood pressure (SBP) and diastolic blood pressure (DBP) by 11% and 12%, respectively, compared, with controls at ambient air temperature. Along with HR and blood pressure (BP), the plasma renin activity, plasma cortisol, and aldosterone concentrations were also lowered by 46%, 34%, and 17%, respectively, while diuresis was increased by 107%.[5]

C. The indirect effects of the temperature on the body are mainly activation of the higher centers to regulate the excess temperature and protect the organs to damage.

Indications

Hydrotherapy, the use of water as a physical modality for health promotion and treatment of various diseases with different level of temperature has been used widely in ancient culture including India, Egypt, and China.[6]

1. **Cerebral Palsy Children** – Hydrotherapy is highly effective form of treatment for cerebral palsy children and adolescents. The buoyancy effect of water relieves load on the lower extremities, whereas, the optimal temperature of the water reduces the spasticity. These effects of water facilitate the voluntary movements. The water offers resistance against the movements during the gait training that further facilitates the voluntary control and balance of the patient. Blohm D[7] conducted the review to evaluate the effectiveness of aquatic interventions for children or adolescents with cerebral palsy. All eight studies reported that aquatic interventions, either as a major component or as a stand alone intervention, were beneficial for children and adolescents with cerebral palsy. Blohm D found improvements in activity for gross motor skills; maintenance of improvement in gross motor function; and increased swimming skills for kindergarten children. The study also reported increases in lower-extremity muscle strength[8] and balance; better respiratory function and reduced spasticity in adolescents. Improvements were also

reported for range of motion with an increase in passive range of motion of lower-extremity joints (one study), and improved active and passive range of motion.

2. **Osteoarthritis** – Exercises in the hydrotherapy pool for Knee, ankle and hip osteoarthritic patients with the complaint of pain, lack of confidence, and have high risk of falling may be an excellent alternative to land exercise.[9] Water buoyancy force which is in upward direction against the gravity reduces load or weight of the body on the joints.[10] The warmth water reduces muscle guarding and hydrostatic pressure of water also reduce swelling. These effects promote muscle relaxation and reduces swelling.[11]

3. **Inflammatory Arthritis** - In patients with ankylosing spondilitis (AS), balneotherapy statistically improved pain; physical activity; tiredness and sleep score; on Bath Ankylosing Spondilitis Disease Activity Index (BASDAI). It indicates the effect of balneotherapy in improving disease activity and functional parameters in patients with ankylosing spondylitis.[12] Infrared sauna, a form of total-body hyperthermia was well tolerated; no adverse effects; and no exacerbation of disease were reported in patients with rheumatoid arthritis (RA) and AS in whom pain, stiffness, and fatigue showed clinical improvements during the 4 weeks treatment period.[13] Hydrotherapy is highly valued by RA patients who were treated with hydrotherapy (30-min session/week) reported feeling much better/very much better than those treated with land exercises (similar exercises on land) immediately on completion of the treatment program (6 weeks).[11]

4. **Fibromyalgia** - A systematic review on management of fibromyalgia syndrome (FMS) through hydrotherapy described as "there is strong evidence for the use of hydrotherapy in the management of FMS" and it showed positive outcomes for pain; tender point count; and health-status. Combination of ST (once daily for 3 days/week) and underwater exercise (once daily for 2 days/week) for 12 weeks significantly reduced pain and symptoms (both short- and long-term); and improved QOL in patients with FMS. Pool-

based exercise using deep water running three times/week for 8 weeks is safe and effective intervention for FMS because it showed significant improvement in general health and QOL compared with control; and significant improvement in fibromyalgia impact questionnaire score, incorporating pain; fatigue; physical function; stiffness; and psychological variables.

5. **Muscle soreness and fatigue** - Leg immersion in warm water ($44 \pm 1°C$) for 45 min before stretch-shortening exercise reduced most of the indirect markers of exercise-induced muscle damage, including muscle soreness, creatine kinase activity in the blood, maximal voluntary contraction force, and jump height. Immersion of extremities of body in the water with the temperature below $15°C$ lowers ratings of fatigue and potentially improves ratings of physical recovery immediately after immersion with reduction in delayed onset muscle soreness compared with the passive stretching.

Contraindications

I.   Pyrexia
j.   Active bleeding
k.   Acute vomiting or diarrhea
l.   Cardiac insufficiency, Recent heart attack or resting angina
m.   Wound infection
n.   Recent neurological event
o.   Recent chemotherapy
p.   Present history of deep venous thrombosis or pulmonary embolism
q.   Stress incontinence
r.   AIDS
s.   Shortness of breath at rest
t.   Uncontrolled epilepsy

Hydrotherapy Pool

Hydrotherapy pool is of different sizes and shapes from a standard pool to large sized to provide therapeutic exercises to treat various musculoskeletal, neurological and sports related injuries. Hydrotherapy is the use of physical properties of water such as temperature and pressure, for therapeutic purposes. The construction and design of the pool depends upon the need of the department.

A **Butterfly Tank** – It is a butterfly shaped hydrotherapy unit designed for arms and legs exercises to be carried out in the unit. It is ideal for the cerebral palsy children. The recessed area at the head and sides of the bath provide good access for the therapist commanding and encouraging the patient for the exercises. The tank is designed for permanent installations with direct connections to hot and cold water supply, overflow and drainage. It is constructed of heavy gauge stainless steel sheet electrically Argon welded tank is shaped to Butterfly.

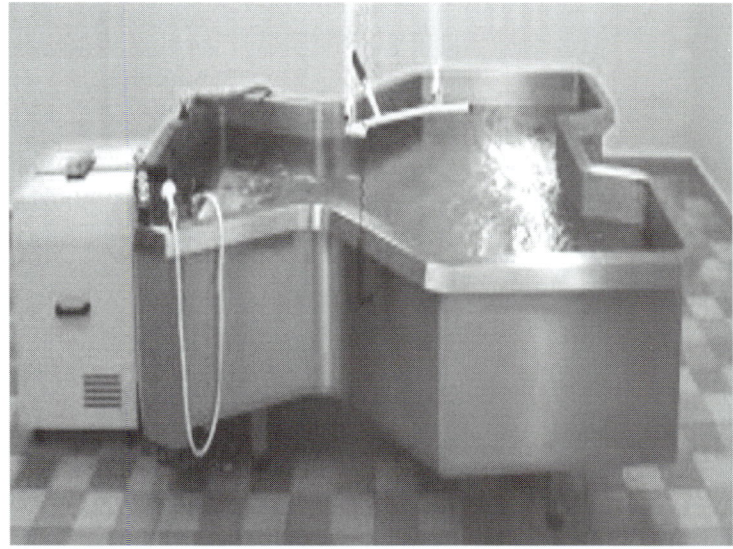

Fig. 11.1 Butterfly Unit (Hubbard's tank)

Whirl Pool – Whirl pool bath made of heavy gauge stainless steel is sturdily fabricated with bright finish inside. The unit is fitted with a motorized turbine ejector and aerator on a spring loaded turbine elevator. The jets are strategically directed at the key muscle groups that are vulnerable to stress and soreness. Ten minutes of immersions in whirlpools produce increase in pulse and finger temperature with increased feelings of well-being and decreased state of anxiety.[14] Whirl pool immersion increases metabolic rate, oxygen intake, and removes metabolites and wastages from the body. It accelerates the healing process.

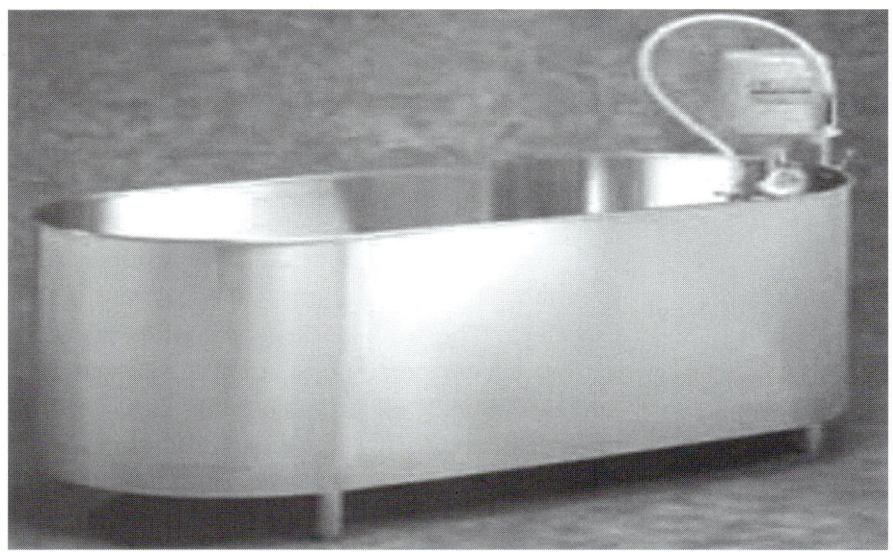

Fig. 11.2 Whirl Pool

B. Hydrotherapy Pool – Different sizes , shapes, and depths of hydrotherapy pool according to the number of the patients are constructed in the physiotherapy department. Three types of pools are commonly constructed in the department

    a.   Below ground

    b.   Below ground deck level and

    c.   Semi raised or raised

Below Ground with or without deck pool - Below ground pool with or without deck level is generally advised to construct. The floor of the pool may be of height adjustable with the motorized system. The advantage of the height adjustable pool is that the wheel chair bound patients would enter easily into the pool as the floor is lifted at the ground level and then it is lowered to the desired depth.

Size - In the daily practice the size of the pool should be of 9.24 meter length and 4.57 in the width. This size of pool provides a good working space for approximately eight people at a time and is used for the most of therapeutic activities. However the size may be kept small if the number of patients on pool therapy are not in large size. **Shape –** Rectangular shape of pool is strongly recommended. **Depth –** The depth of the pool also varies from .84 meter to 1.42 meter. **Floor –** The floor may be uniform or stepped. Stepped floor is having advantages of providing several depth. To avoid fear of stepped floor, the edge of each step must be clearly marked. The steps used in the hydrotherapy pool should have height of 150mm, depth 300mm and width 600mm to avoid any inconvenience. Patients may enter into the pool with the help of stairs or they may be shifted into the pool by hoists (a mechanical hydrolytic and electrical). Recently height adjustable floors are introduced to maintain the desired depth and to provide barrier free access to the wheelchair bound patients. However, these pools cost little bit high than the other pools. Parallel bars are installed at appropriate side of the pool with an appropriate height. The handrails at both the side of the stairs are also installed. The assistive devices such as turbulence, underwater jets floats for the activities and to facilitate exercise should be available.

Temperature of Pool – The temperature of pool depends on the condition of the patient. Different authors have suggested different temperature for various conditions. Two main factors affecting oxygen transport during immersion are temperature and hydrostatic pressure. Oxygen transport was improved above neutral temperature, because of increase in cardiac output resulting from the combined actions of hydrostatic counter pressure and body heating. Below neutral temperature, oxygen transport is altered. At any of the temperatures tested, the pulmonary tissue volume and arterial blood gases were not significantly affected

Exercises in water can performed in wide range of temperature, but warmer temperature appear to be more favorable for therapeutic activities.[15] Heat is lost from the body much faster in water than when exercising elsewhere, even though the ambient temperature in a gym is likely to be much less than the water temperature. The thin people lose heat more quickly because they do not have such a good layer of subcutaneous fat. On the other hand, obese people have too much insulation, and could theoretically be at risk from overheating. An ideal temperature for exercising with chronic arthritis would be thermoneutral. Some authors believe a pool temperature of 30.5 to 33.3° (87 to 92° F) is ideal for therapeutic exercise and general physical programmes providing both sedative and stimulating effects. In the United Kingdom it is not recommended that therapeutic activity takes place if the water is less than 27^0C, whereas, in the United States, pool water is generally kept lower than, at about 24^0C. In view of the above it can be inferred that the temperature between 32^{0}C (89.6^{0}F) and 35^{0}C (95^{0}F) is suitable for the therapeutic activities. This range of temperature caters all conditions.[16]

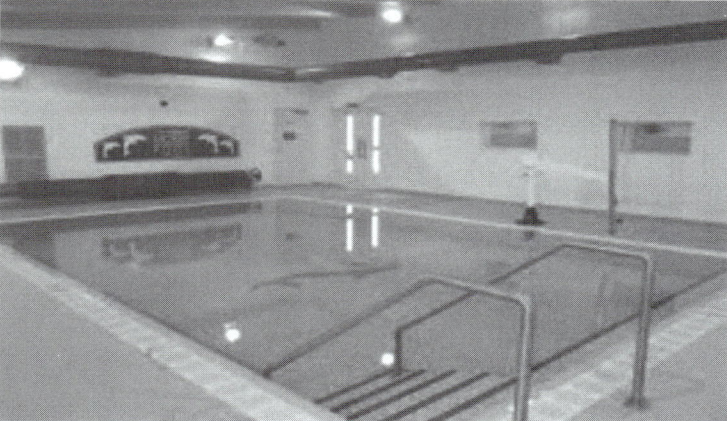

Fig. 11.3 Hydrotherapy pool (Below Ground)

Ventilation – The temperature of room should be lower than that of the temperature of water to allow gently cooling. It is maintained at 25^{0}C. A dehumidifier decreases the humidity of the room and maintains humidity at the appropriate level.

Changing Room – There should a separate room for changing cloth before and after the pool therapy. This should have direct access to the pool. Sometimes it is constructed inside the pool. The privacy of the patient should be the priority of the therapist. The changing room temperature should be maintained 4^{0}C lower than the temperature of the pool.

Preparation of the patient

- Patient should be examined thoroughly for the contraindication especially for the contaminated diseases.

- Treatment should not be given immediately after meals, nor it is wise to give them too longer after meals.

- The patient should be asked to empty his or her bladder before immersion, since a warm bath often has a diuretic action.•

- The patient should be asked to put on shorts or in the case of female patients a proper bathing suit is given

- Before entering into the pool the patient is asked to take a bath

- Non ambulatory patients are transferred into the pool with the assistance or electrically or hydraulically operated hoist. The ambulatory patients may walk down the steps if the pool is below ground. If the pool is raised above the ground all the patients can be transferred by the hydraulically or electrically operated hoist.

- Adjustable floor, if available, provide direct access to the pool.

- The temperature of the pool should be as per the condition of the patient

- The treatment should not exceed the appropriate time.

- After completing session the patient is transferred to the changing room immediately. He or she should be given plenty of water. The patient should leave the room after half an hour of the therapy.

Strengthening Exercises in Pool

Strengthening exercises are carried out in the hydrotherapy pool to strengthen the muscles of lower and upper extremity. The proper assessment of the muscle strength of each muscle needs to be done before starting the exercises. Muscles those are grade 2 are strengthen by using the buoyancy effect. However, grade 3 and grade 4 muscles may be strengthen with resistance offered by the water. The therapist should instruct the patient with an appropriate verbal commands. Free exercises such as mini squat, step up and step down active range of motion against the resistance of water help in improving the strength of the muscles. The progression of exercises in water should be based on the improvement in the strength and balance of the muscle.

Oxford Scale for Muscle Power Grading – Modified for Water

This scale is used to grade the strength of the muscle in water but it is limited to the muscles which retain little power but range of movement. The scale of muscle power on land is graded from 0 to 5 where 0 has no contraction and 5 is the normal. In water the scale commences from 1 and continues to 5 but it must be recognized that grade 5 in water is not normal as such function cannot be tested there.

The scale of muscle power modified for water is as under –

1. Contraction with buoyancy assistance.

2. Contraction with buoyancy counter balanced and contraction against buoyancy.

3. Contraction against buoyancy at speed

4. Contraction against buoyancy and light float

5. Contraction against buoyancy and heavy float.

Gait Training in Pool

Hydrotherapy can reduce weight-bearing to 20%, enabling re-education of gait to commence very early in a patient's recovery. The buoyancy force, hydrostatic pressure and temperature of water reduce pain and swelling. These effects of pool therapy increase the confidence of the patient and encourages for the exercises. The studies found that the patients who find difficulty in standing and walking on the ground have improved the balance, coordination and gait after the pool therapy.

The patient is transferred into the pool manually or by the hoist. To improve standing balance, non-ambulatory patients are made stand in the pool and asked to hold the railings of parallel bar. As the balance improves, patient is asked to raise one hand above the shoulder. Both the hands are raised alternately. In the progression the patient is asked to stand without the support of the railings. Both the hands are raised above the shoulder simultaneously. As the patient gains confidence he or she is asked to throw the ball and catch it. The therapist should throw the ball to the patient little away from the midline.

Once the patient gains confidence in standing he or she is asked to place heel of one leg forward. The same is repeated on the other leg also. An appropriate size of the step is placed before the patient. He or she is instructed to place one foot over the step and then take it down. It is repeatedly performed on both the legs. Three sets of thirty repetitions of mini squat (30 flexion) are done daily. If the patient gains confidence in doing mini squat and step up and down without the support, he or she is asked to ambulate in the pool without the support of the parallel bar. If the patient gains confidence on walking in the pool then he or she should practice gait training on land with the help of parallel bars.

Foot Baths

There are two types of foot baths - cold foot bath and warm foot bath. For cold foot bath, a small tub is used with the cold water up to the level of calf muscles. The temperature of the water should not exceed 18°C. Cold foot bath is indicated to the patients with varicose vein, headache, low blood pressure, sweaty foot, contused ankles and circulatory impairment. Both the feet are placed into the water up to the level of calf muscles for at least 15 minutes. Cold bath should be avoided to the patients with cold feet, hyper tension, irritable bladder, urinary tract infection, and diabetes. The large size of the foot can also be used if the aim of the treatment is exercises in the tub. The warm foot bath is indicated to the patients with cold feet. A small size tub of warm water with the temperature of 97°F is taken. The feet are immersed into the bath and hot water is gradually added till it reaches to the 103°F-104°F. The temperature of the tub is maintained at this level by adding more warm water and procedure should last 10-15 minutes. The procedure can be repeated daily for at least two weeks. The warm foot bath should be avoided to the patients with varicose veins, lymphostasis or edema.

Sitz Bath

The small tub with the warm water with the temperature of 103 - 104°F is suitable for the sitz bath. The size of the tub should be appropriate so that patient can sit easily on it. Patient sits in the tub and the water covers the glutei. The patient maintains the sitting position for 15 -20 minutes. Hot water may be added during the procedure to maintain the temperature of the water at 103°F to 104°F. The sitz bath are indicated to the patient with anal fissures, piles, difficulty in voiding the bladder, and irritable bladder, inflammation or infection of the prostate and preparation for the pregnancy.

Body wraps

Wrap is primarily used as supportive measure for treating fever and local inflammation. For the therapeutic purposes hot wraps and cold wraps are basically used. The treatment period lasts around 45 to 60 minutes sometimes up to three hours. Patient is placed in a comfortable position. A linen cloth is moisturized with cold or hot water. Patient is wrapped with the hot or cold linen for an appropriate time. The cold water wraps are advised for pyrexia and hot packs are for respiratory diseases. They are wrapped properly around the part or body which is being treated. The patient is wrapped in a blanket or another cloth for 45 to 60 minutes. Cold wraps are advised to the rheumatoid arthritis and pyrexia, whereas, hot wraps are advised to the bronchitis, lung diseases, neuralgia, prostatitis, vaginitis, and inflammation in the pelvic cavity.

References

I.   A Mooventhan and L Nivethitha, Scientific Evidence-Based Effects of Hydrotherapy on Various Systems of the Body, N Am J Med Sci. 2014 May; 6(5): 199–209.

ii.   Kreighbaum E, Barthelss KM (1996) Biomechanics: a Qualitative Approach to studying Human Movement. Allyn and Bacon, pp98-99.

iii.   Alain – Yvan Belanger, therapeutic Electrophysical agents evidence Behind Practice, third edition, Wolters Kluwer, pp126.

iv.   Weston M, Taber C, Casagranda L, Cornwall M. Changes in local blood volume during cold gel pack application to traumatized ankles. J Orthop Sports Phys Ther. 1994;19:197–9. [PubMed]

v.   Srámek P, Simecková M, Janský L, Savlíková J, Vybíral S. Human physiological responses to immersion into water of different temperatures. Eur J Appl Physiol. 2000;81:436–42. [PubMed].

vi.   Fleming SA, Gutknecht NC. Gutknecht. Naturopathy and the Primary Care Practice. Prim Care.2010;37:119–36. [PMC free article] [PubMed].

vii.   Blohm D effectiveness of aquatic interventions for children with cerebral palsy: systemic review of the current literature. University of York, Centre of Reviews and Dissemination 24.04.2013

viii. Gorter JW, Currie SJ,Aquatic exercise program for children and adolescents with cerebral palsy: why do we know and where do we go?, University of York, Centre of Reviews and Dissemination 24.07.2014)

ix. Arnold CM, Busch AJ, Schachter CL, Harrison EL, Olszynski WP. A Randomized clinical trial of aquatic versus land exercise to improve balance, function, and quality of life in older women with osteoporosis. Physiother Can. 2008;60:296–306. [PMC free article] [PubMed].

x. Biscarini A, Cerulli G. Modeling of the knee joint load in rehabilitative knee extension exercises under water. J Biomech. 2006;17:1–11. [PubMed].

xi. Eversden L, Maggs F, Nightingale P, Jobanputra P. A pragmatic randomised controlled trial of hydrotherapy and land exercises on overall well being and quality of life in rheumatoid arthritis. BMC Musculoskelet Disord.2007;8:23. [PMC free article] [PubMed].

xii. Altan L, Bingöl U, Aslan M, Yurtkuran M. The effect of balneotherapy on patients with ankylosing spondylitis.Scand J Rheumatol. 2006;35:283–9. [PubMed]

xiii. Oosterveld FG, Rasker JJ, Floors M, Landkroon R, van Rennes B, Zwijnenberg J, et al. Infrared sauna in patients with rheumatoid arthritis and ankylosing spondylitis. A pilot study showing good tolerance, short-term improvement of pain and stiffness, and a trend towards long-term beneficial effects. Clin Rheumatol. 2009;28:29–34. [PubMed.

xiv. Robiner WN. Psychological and physical reactions to whirlpool baths. J Behav Med. 1990;13: 157–73. [PubMed].

xv. Becker, B. and Cole, A. Comprehensive Aquatic Therapy. Butterworth Heinemann. Woburn MA, 2003.

xvi. Sova, Ruth. "Exercising in Hot Weather," The AKWA Letter, Vol. 3, #2, (July 1989).

Chapter 12

Light Amplification By Stimulated Emission Of Radiation

The term laser is an acronym for light amplification by stimulated emission of radiation.[1] Laser technology is rapidly advancing and its application to medical fraternity is constantly growing. Laser is a form of light and the healing properties of the light have been described since ancient Roman times.[2] A laser is generally used as a source or generator of radiation.[3] Radiation is the process by which energy is propagated through space. The direction of propagation of radiant energy is normally a straight and absorbed by the medium through which it travels. The velocity of travel remains equal in a vacuum, but may vary within different media. This radiating energy is collectively known as electromagnetic radiation.

Initially lasers used in surgery and, ophthalmic surgeons were the first especially to use the first ruby laser successfully for the treatment of detached retina in humans.[4] The major use of the laser in medicine is based on the photothermal and photoablative interactions of laser with tissues such as cut, weld and even destroy tissues.

A low power laser was introduced in the United States with the claim that the device could help in reducing pain, spasm, and inflammation and prompt healing.[5] The use of low levels of visible or near-infrared light for reducing pain, inflammation and edema, promoting healing of wounds, deeper tissues and nerves has been known for almost forty years since the invention of lasers.

Production

The laser light produced in a lasing cavity, containing a medium such as CO_2 (high powered laser), or helium-neon (low powered laser). The lasing cavity or chamber has two mirrors on each side. One side mirror is 100 percent reflect mirror and other side mirror is a semi-permeable. The semi-permeable mirror reflects only a predetermined quality of photons.

A high intensity flash lamp is used to raise the atoms, ions, or molecules of the medium to from their ground state (E_1) to one of several tiers of upper energy state (E_2), creating a condition known as population inversion.[6] It is the precondition for laser light. It is not achieved with spontaneous emission because the lifetime of the electrons in the excited state is insufficient to take them beyond the second energy tier. Once the electron shifts to its high energy orbits, the electron are inherently unstable and fall spontaneously within a short period of time to lower energy levels and in so doing release their extra energy as photon of light.[7] It is called spontaneous emission. It is the quantum of energy representing the difference between the ground state (E_1) and excited state (E_2).

If an unstable atom allowed to reach its end, this process will prevent the energy transfer level necessary for laser radiation. If; however, a photon of appropriate energy strikes an atom while it is maintained in an excited state, the atom is immediately stimulated to emit its excess energy and make its transition to the ground state. This process is called stimulated emission.[8] The photon of an excited state are aligned in a lasing chamber they hit the semi-permeable silver resonating mirror, and then reflect to the reflecting mirror. The reflection of the portion between two mirrors back and forth in the lasing chamber through the medium further amplifies the light. This produces intense photon resonance. The semi-permeable reflecting mirror (surface) also known as output coupler allows photons to eject from the chamber into the fiber optic cable. The fiber optic cable is a threadlike filament composed of glass that guides the stimulated photons by directing them to the treatment surface.

Laser light is located in a narrow spectral band of visible and invisible radiation. The He Ne laser beam is visible at 632.8 nm and is continuous while the Infra Red Laser light is invisible at 904 nm and is pulsed. Laser energy is measured in joules per square centimeters of tissue area, and laser power is expressed in milliwats. Cold lasers have an average power output of 1-2 milliwatts.

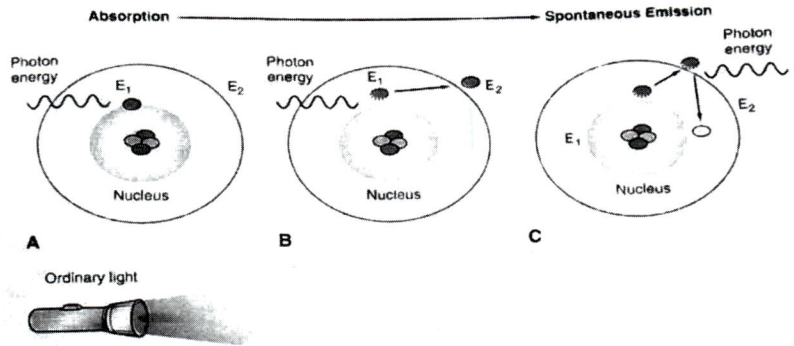

Fig: 12.1a Production of LASER

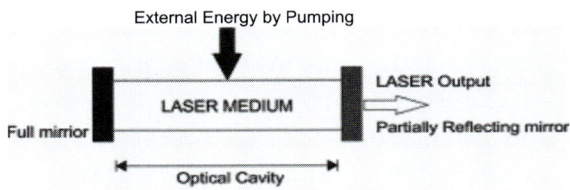

Fig: 12.1b Production of LASER

Physical Characteristics

There are three properties of laser that distinguishes it from incandescent and fluorescent light source: - Coherence, Monochromatic, and Collimated Beam. **Coherence** - all of the photons of light emitted from individual gas molecules are of the same wavelength. The individual light waves are located in step with another. All the waves having same phase and same wavelength travel in the same direction. Coherent temporal- when the waves have same phase. Spatial Coherence – when the wave travel in the same direction. Spatial coherence allows the light to be directed through a focusing lens and directly propagated to targeted tissues because of its directional stability. **Monochromatic:-** it is of a singular wavelengths and is of one color. For example HeNe produces a red light. Because of its wavelength specificity, laser light is characteristically pure. Light purity is inversely related to its wavelength. The shorter the wave length, the greater the purity of the light. **Collimated Beam: -** collimation refers to the minimal divergence or moving apart of the

Light Amplification by Stimulated Emission of Radiation

photons in a laser beam. Laser beams can be produced by applying electrical, mechanical or chemical energy to various forms of matter. The spatial and temporal coherence minimizes divergence and focus the energy so that it is concentrated on one area. To achieve temporal and coherence, the photons are aligned in a reflecting chamber. The photons are then reflected back and forth between mirrors to achieve amplification before being ejected through a fibroptic cable or a diode to reach the area to be treated.

When the laser contacts with the skin it can be reflected, absorbed or dispersed. The absorption and depth of penetration depends upon the tissue contents and laser wave length. The thickness of the dermis, the presence or absence of muscular, adipose, or osseous tissues are all important when considering the penetration of tissues by laser radiation. A prerequisite for absorption is that the wavelength of the irradiated light is suited to the absorbing material. The resonance of human tissue is such that it absorbs the light of laser quite well. This is based on the theory that human tissue cells oscillate at a frequency that is very similar to that of laser light.[48]

The depth of penetration of He Ne – laser directly occurs at approximately 3 mm of soft tissue thickness and that indirect penetration can occur up to 1 cm. Since the light of the He Ne - is of a red color, it will penetrate deeper into pale tissues than into red tissues (i.e. oral cavity). The He Ne laser is, therefore, primarily used for direct skin stimulation and for the stimulation of acupuncture points that have a superficial location.

The pulsed infra red laser appears to penetrate to depths of 1-5 cm in soft tissues. It is therefore, less absorbed in the dermis and more in the deeper and dense tissues, such as ligaments, tendons, and muscle and may be in the periosteum. Infra red laser irradiation as a power of 10 milliwatt will result in a penetration depth of 18 mm in the bone axis direction and 6 mm in the cortico-medullar direction.[49,50]

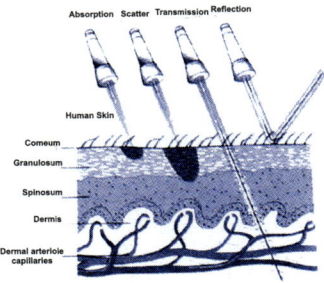

Figure 12.2 characteristics of Laser - Absorption,, scatter, transmission, and reflection.

Light Amplification by Stimulated Emission of Radiation

Classification

The laser is classified with reference to power, wavelength, and effects into five classes.

Class I: - The laser with power of less than .5 milli-watt in the visible and invisible range has no therapeutic effects. It is used primarily for the black board pointers and barcoding reading at shopping centers, CD players and laser printers. These lasers typically enclosed and pose no danger to use.

Class II: - The laser with power output up to 1 milli-watt has limited effects.

Class III: - The laser with power output of 1 milli watt to 500 milli-watt has sub classified in to 3A and 3B. These lasers have significant therapeutic effects in the tissues. The food and drug administration (FDA), USA allowed class 3 laser to use in the physiotherapy clinics; however, certification is needed before applying to the patient. The class three laser is a form of electromagnetic energy with a wavelength of 600 to 1000nm, falls within the visible or infrared section of the electromagnetic spectrum. This class of laser has adverse effects on naked eyes, it is, therefore; necessary for the clinician and the patient to put on protective goggles, during application of the laser. HeNe (Helium-Neon) and GaAs (Gallium-Arsenide) with wavelength of 632.8nm and 910nm respectively produce class three (low power) lasers. Class 3a lasers such as HeNe lasers (not exceeding 5miliwatt) energy does not produce injury with momentary viewing. Class 3b lasers (HeNe) lasers above 5miliwatt energy but not exceeding 500miliwatt) may cause injury with direct viewing of the beam or specular reflection; however; do not cause danger to the skin. The low power lasers are also known as cold lasers.

Class IV and V: - The lasers with the power of more than the 500miliwatt are categorized into these classes. These types of lasers posses eye, skin and fire hazards and cannot be operated without the goggles. The common use of class IV and V is in the surgical interventions.

Types

Ruby Laser: - The first working laser was ruby laser made by Theodore H. "Ted" Maiman at Hughes research laboratories on May 16, 1960.[9] A ruby laser is a solid state laser that uses a synthetic ruby crystal as its gain medium. These lasers produce pulses of coherent visible lights of at a wavelength of 694.3nm, which is a deep red color. Typical ruby laser pulse lengths are on the order of a millisecond. Ruby laser most often consists of a synthetic rod that is energized through optical pumping, typically by a xenon flashtube. Electrical stimulation to the flashtube causes the excitation of the ruby molecules that raises the electrons to a higher energy level (stimulated emission). The electrones stay in the higher level for a short time, before falling to the metastable level where they stay for longer time.[10] Population inversion occurs as the electrons increases in the metastable level than the ground level. This whole process occurs in the lasing chamber which contains total reflection and partly reflection mirrors. The semipermeable (partial) mirror allows some of the photons to emit from the chamber into the fiber optic cable in the form of red light of 694.3nm wavelength.

Helium Neon Laser: - Helium-neon laser is produced by a tube containing atoms of helium and neon. The helium gas atoms are elevated or excited from the ground state by application of electrical stimulation called a flesh gun. The excited level of helium atom very closely approximate ground level of the neon atom. When excited helium atom collides with a ground state neon atom, the energy produced is transferred to the neon atom, and the helium returns to the ground state. The concentration of the photons in the excited level increases than the ground level that leads to spontaneous emission. The photons reflect to and fro between mirrors along the tube. The semipermeable mirror allows photons to emit form the tube into the fiber optic cable in the form of red light of 632.8nm wavelength.

Gallium Arsenide Laser: - Gallium Arsenide laser is the first semiconductor laser, used in 1962. This laser has the wavelength of 850nm. This laser housed in a diode. Diode a electrical component allows electrical current to pass in one direction through the device offering high level electrical resistance in the reverse direction. A junction diode is formed by depositing a thin coating of zinc in the device, that allows electric current to flow more readily in the direction from zinc to Gallium Arsenide. The laser reaction occurs in this junction region and energy is delivered in the pulsed mode. The indirect depth of penetration of this type of laser is 5cm.

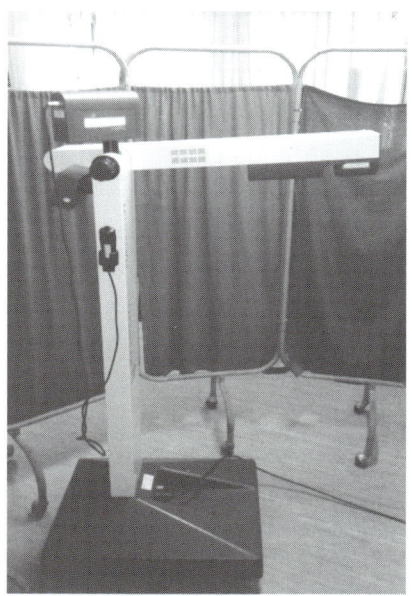

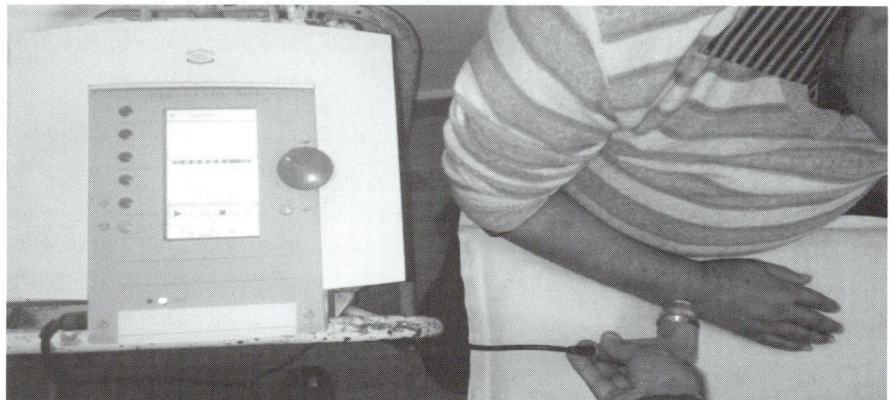

Figure:12.3. A. Scanner Lase, B probe Laser.

Physiological Effects

The investigation in to the biologic and physical effects of cold laser radiation is still in its early stages.[11] The effects of laser on biological tissues are directly related to the wavelength of the beam, the depth to which it penetrates, and the dosage, (the intensity and duration of the treatment).[5] The human skin absorbs as much as 99 percent of the radiation, dark skin absorbs more than light.[12] Some of the physiological effects attributed to the low power laser include acceleration in collagen synthesis, an increase in vascularization of healing, a decrease in microorganism, and reduction in pain. In vitro studies using low level radiation of 633 nm and 904 nm demonstrated cellular ATP synthesis and activation of calcium (C^{++}) at the cell membrane level.

Would Healing: There are several animal studies employing rabbits, mice, rats and guinea pigs, that show low power laser has a stimulating effect on wound healing.[13,14,15,16,17,18] The common findings of all these studies are that the irradiated animals form granulation tissue up to 25 percent more than the non radiated animals with enhanced epithelialization and increased phagocytosis. The irradiation may activate the vessels adjacent to the wound, it may increase the phagocytic capacity of macrophages, accelerating their activity to clear the way for the advancing vessels, or it may loosen the fibrin network of the clot.[19] These findings suggest that the low power laser seems to have a stimulating effect on regenerating epithelium.

Inflammation, edema and Pain: - Following injury many inflammatory agents generate at the site of wound in response to phagocytic processes and other irritants. Among these are highly reactive superoxide radicals. These combine with local arachidonic acids to produce prostaglandin-E. Prostaglandin-E is a fatty acid that causes the breakdown of ATP to cyclic AMP and induces changes in nociceptor membrane potentials.[51] This change increases the sensitivity threshold of the nociceptor and thus lead to an increase in its firing rate[20]. In addition to involved in pain production, prostaglandins also cause increased vasodilatation and further propagate the inflammatory process. A study of Helium-Neon laser effect upon mouse skin was conducted. The mouse skin was injured to investigate the superoxide dismutase activity of irradiated tissues.[21] The study found that successive daily helium-neon exposure resulted in a significant increase in superoxide dismutase activity. Superoxide dismutase exerts protective effects against a variety of inflammatory agents or events by acting as a scavenger of superoxide radicals. Therefore, superoxide dismutase inhibits prostaglandin formation it may not only be effective as an anti-inflammatory agents but also may be involved in the reduction of pain and edema.

Collagen Metabolism

The low power laser irradiation to the fibroblast, produces mitochondrial and rough endoplastic reteticulum hypertrophy with enlarged cisternae. Numerous microfibrils were present, especially close to the Golgi apparatus following exposure to the laser.

Clinical Uses

The use of low levels of visible or near-infrared (NIR) light for reducing pain, inflammation and edema, promoting healing of wounds, deeper tissues and nerves, and preventing tissue damage has been known for almost forty years since the invention of lasers.

In 1967, a few years after the first working laser was invented, Endre Mester in Semmelweis University, Budapest, Hungary wanted to test if laser radiation might cause cancer in mice.[22] He shaved the dorsal hair, divided them into two groups and gave a laser treatment with a low powered ruby laser (694 nm) to one group. They did not get cancer, and to his surprise the hair on the treated group grew back more quickly than the untreated group. This was the first demonstration of "laser biostimulation". Since then, medical treatment with coherent-light sources (lasers) or noncoherent light (light-emitting diodes, LEDs) has passed through its childhood and adolescence.[23] The following common conditions are effectively managed with the low level laser therapy -

i. Chronic open wound.[24]
ii. Non healing fractures
iii. Bursitis – subacromial bursitis, prepatellar bursitis, infrapatellar bursitis,
iv. Tendinitis- supraspinatus tendinitis, infraspinatus tendinitis, subscapular tendinitis, bicipital tendinitis,
v. Ligamentous Sprain- anterior cruciate ligament sprain, medial collateral ligament sprain, lateral collateral ligament sprain, anterior talofibular ligament, coracohumeral ligament, deltoid ligament
vi. Muscle Strain- extensor carpi radialis brevis, gluteus maximus, minimus and golfers elbow.

Precautions

Laser unlike ordinary light emits a beam that is completely focused on a fovea of the eye. Absorption of laser energy by the eye can produce a burn, causing partial or complete loss of vision. For a precautionary measure, the therapist should wear goggles of an appropriate optical density. The practitioner must ask for the goggles to manufacturer while purchasing the laser equipment. The manufacturer or dealer provides the set of goggles for the patient as well as for the clinician. However; single pair of the goggles may not be appropriate for all the wavelengths of laser. The patient should not be allowed to see the laser beam during the treatment session or he or she may be given goggles to wear during the entire session.

Contra-indications

i.   Pregnant women
ii.   Unclosed fontanelles of children
iii. Cancerous lesion, infected tissues. Malignancy.
iv.   Cornea
v.   Endocrine glands
vi.   Hemorrhagic area
vii. Areas of deficit sensation
viii. Epiphyseal plates of children
ix.   Sympathetic ganglion
x.   Vagus nerve
xi.   Mediasternum.

Procedure

Check all the contraindications and take necessary precautions needed before commencing the treatment. Place the patient in a comfortable position. The part which is being treated should be well supported and exposed. Explain the procedure to the patient and also instruct not to see the beam of the laser. most of the laser equipments are designed to have list of conditions with the preset of frequency, time and energy according to the conditions; however manual setting options will also be available if the therapist wants to modify it. The time and frequency required for pain relief is 16-20seconds and 5-20 pulses per second respectively and for wounds 20-30 second and 20-80 pulses per second.[25] There are only three valid irradiation techniques for LLLT in tendinopathies: a) direct irradiation of the tendon, b) irradiation of trigger points and c) irradiation of acupuncture points. Direct the laser beam in case of scanner laser to the treatment area and then activate the laser by pressing the start button. A light will stay on for the duration as selected. In case of probe laser the probe is paced directly over the treatment area and remain constant throughout the session.

Subacromial Impingement Syndrome and supraspinatus tendinitis

Shoulder pain is a common musculoskeletal condition that affects up to 25% of the general population.[26] Pain in the shoulder is one of the major concerned in the clinical practice. The most frequent cause of shoulder pain is subacromial impingement syndrome.[27] The subacromial bursa, tendon of supraspinatus and long head of biceps get impinged between the head of humerus and acromial arch during the overhead activities. The syndrome is associated with the repetitive overhead activities such as tennis, base ball, throwing, cricket bowling and swimming, This painful condition leads to decreases in muscle strength and range of motion (ROM) of the shoulder which adversely affect the patients' quality of life.[28]

The SAIS causes edema, inflammation and can become chronic if adequate treatment is not administered. The conservative treatment approaches such as analgesic and nonsteroidal antiinflammatory drugs, resting, modification of daily activities, physical therapy approaches, range of motion and strengthening exercises, subacromial local anesthetic or corticosteroid injections[29,30,31] can be used to reduce pain, improve joint stiffness, impaired muscle strength and quality of life in patients with SAIS. Recently, low level laser therapy (LLLT) is widely used in various rheumatologic and musculoskeletal disorders which have analgesic, anti-inflammatory and biostimulating effects. The LLLT induces cell proliferation, collagen synthesis, protein synthesis, tissue reparation, wound healing and pain relief through direct irradiation without thermal response.[32,33,34,35,36,37]

Kelle B, and Kozanoglu E conducted a controlled clinical trial to investigate the effectiveness of low-level laser treatment and local corticosteroid injection in patients with subacromial impingement syndrome.[38] They recruited one hundred thirty-five patients with subacromial impingement syndrome into their study. The patients were allocated to three groups: local corticosteroid injection (group I); sham laser treatment (group II); and low-level laser treatment (group III). Low-level laser treatment was performed three times per week for a total of nine sessions. Local corticosteroid injections were administered twice, with an interval of 10 days between each. The patients were assessed at pre-treatment, post-treatment and three and six months after the first visit. They found that the effectiveness of low-level laser treatment was similar to that of local corticosteroid injection in patients with subacromial impingement syndrome, and concluded that both low-level laser treatment and corticosteroid injection were more effective than sham laser treatment.

The Gallium-Aluminum-Arsenide (GaAlAs, infrared laser) diode laser device (Chattanooga group, USA) with a wavelength of 850nm, power output of 100mV, continuous wave and $0.07cm^2$ spot area laser were used for the laser therapy. The laser was applied with a dosage of 5 $joule/cm^2$ (totally 15-20 joule) at maximum 5-6 painful points for 1 minute at each point over subacromial region of the shoulder.[39] Haslerud S, Magnussen LH,and et. al. conducted a systematic review and meta-analysis of randomized controlled trials to see the efficacy of low-level laser therapy for shoulder tendinopathy.[40] This review shows that optimal LLLT can offer clinically relevant pain relief and initiate a more rapid course of improvement, both alone and in combination with physiotherapy interventions.

The low level laser therapy is incorporated with the strengthening exercises of the scapular and parascapular muscle because weakness of these muscles is one of the major causes of subacromial impingement syndrome, especially if the patient is involved in the overhead activities. The house wives with protracted shoulders also develop SIS. Low level laser therapy definitely helps in improving the symptoms of pain, swelling and healing but does not contribute to the strengthening. Therefore, other symptoms such as range of motion (glenohumeral rhythm) would not be improved unless and until the therapist strengthens the rotator cuff muscles and scapula stabilizers (serratus anterior, rhomboid and middle fibers of the trapezius).

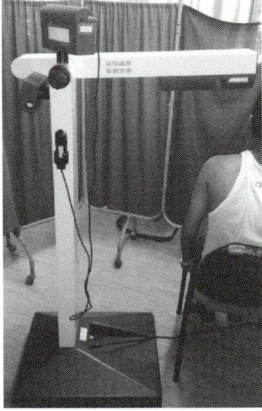

Figure 12.4 application of laser on subacromial space.

Light Amplification by Stimulated Emission of Radiation

Extensor Carpi Radialis Brevis Tendinitis or Tennis Elbow

Lateral elbow tendinopathy (LET) or "tennis elbow" is a common disorder with a prevalence of at least 1.7%[41] and occurring most often between the third and sixth decades of life. Physical strain may play a part in the development of LET, as the dominant arm is significantly more often affected than the non-dominant arm. The condition is largely self-limiting, and symptoms seem to resolve between 6 and 24 months in most patients.[42]

A number of methods such as steroid injections, non-steroidal anti-inflammatory drugs and a regimen of physiotherapy with various modalities, seem to be the most commonly applied treatments. Despite of availability of the several therapeutic methods the patients with tennis elbow do not show long term improvements. Bjordal J, and et al shown in a systematic review of tendinopathy that the effect of low level laser therapy is a dose dependant.[44]

Low level laser therapy has been suggested by many authors as an effective method of treating the patients with tennis elbow. The low level laser therapy has an anti-inflammatory and a biostimulatory effect on collagen production.[45] Both of these effects were dose-dependent and could be induced by all wavelengths between 630 and 1064 nm with slight variations in therapeutic dose-ranges according to the wavelength used. The anti-inflammatory effect was seen in higher therapeutic dose-ranges than the biomodulatory effect on fibroblast cells and collagen fiber

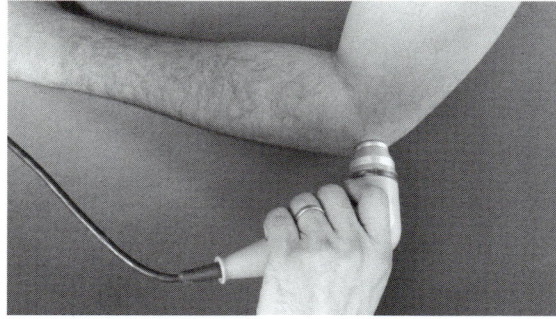

Figure 12.5 Probe laser on lateral epicondyle, the optical head is directed on the treatment area.

Carpel Tunnel Syndrome

A Swedish study found that 3.8% of the population have a clinical diagnosis of CTS, and 4.9% have electrophysiologic evidence. A total of 2.7% of the population were found to have both.[46] CTS of a severity indicating surgery has been found in 0.7% of a general population.[47] The borders of the carpal tunnel are wrist carpal bones on the medial, lateral and dorsal aspect and the transverse carpal ligament on the volar aspect. The median nerve and nine of the finger and thumb flexor tendons pass through this space. CTS is characterized by symptoms of numbness, tingling and paraethesias, which are not always limited to the median nerve distribution. Conservative treatment may include ultrasound, cryotherapy, exercises, bracing, and steroid injections. However, surgical decompression (carpal tunnel release) is often elected.

Laser therapy can highly be effective for carpel tunnel syndrome, when correctly diagnosed. In such a compression neuralgia, low level laser acts by reducing edema and eliminating pain. If treated early, complete remission of symptoms can be achieved with laser alone. Although each case will differ depending on the individual and the stage of the condition, in general treatment every 3 or 4 days would be advised to a total of approximately 10 sessions. The studies have observed beneficial effect from real laser, higher laser dosages (9 Joules, 12-30 Joules or 32 J/cm^2, 225 J/cm^2) were used at the primary treatment sites median nerve at the wrist.

Naeser MA, et al[52] investigated whether real or sham low level laser therapy plus microamperes transcutaneous electric nerve stimulation (TENS) applied to acupuncture points significantly reduces pain in carpal tunnel syndrome (CTS). Red-beam laser (continuous wave, 15mW, 632.8nm) on shallow acupuncture points on the affected hand, infrared laser (pulsed, 9.4W, 904nm) on deeper points on upper extremity and cervical paraspinal areas, and microamps TENS on the affected wrist. Devices were painless, noninvasive, and produced no sensation whether they were real or sham. The hand was treated behind a hanging black curtain without the patient knowing if devices were on (real) or off (sham). Significant decreases in McGill Pain Questionnaire (MPQ) score, median nerve sensory latency, and Phalen and Tinel signs after the real treatment series but not after the sham treatment series. Patients could perform their previous work (computer typist, handyman) and were stable for 1 to 3 years.

Elwakil TF, Elazzazi A, Shokeir H[53] conducted the study to evaluate the effectiveness of low level laser treatment (LLLT) for CTS in comparison to the standard open carpal tunnel release surgery. 60 symptomatic hands complaining of CTS were divided into two equal groups. Group A, was subjected to LLLT by Helium Neon (He-Ne) laser (632.8 nm), whereas group B was treated by the open approach for carpal tunnel release. The patients were evaluated clinically and by nerve conduction studies (NCSs) about 6 months after the treatment. LLLT showed overall significant results but at a lower level in relation to surgery. LLLT showed significant outcomes in all parameters of subjective complaints (p < or = 0.01) except for muscle weakness. Moreover, LLLT showed significant results in all parameters of objective findings (p < or = 0.01) except for thenar atrophy. LLLT has proven to be an effective and noninvasive treatment modality for CTS especially for early and mild-to-moderate cases when pain is the main presenting symptom. However, surgery could be preserved for advanced and chronic cases.

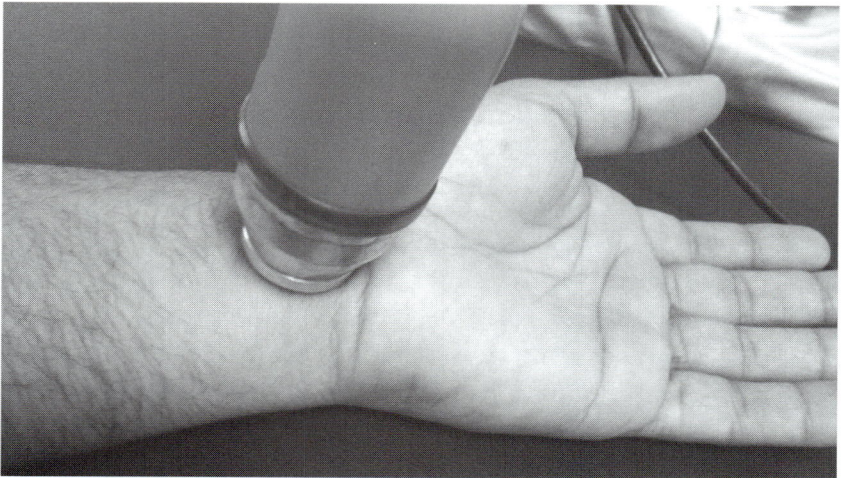

Figure: 12.6a probe laser beam on the carpel tunnel,

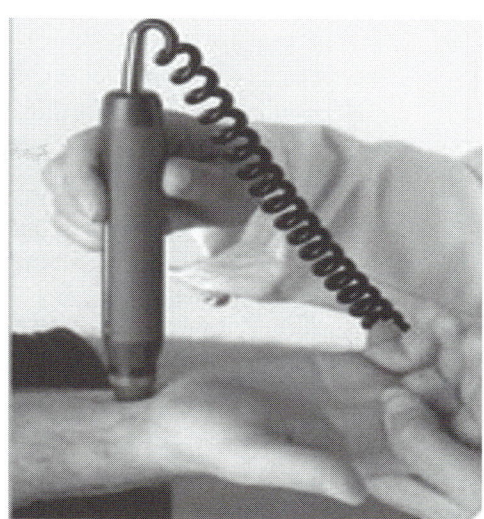

Figure: 12.6b probe laser beam on the carpel tunnel,

References

1. Kleinkort JA and Rolly JA; Laseer Accupuncture: its uses in physical therapy. Am J Accupuncture 12:51,1984

2. Thermal agent in Rehabilitation, Susan L. Michlovitz, 3rd edition, CPR, PP255.

3. Bloom AL: Gas Laser John Wiley and Sons, New York, 1971, pp 1-24.

4. Electrotherapy, Endurance Based Practice, edited by Sheila Kitchen, 11th edition, curchil Livingstone, pp 171.

5. Physical agents, A comprehensive Text book for Physicla Therapist, Bernadette Hecox, Tsega Andemicael Mechreteab, Jooseph Weisberg, Appleton and Lange Norwalk, Connecticut, PP391.

6. Susan L, Michlovitz, Thomas P. Nalan Jr., Modalities for therapeutic intervention, 4th edition, CPR, Jaypee Brotheers, New Delhi, pp145.

7. Electrotherapy, Endurance Based Practice, edited by Sheila Kitchen, 11th edition, curchil Livingstone, pp 172.

8. Susan L Michlovitz, Thermal agents in rehabilitation, 3rd edition, CPR, FA Davis company, Philadelphia, pp. 257-258.

9. Laser Fundamentals by William, Thomas Silfvast-Cambridge University Press 1996 pp 547-549.

10. Basant Kumar Nanda, Electrotherapy Simplified 2nd edition, Jaypee, New Delhi, pp425.

11. Thermal agent in Rehabilitation, Susan L. Michlovitz, 3rd edition, CPR, PP262.

12. Goldman L, Rockwell JR, Laser in Medicine. New York; Gordan & Breach 1971

13. Mester E, Mester AF, Mester A. The biomedical effect of laser application. Laser in surgery and medicine. 1985;5;31-39.

14. Haina D, Brunner R, Landthalet M, et al. Animal experiments on light-induced wound healing. Laser in bio-medical Research 1973;4:1-3.

15. Mester E. Spiry R, Azende B, at al. Effect of laser rays on wound healing. Am J Surg 1971; 122:532-535.

16. Surinchak J. Alago M, Bellamy R, et al. Effects of low level energy laser on the healing of full thickness skin defects. Lasers in Surg Med 1983;2:267-274.

17. Kana J, Hutschenreiter G, Haina D, et al. Effects of low density laser on healing of open skin wounds in rats. Arch Surg 1981; 116: 293-296.

18. Kovscs I, Mester E, Gorog P. laser induced stimulation of the vascularization of the healing would- an ear chamber experiment. Experimentia 1974;30:341-343.

19. Kovscs I, Mester E, Gorog P. laser induced stimulation of the vascularization of the healing would- an ear chamber experiment. Experimentia 1974;30:341-343).

20. Castel MF. A clinical guide to low power laser therapy, Physio Technology Ltd- Medelco, Downsview, 1985).

21. Essman WB. Studies of helium-neon laser effect upon mouse skin and mouse skin injury. Queen Collage of the City University of New York, Flushing, NY, unpublished, 1984.

22. E. Mester, B. Szende and P. Gartner, The effect of laser beams on the growth of hair in mice, Radiobiol Radiother (Berl) 9 (1968) 621-6.].

23. Michael R. Hamblin, Department of Dermatology, Harvard Medical School, BAR 414, Wellman Center for Photomedicine, Massachusetts General Hospital, 40 Blossom Street, Boston MA 02114).

24. Mester E. Effect of laser rays on wound healing. Am J Surg. 1971; 122. Shaw CJ. The effects of low power laser on wound healing: a review of literature. Student paper, New York University Physical Therapy Program, December 1982.

25. Shaw CJ. The effects of low power laser on wound healing: a review of literature. Student paper, New York University Physical Therapy Program, December 1982.

26. Thornton AL, McCarty CW, Burgess MJ. Effectiveness of low-level laser therapy combined with an exercise program to reduce pain and increase function in adults with shoulder pain: a critically appraised topic. J Sport Rehabil. 2013 Feb;22(1):72-8. Epub 2012 Oct 11).

27. Mohtadi NG, Vellet AD, Clark ML, Hollinshead RM, Sasyniuk TM, Fick GH, et al. A prospective, double-blind comparison of magnetic resonance imaging and arthroscopy in the evaluation of patients presenting with shoulder pain. J Shoulder Elbow Surg. 2004;13:258–65. 10.1016/j.jse.2004.01.003[PubMed].

28. MacDermid JC, Ramos J, Drosdowech D, Faber K, Patterson S. The impact of rotator cuff pathology on isometric and isokinetic strength, function, and quality of life. J Shoulder Elbow Surg. 2004;13:593– 8.10.1016/j.jse. 2004.03.009 [PubMed)

29. Kromer TO, Tautenhahn UG, de Bie RA, Staal JB, Bastiaenen CH. Effects of physiotherapy in patients with shoulder impingement syndrome: a systematic review of the literature. J Rehabil Med. 2009;41:870–80.10.2340/16501977-0453 [PubMed].

30. Celik D, Atalar AC, Güçlü A, Demirhan M. The contribution of subacromial injection to the conservative treatment of impingement syndrome. Acta Orthop Traumatol Turc. 2009;43:331–5.10.3944/ AOTT. 2009.331 [PubMed]

31. Camargo PR, Haik MN, Ludewig PM, Filho RB, Mattiello-Rosa SM, Salvini TF. Effects of strengthening and stretching exercises applied during working hours on pain and physical impairment in workers with subacromial impingement syndrome. Physiother Theory Pract. 2009;25:463–75. [PubMed

32. Michener LA, Walsworth MK, Burnet EN. Effectiveness of rehabilitation for patients with subacromial impingement syndrome: a systematic review. J Hand Ther. 2004;17:152–64. 10.1197/j.jht.2004.02.004[PubMed].

33. Enwemeka CS, Parker JC, Dowdy DS, Harkness EE, Sanford LE, Woodruff LD. The efficacy of low-power lasers in tissue repair and pain control: a meta-analysis study. Photomed Laser Surg. 2004;22:323 9.10.1089/pho. 2004.22. 323 [PubMed].

34. Kulekcioglu S, Sivrioglu K, Ozcan O, Parlak M. Effectiveness of low-level laser therapy in temporomandibular disorder. Scand J Rheumatol. 2003;32:114–8. [PubMed].

35. Khadra M. The effect of low level laser irradiation onimplant-tissue interaction. In vivo and in vitro studies. Swed Dent J Suppl. 2005;172:1–63. [PubMed].

36. Woodruff LD, Bounkeo JM, Brannon WM, Dawes KS, Barham CD, Waddell DL, et al. The efficacy of laser therapy in wound repair: a meta-analysis of the literature. Photomed Laser Surg. 2004;22:241–7.10.1089/ 1549541041438623 [PubMed].

37. Ezzati A, Bayat M, Taheri S, Mohsenifar Z. Low-level laser therapy with pulsed infrared laser accelerates third-degree burn healing process in rats. J Rehabil Res Dev. 2009;46:543–54.10.1682/JRRD.2008.09.0121 [PubMed].

38. Kelle B, and Kozanoglu E Low-level laser and local corticosteroid injection in the treatment of subacromial impingement syndrome:Clin Rehabil. 2014 Feb 11;28(8):762-771. [Epub ahead of print

39. Sebnem Koldas Dogan, Saime AY, and Deniz Evcik conducted a randomized placebo controlled double-blind prospective study to know the effectiveness of low laser therapy in subacromial impingement syndrome).

40. Haslerud S, Magnussen LH, Joensen J, Lopes-Martins RA, Bjordal JM. The efficacy of low-level laser therapy for shoulder tendinopathy: a systematic review and meta-analysis of randomized controlled trials.Physiother Res Int. 2015 Jun;20(2):108-25. doi: 10.1002/pri.1606. Epub 2014 Dec

41. Shiri R, Viikari-Juntura E, Varonen H, Heliovaara M. Prevalence and determinants of lateral and medial epicondylitis: a population study. Am J Epidemiol. 2006;164: 1065–74. doi: 10.1093/aje /kwj325. [PubMed] [Cross Ref],

42. Smidt N, Lewis M, DA VDW, Hay EM, Bouter LM, Croft P. Lateral epicondylitis in general practice: course and prognostic indicators of outcome. J Rheumatol. 2006;33:2053–59. [PubMed].

43. Peterson M, Elmfeldt D, Svardsudd K. Treatment practice in chronic epicondylitis: a survey among general practitioners and physiotherapists in Uppsala County, Sweden. Scand J Prim Health Care.2005;23:239–41. doi: 10.1080/02813430510031333. [PubMed] [Cross Ref].

44. Bjordal J, Couppé C, Ljunggreen A. Low level laser therapy for tendinopathy. Evidence of a dose-response pattern. Physical Therapy Reviews. 2001;6:91–99).

45. Lopes-Martins R, Penna SC, Joensen J, Iversen VV, Bjordal JM. Low level laser therapy (LLLT) in Inflammatory and Rheumatic Diseases: A review of Therapeutic Mechanisms. Current Rheumatology Reviews. 2007;3:147–54. doi: 10.2174/157339707780619421. [Cross Ref].

46. Atroshi I, Gummesson C, Johnsson R, Ornstein E, Ranstam J, Rosen I. Prevalence of carpal tunnel syndrome in a general population. JAMA. 1999;282:153–158. [PubMed].

47. Atroshi I, Gummesson C, Johnsson R, McCabe SJ, Ornstein E. Severe carpal tunnel syndrome potentially needing surgical treatment in a general population. J. Hand Surg. Am. 2003;28:639–644. [PubMed].

48. Aubry JR. Clinical low power laser therapy, Montreal Nov. 1985.

49. Castel MF, A clinical guide to low laser therapy. Physio technology Ltd. – Medilco, Downsview, 1985.

50. Mester E, Mester AF, Mester A. the biomedical effects of laser application, Lasers in Surgery and Medicine. 1985; 5:31-39.

51. Haymo Thiel, DC, Low Power Laser Therapy- and Introduction and a review of some biological effects. The Journal of the CCA/ Volume 30 no.3, September 1986.

52. Naeser MA, Hahn KA, Lieberman BE, Branco KF, carpal tunnel syndrome pain trated with low level laser and microamperes transcutaneous electric nerve stimulatin: a controlled study,Arch Phys Med Rehabil 2002 (Jul); 83 (7): 978-988.

53. Elwakil TF[1], Elazzazi A, Shokeir H: Treatment of carpal tunnel syndrome by low-level laser versus open carpal tunnel release. Lasers Med Sci. 2007 Nov;22(4):265-70. Epub 2007 Mar 3.

Chapter 13

Pneumatic Intermittent Compression Therapy

The concept of compression in relieving swelling and symptoms has been using by the physiotherapist for many years. Traumatic injury to the extremities in sports practice may cause insult of the blood vessels and muscle fibers that increases bleeding and swelling. In order to prevent and improve bleeding and swelling in the local area, the local area is compressed with the elastic crepe bandage combined with elevation and ice.

Intermittent compression units are the mechanical pressures to encourage venous and lymphatica return from the extremities. The application of pressure intermittently through mechanical device into the tissues to improve edema has become usual practice in the rehabilitation field. Intermittent pneumatic compression, that results an increase and decrease pressure on the vessels, is similar to the cryotherapy which produces vasoconstriction and vasodilatation, however, IPC does not change the temperature of the tissues significantly, but hunts the vessels. The increase and decrease pressure on the vessels not only helps in mobilizing the fluid but also helps in improving many other conditions such as peripheral vascular ailments, including traumatic edema (sub acute and chronic), venous insufficiency, arterial insufficiency, lymphedema, leg ulcers, amputed limbs, and would healing.

The intermittent compression applies to the extremities may either be circumferential or sequential. Circumferential is the application of an equal amount of pressure to all the parts of the extremity simultaneously, whereas, the sequential involves the application of pressure from the distal parts to the proximal. The distal chamber or most distal chamber inflates, followed by the next, and so on, until pressure is applied to the length of the appliance. The increase in pressure first in distal chamber and progressively to the proximal part forces the edematous fluid back into the heart and reduces swelling.

Mechanism of Edema Formation

An excessive collection of the fluid in the local or generalized area is termed as edema which results from increased permeability of the capillary walls, increased capillary pressure due to venous obstruction or lymphatic obstruction or renal impairment. The aberrant change in the hydrostatic and oncotic pressure acting across the capillary walls can cause extracellular matrix or interstitial edema. Hydrostatic edema refers to accumulation of excessive interstitial fluid in the tissues which results from elevated capillary hydrostatic pressure. Permeability edema refers to accumulation of an excessive fluid in the interstitial space as a result from disruption of the physical structure of the pores in the microvascular membrane such that the barrier is less able to restrict the movement of macromolecules from the blood to the interstitial space. Lymphedema represents a third form and may result from impaired lymph pump activity, an increase in lymphatic permeability favoring protein flux from lumen to interstitial fluid, lymphatic obstruction (e.g. microfiliarisis), or surgical removal of lymph nodes as occurs in the treatment of breast cancer.

The expansion of the excessive fluid is prevented by the certain anatomical structures such as kidneys are enveloped by a tough fibrous capsule, the brain is surrounded by the cranial vault, skeletal muscles are in the volar and anterior tibial compartments are encased in tight fascial sheath. As a consequence of the inability of these tissues to readily expand their interstitial volume, relatively small increments in transcapillary fluid filtration induce large increase in interstitial fluid pressure. This in turn, reduces the vascular transmural pressure gradient and physically compresses capillaries, thereby reducing nutritive tissue perfusion.[1]

Mechanism of fluid exchange

There is a difference between the hydrostatic pressure (within the capillaries generated by systolic force of the heart) and interstitial pressure (in the tissues). The hydrostatic pressure at the arteriole end of a capillary is 25mmHg and at the venule end of the capillary is 10mmHg. Whereas; the interstitial pressure is normally negative, averaging approximately -5.3 mm Hg. The negative interstitial pressure acts as suction. This difference in pressure between

Pneumatic Intermittent Compression Therapy

hydrostatic and interstitial forces the fluid out of the capillary into the interstitial space (into the tissue).

The fluid potential is created due to the inability of large molecules of plasma proteins mostly serum albumin to pass through the walls of capillaries. The accumulation of these proteins within the capillaries membrane induces osmosis. This creates osmotic pressure of approximately 19 mm Hg, also known as Osmotic Pressure (OP) or colloid osmotic pressure (COP) which helps in drawing the fluid into the capillaries from the interstitial space. The plasma colloid osmotic pressure is augmented approximately 50% by the so called "Donnan effect," which explains that the negative protein molecules attract the large number of positive ions, mainly sodium ions. Therefore, accumulation of large plasma protein in the capillary membrane attracts the sodium ions which increase the total PCOP by 9 mm Hg, making the total PCOP 28 mm Hg, which tends to force fluid into the capillaries.

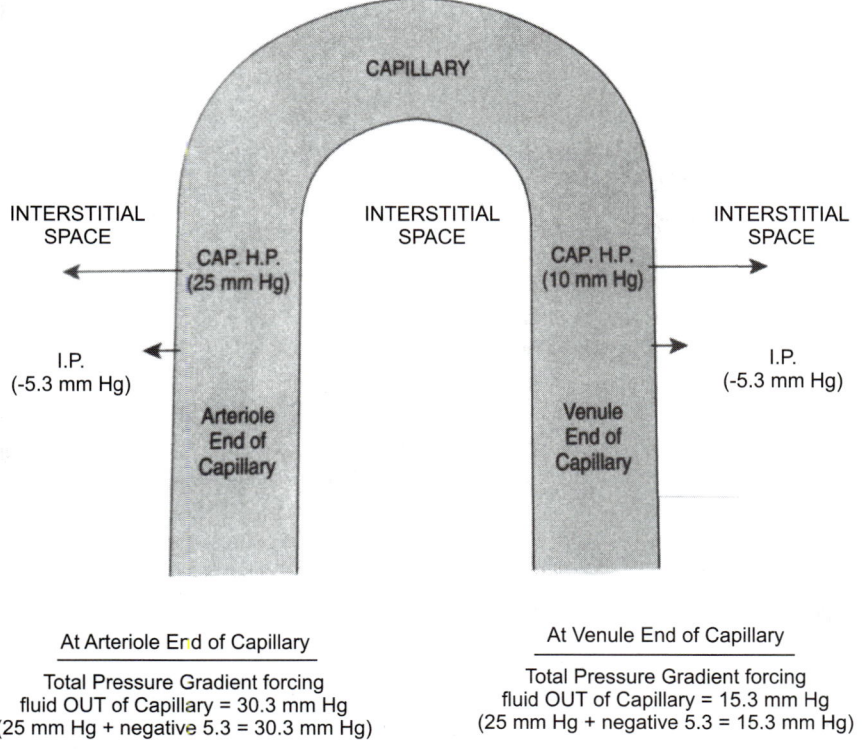

Figure 13. 1 hydrostatic pressure, interstitial pressure and osmotic pressure.

Intermittent Pneumatic Compression Mechanism

The application of intermittent air pressure through the inflatable sleeve into the tissues of extremities increases pressures in the interstitial spaces. When the pressure in the interstitial spaces reaches higher than the lymph and blood vessels, resulting pressure gradient encourages the fluid to draw into the venous and lymphatic vessels. The intermittent compression which involves increase and decrease of the interstitial pressure either circumferentially or sequentially forces the fluid into the venous system, that eventually is absorbed by the lymphatic ducts. The lymphatic uptake and return is assisted by spreading the edema over a large area usually proximal, allowing more lymphatic ducts to absorb the solid matte.[2]

Equipment

The intermittent pneumatic compression unit consists a control box, pump, the hoses, and the compression sleeves. The control unit controls the on and off time as well as pressure on the sleeves. The hose connects the control unit with the air chambers or sleeves. The number of hoses depends on the chamber pumps. The single chamber requires only single hose. The multi – chamber pumps require multiple hoses, usually three which may be color coded to ensure proper sequencing of the inflation. The multi chamber pumps inflate the distal chamber of the sleeve and then sequentially to the proximal. This sequential inflation of the chambers from distal to the proximal enhances the return of the fluid proximal into the heart.

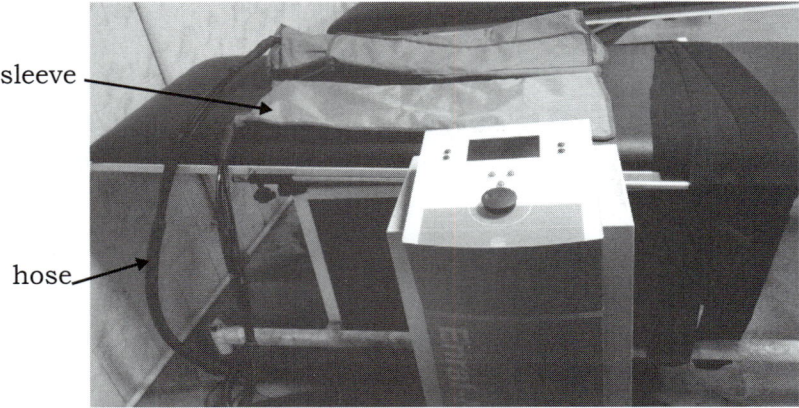

Fig 13.2a Pneumatic Compression therapy with sleeves for upper and lower extremity

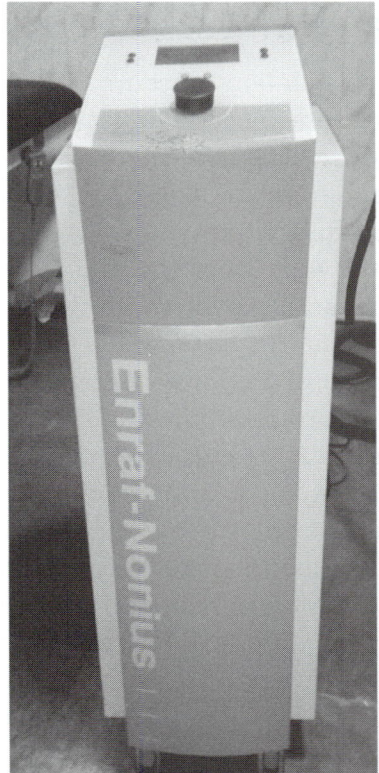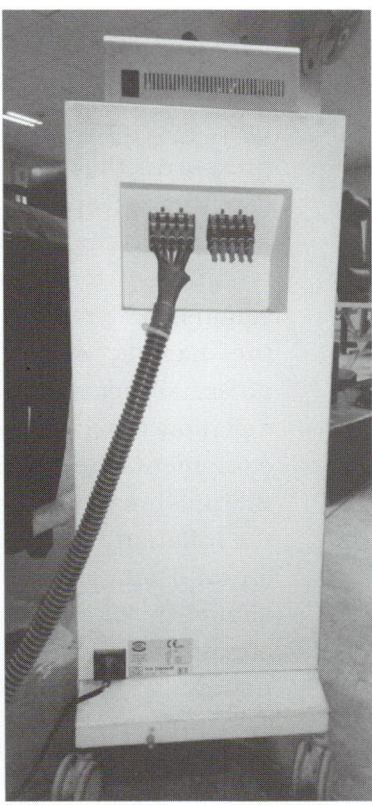

Fig 13.2bPneumatic Compression Therapy front and back

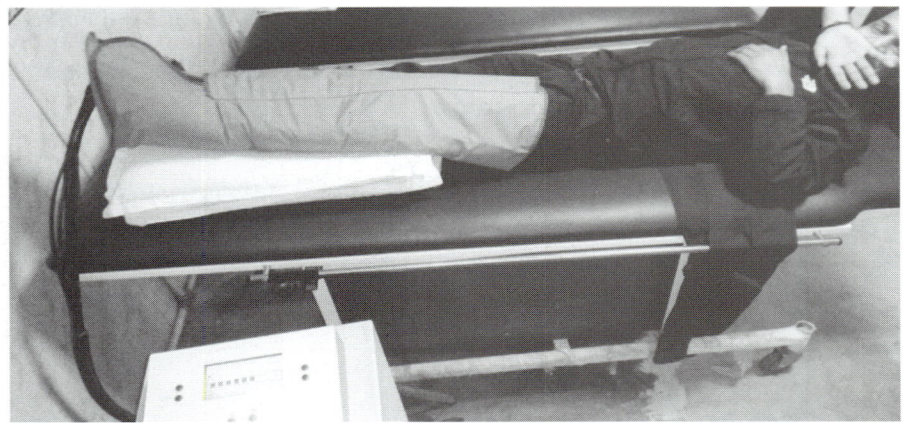

Figure 13.2c Application of intermittent pneumatic compression
therapy unit for lower extremity.

Parameters

The parameters such as inflation pressure, inflation and deflation time, and total treatment time need to be set carefully. The inflation pressure is the pressure created in the interstitial spaces. The arterial capillary pressure is usually about 30 mm Hg. The inflation pressure higher than the arterial capillary pressure between 30 and 35 mm Hg is sufficient to drain the fluid from the interstitial space into the venous and lymphatic vessels. Anyhow; the inflation pressure above the diastolic minus 10mm Hg is not recommended as this can potentially cause collapse of the blood vessels. The inflation and deflation time are set according to the conditions. Now a days the equipments are supplied with the preset on and off time; however, the therapist may manually set the on and off time as required. Usually the inflation time should be three to four times of the deflation time, for an example if the inflation time is 80 seconds the deflation time should be 25 seconds. The total treatment time also depend on the conditions and it may vary from 45 minutes to the four hours; however it is usually kept between 45 minutes and one hour.

Doses

Treatment guidelines recommended by the Jobst Institute as mention on the table. The therapist can change the parameters as required for the conditions. The initial treatment should be intensive and is reduces as patient shows improvement in the sign and symptoms

Table 1: Jobst dosimetery of intermittent pneumatic compression therapy

Indications	Pressure mm Hg	Total treatment time	Inflation time	Deflation tiem
Postmastectomy Lymphedema	30-50 mm Hg	2 treatment periods a day for 3 hours	80-100 seconds	25-35 seconds
Edema of lower extremities	30-60 mm Hg	2 treatment periods a day for 3 hours	80-100 seconds	25-35 seconds
Peripheral edema and venous stasis ulceration	85 mm Hg	1 treatment period for 2 ½ hours 3 times a week	80-100 seconds	30 seconds
Stump reduction	30-60 mm Hg	Three treatment periods a day for 4 hours	40-60 seconds	10-15 seconds
Hand edema	30-50 mm Hg	2 treatment periods a day of 30 minute to 1 hour each	Flexion position 5-10 minutes	Flexion position 5-10 minutes

Indications

I. Sub-acute and chronic traumatic edema
ii. Shoulder hand syndrome and hand edema
iii. Amputed limbs
iv. Lymphedema
v. Stasis ulcer
vi. Arterial insufficiency
vii. Renal insufficiency
viii. Prevention of thrombophlebitis
ix. Wound healing

Contraindications

I. Acute traumatic injury
ii. Acute pulmonary edema
iii. Acute deep venous thrombosis
iv. Immediately after fracture
v. Congestive heart failure
vi. Acute dermatological infections

Procedure

I. The patient is placed in a comfortable position

ii. The blood pressure is measured to be in the safe side. High BP patients are not put on the IPC unit.

iii. Explain the procedure to the patient, especially time of treatment as it requires patient to be in the same position for one hour. He or she should be asked to empty the bladder.

iv. Expose the extremity which is being treated. Remove jewelry. Inspect the area, any wound or open cut should be covered with sterile gauze.

v. Place the stockinette on the part being treated and smooth out all wrinkles, when an amputed limb is treated, the stockinette is often placed over the elastic bandage used to shape the stump.

vi. Place the extremity into the sleeve, secure it with the zip.

Pneumatic Intermittent Compression Therapy

vii. Elevate the extremity above the heart level to facilitate in draining the fluid into the proximal. Two and three or more pillows may be placed under the ankle and thigh respectively. Avoid placing pillows under the calf muscles as it may obstruct the fluid return; however, patients comfortable should be the priority.

viii. The sleeve is connected with the control unit via hose (s).

ix. Set the inflation pressure, inflation and deflation (on and off) time, and total treatment time.

x. The intermittent compression applies to the extremities may either be circumferential or sequential. Circumferential is the application of an equal amount of pressure to all the parts of the extremity simultaneously, whereas, the sequential involves the application of pressure from the distal parts to the proximal. The distal chamber or most distal chamber inflates first, followed by the next, and so on, until pressure is applied to the length of the appliance.

xi. Turn the power on.

xii. Observe any discomfort or tingling or overpressure. Instruct the patient to alarm any uncomfortable to the therapist.

xiii. At the end of treatment, turn the sleeve off when it is fully deflated.

xiv. Turn the power off and remove all the garments and stockinette.

xv. Inspect the skin for discoloration and ulceration.

xvi. Active and resistive exercises are performed in elevated position to further drain the fluid. Compression garments are applied after the exercises if required.

Intermittent pneumatic compression therapy in venous and lymphatic edema

Conventional compression stockings and bandages impede leg swelling but are less efficient in supporting the deficient veno-lymphatic pump when patients are unable to move. In this situation, actively compressing the limb using intermittent pneumatic therapy is a very meaningful and effective treatment option. intermittent pneumatic therapy is a very effective although underused treatment modality, especially in immobile, wheelchair-bound patients. By inflation and deflation of the air-filled garments, intermittent pneumatic therapy produces cycles of pressure waves on the leg, thus mimicking the working and resting pressures applied by compression bandages. Intermittent pneumatic therapy not only reduces leg swelling but also augments the veno-lymphatic pump, which is essential for the restoration of the damaged microcirculation of the skin.[3] The IPC treatment influenced both the amount of edema and the density of tissue compartments.[4] Post-traumatic oedema after 6-12 weeks immobilization in a cast was treated using intermittent pneumatic compression. The study group comprised 18 patients with 19 distal fractures of the lower leg. They were given compression treatment on five consecutive days for about 1 hour daily. Reduction in oedema was assessed by measuring leg circumferences at three levels: the malleolus; 20 cm proximally from the malleolus; and the Chopart joint. The untreated control group consisted of five patients. Changes in oedema were followed daily for one week. A significantly greater reduction in oedema occurred in the study group at all three measurement levels as compared with the control group.[5]

Grieveson found that the highest mean reduction in limb volumes was recorded for a pressure of 40 mmHg, 10 second deflation time and 15 second inflation time. Other significant results were obtained by the 30 mmHg pressure, 35 second deflation time, and 5 and 45 second inflation times (respectively). For many setting combinations no significant differences were observed between the limb oedema seen in the control and experimental groups. In addition adverse effects were observed in six out of nine subjects at 70 mmHg pressure and this pressure was discontinued. One subject suffered cramp at 60 mmHg pressure. Lower pressures together with shorter inflation and deflation times appear to be more efficient than higher pressures and long inflation/deflation times. In addition the lack of significant reduction in oedema at pressures above 40 mmHg suggests that the higher pressures cause a tourniquet effect.[6]

Tonometry studies showed that elasticity of lower limbs tissue is lower in the calf with more hard skin than in the thigh, and that most efforts for improvement using intermittent compression therapy should be directed at the regions above the ankle, the site of common dermatitis, ulcers, and lymphorrhea. Indeed, the pre-and post intermittent compression therapy recordings showed most decrease of stiffness (or increase in elasticity) in the calf in 100% of patients, including the 3-year follow-up patients. Thus, tonometry provided objective evidence of the effectiveness of long-term IPC.[7]

References

1. Abtahian F et al. Regulation of blood and lymphatic vascular separation by signaling proteins SLP-76 and syk. Science 299:247-251,2003.

2. Chad Starkey, Therapeutic Modalities, third edition, FA Davis Company, Philadelphia, pp280.

3. Partsch H, Intermittent pneumatic compression in immobile patients. Int Wound J. 2008 Jun;5(3):389-97.

4. Airaksinen O, Partanen K , Kolari PJ , Soimakallio S, Intermittent pneumatic compression therapy in posttraumatic lower limb edema: computed tomography and clinical measurements.Archives of Physical Medicine and Rehabilitation [1991, 72(9):667-670].

5. Airaksinen O, Kolari PJ, Herve R, Holopainen R. Treatment of post-traumatic oedema in lower legs using intermittent pneumatic compression. Scand J Rehabil Med. 1988;20(1):25-8

6. Grieveson S Intermittent pneumatic compression pump settings for the optimum reduction of oedema. J Tissue Viability. 2003 Jul;13(3):98-100, 102, 104 passim.

7. Marzanna Zaleska, Waldemar L. Olszewski, and Marek Durlik. The Effectiveness of Intermittent Pneumatic Compression in Long-Term Therapy of Lymphedema of Lower Limbs. Lymphat Res Biol. 2014 Jun 1; 12(2): 103–109.

Chapter 14

Traction

Traction is an application of mechanical or manual force that separates the vertebrae and increases the inter-vertebral and facet joint space in the physiological range for the therapeutic purposes. The increased inter-vertebral space reduces pressure on the inter-vertebral discs, increases inter-vertebral foramen space, and elongates the ligaments and other soft tissue structures. The use of gravity as the traction force has been refined and techniques for spinal traction such as positional traction, inversion traction, Goodly polyaxial traction, Goodly-Shement lumbar lift, the Cotterell 90/90 Backtrac, and autotraction have been developed.[1]

Traction is an ancient therapeutic tool that was described at the time of Hippocrates. Cyriax in 1950 popularized the use of traction for treatment of lumbar disc lesions, causing sciatica.[2] The traction is used to distract the articular surfaces for reduction of the dislocated joints and fractured segments for reduction of the fractures. Cyriax advocated traction forces of at least half the weight of the body when applying to the lumbar spine.[3] He believed that the static traction would effectively reduce bulging or herniated intervertebral discs.

Several forms of traction such as continuous, sustained and intermittent are being used in the physiotherapy practice and the studies claim their effectiveness in patients with radiculopathy, facet hypomobility, disc degeneration and soft tissue shortening (ligaments and capsule). The studies found that the sustained prolong stretching with low weight are more effective than the short period with heavy weight. Contrary to that the intermittent mechanical traction is found more effective than the continuous traction.[4] Several studies have used diagnostic imaging to document changes in disc herniation. Mathews administered epidural injection of contrast medium to 611 patents of sciatica and limited SLR. Radiographic findings included reduction of disc prolapsed, vertebral separation, and flow of contrast material into the disc spaces.[5] Despite of substantial evidence to support mechanical effects the clinicians have different opinions on the lumbar pelvic traction. Cheatle and Esterhai surveyed 534 orthopedic surgeons and physiotherapist to evaluate their decision making process in considering use of lumbar pelvic traction, of 213 completed questionnaires, 28% responded they would prescribe traction for radicular low back pain, 54% indicated that their rationale for using traction was to ensure bed rest, whereas, 17% reported that the purpose of traction was to decrease nerve root or disc pressure.[6] Despite of the controversies, basically because of variability of in current practice, it is concluded that the traction is one of the oldest physical therapy modalities which has mechanical effects in the tissues that helps in removing the pressure on the nerve roots by increasing the intervertebral joint space.

Principles

The application of mechanical or manual force to distract the vertebral joint must be sufficient to overcome the sum of resistance of the weight of the body parts, the tension of the surrounding soft tissues, the force of the friction between the patient and table, and the force of gravity.

Position of Patient – Traction can either be given in the sitting or in lying position. The lying position is preferred over the sitting because in this position there is greater separation or opening of the intervertebral space and posterior pillars like facet joints, patient feels more comfortable because of relaxation of the muscles, decrease muscle guarding, and less force is required to overcome the soft tissues. In addition to that the traction may also be given in different lying positions such as supine, prone, side lying & crook lying.

Surrounding soft tissue tension - The manual or mechanical force usually applied in the longitudinal direction which is parallel to the spine and resisted by the muscles. Minimal soft tissue stretching or no distraction would occur if there is muscle contraction during the traction. However, significant stretching of ligament, facet joint capsule can be achieved secondary to creep. This leads to distraction of the vertebral bodies, and increase in the intervertebral joint space. A drop in pressure in the intervertebral space may be sufficient to draw any bulging or herniated disc material back toward the center of the space.[7]

Friction Force - Friction is a resistive force which opposes the traction force and lies parallel to the articular surfaces. The traction tables are split to allow the movement of the table surface with the particular lumbar segment which reduces the friction force. The friction force in the lying position is negligible for the cervical spine. The force of friction is dependent on the magnitude of the force compressing the two objects together, the greater the weight of the body part being pulled, the higher the friction force.

Angle of Pull – The angle of pull refers to the angle of the rope or bar attaching the halter or device or belt to the traction machine with the proper position of the head or lumbar spine. The angle of pull (the long axis of the vertebral column) must be appropriate for the pathology being treated.

Gravitational force – The force of the gravity acts on the vertebral bodies against the traction pull if the position of the patient is anti gravity. The force of gravity against the traction is higher in the sitting position, whereas, it is negligible in the supine position.

Types

There are several types of the traction used to distract the joint surfaces of the spine and peripheral joints. The most commonly tractions used in the physiotherapy practice are-

Continuous Traction – The traction is advised continuously with constant force and small amount of weight for several hours usually for 10-14 hours. The traction may be applied in the hospital or at home. The aim of the continuous traction is to stretch the soft tissue structures, increase the intervertebral foramen and to reduce pressure on the spinal nerve roots. This type of traction is rarely used now days.

Sustained Traction – The sustained traction is also known as static traction which is similar to the continuous traction in which force is applied continuously but not more than 45 minutes.[1] Cyriax believed that the static traction would effectively reduce bulging or herniated intervertebral discs.[8] The more weight is applied with short period of time than the continuous traction. The aim of the static traction is to stretch the soft tissue structures, increase the intervertebral joint space and remove pressure from the disc on the nerve roots.

Intermittent Traction – There is a brief cyclical interval between the traction forces. It means the traction force increases and decreases intermittently. The period between the two successive forces is known as rest period or hold time which can be increased or decreased according to the condition and symptoms of the patient. The ratio of hold and rest period is usually set at 1:1 or 2:1, although the most effective ratio has not been determined.[8] The intermittent traction is usually applied for ten to thirty minutes, and this traction is also known as mechanical traction as the intermittent force is delivered by the machine, however, intermittent traction can also be delivered manually but the release force, and hold time cannot be as accurate as the force applied by the machine. Moreover the intermittent traction applied manually cannot be for longer than ten minutes due to fatigue.

Mechanical Effects

Cyriax described three beneficial effects of traction i) distraction to increase the intervertebral space, ii) tensing of the posterior longitudinal ligament to exert centripetal force at the back of the joint, and iii) suction to draw the protrusion toward the center to the joint.[9] The mechanical effects such as separation of the intervertebral bodies, distraction and gliding of facet joints, widening of the intervertebral foramen, elongation of ligaments and muscles, and straightening of the spinal curves can be achieved with either of traction. The stimulation of proprioceptors and mechanoreceptors are also the major physiological changes occur during the traction.

Methods

There are many methods of traction used to treat patients with cervical and lumbar mechanical pain. These methods of traction can be advised to use at home or in the clinics under the supervision of the physiotherapist. The following methods of traction are described as under –

Bed Traction – The bed traction is an old method of traction recommended to the patients for the longer period of time usually for a day to several days at home with the prescription of physiotherapist or other clinicians. The traction is applied to the patient in a bed by means of attached bars, pulleys, and weights. There is a traction kit comprises of lumbar belt or cervical holder, bars, pulleys, and weights available with the chemist shop may be purchased by the patient for the home traction. This method is rarely used now a days.

Mechanical traction - The mechanical traction is often used as a part of a comprehensive treatment in out patient rehabilitation department. Mechanical traction for the lumbar or cervical spine can either be intermittent or continuous which involves a tractive force applied to the spine via a mechanical system. The mechanical traction is usually applied for the time period of 10 to 30 minutes.

Manual Traction – Manual traction is one of the most effective traction techniques applied with the help of physiotherapist hands. The traction has similar physiological effects of mechanical traction. The advantage is that the manual traction allows the physiotherapist to feel the patients reaction to the application of force to the spine. The disadvantage is that it can only be applied for short period of time seconds to minutes usually 15 to 60 seconds due to fatigue of the muscles. However the traction period can be increased with brief period of rest. The belt can also be used to apply traction force so that less efforts are made with the hands. This can help in applying manual traction for longer period of time with greater force.

Positional Traction – the patient with spinal pain is placed in a position that elongates the short structures, and alleviates the pressure on entrapped spinal nerves by increasing the intervertebral space. The method is mostly used for the lumbar radiculopathy or localized pain. The patient lies on the non painful side with the painful uppermost. An appropriate size of towel roll is placed under the non painful side which causes distraction force on the uppermost painful side. The distraction force opens the facet joints, increases intervertebral disc and foraminal space. The method relieves the pressure on the entrapped nerves.

Gravity Assisted Traction – The gravity is used as a traction force. It is usually recommended for the lumbar spine. The patient lies in a chest harness on a table that can be tilted to a vertical position; the lower half of the body hangs free to provide a distraction force to the spine.

Inversion Traction – The inversion technique is not used now days in the physiotherapy clinics as it may cause temporary rise in blood pressure and ophthalmic artery pressure in young healthy subjects warning additional precautions for using this method. The patient is suspended by the ankles, or thigh and the head down position, allowing the weight of the upper body to act as a traction force. It is applied for 5-15 minutes.

Autotraction – The method utilizes a specially designed table that is divided into two sections that can be individually tilted and rotated. The patient provides the traction force by pulling with the arms and or pushing with the feet.

Indications

Traditionally, lumbar traction has been advocated for the treatment of back and nerve root pain due to herniated nucleus pulposus, degenerative disc disease, and foraminal stenosis.[4] Traction may be used for the joint hypomobility, contracted connective tissues, adhesions, apophyseal joint impingement, and muscle spasm.[10] The studies have shown the effectiveness of the traction in the treatment of radiculopathy following herniated disc, narrowing of the intervertebral foramen, and degenerative disc prolapse.[11-14]

Contraindications and Precautions

Traction is contraindicated to the

I. patients with systemic and local disease affecting the static and dynamic stabilizers of the joints such as infection/tumor like tuberculosis, vertebral basillary insufficiency, osteoporosis, and rheumatoid arthritis (involvement of atlanto axial joint),

ii. Hypermobility or instability of the joint

iii. Cardiac disorders, vascular disease and aortic aneurysm.

iv. Pregnant women (lumbar traction), hiatus hernia, cardiac and pulmonary disease as the harness may increase the pressure in these areas that may cause adverse effects.

v. Vertebral dislocation, vertebra subluxation,

vi. Patients with temporomandibular joint dysfunction (cervical traction) as the halter can put excessive pressure

Following precautions should be taken for safe and comfortable treatment -

I. Acute sprain and strain

ii. Claustrophobia

iii. Mental disorientation

iv. Children and frail elderly patients

v. Spinal surgical intervention

vi. Obesity

vii. Cardiopulmonary problems such as hypertension and difficulty in breathing.

Application

The application of the traction to the cervical, lumbar or any other joint depends on the nature of the condition which is being treated. The parameters of the traction such as time, tension, and angle of pull depend on the level of the spine where the traction force is applied.

A. Cervical Spine

a. Position of Patient – The position of patient may either be supine or sitting with appropriate back support and pillows under the neck. The sitting position is used rarely now days in the physiotherapy practice.

b. Tension or Weight – In supine position the vertebral separation begins when tension equals to the seven percent of the patient body weight[15] The amount of force to be applied depends on the sign and symptoms, goals of the intervention, and the position of the patient during the traction.[16] It is good to start with the low magnitude of force, usually 10 – 15 pounds, for the first treatment session. At least 20 to 30 pounds of force are required to overcome the resistance of the head and soft tissue structures and to produce elongation of the spine in the cervical region.[12] The upper cervical requires less magnitude of force usually between 10 to 15 pounds for the significant distraction than the lower spine.

c. Angle of Pull – The angle of pull is the angle between the rope attaching to the machine and the halter to the head and neck. It is adjusted according to the condition and level of the lesion. The cervical traction may be given in neutral, flexion, and in extension position of the neck. The best position is the comfortable that relieves the symptoms. If the recommended position aggravates the symptoms, it should immediately be changed. Angle of pull for the cervical traction irrespective of its type is usually kept between the 10 degrees to 35 degrees of flexion. However lower angle of pull are also recommended by the clinicians. Susan L. and et al[8] have recommended the following angle of pull for the cervical spine.

Upper cervical spine (C1-C2)	0^0- 05^0
Mid Cervical spine(C-C5)	10^0-20^0
Lower cervical spine (C5-C7)	25^0-35^0

d. Procedure – The patient lies supine with hip and knees flexed. A proper head halter is used that position the head slightly in flexion, enabling the traction pull to be exerted from the occiput, not from the chin. Such halters concentrate the traction force posteriorly, where it is most beneficial. A triangle wedge is used to support the neck and to keep the neck flexed, however, if flexion angle of pull is not required the edge is removed and a small towel roll is placed under the neck. The angle of pull is increased or decreased with height of the bar through which a rope is passes and attached to the halter. The angle of pull for the acute cervical radiculopathy should be at neutral or slightly be in the extended position as this position would open the anterior intervertebral joint space and closes the posterior intervertebral joint space that forces the protruded soft disc back into the intervertebral joint space. To treat the facet hypomobility the triangle wedge is used to bring the neck into the flexion as it opens the posterior pillars. The flexion angle of pull should be as per the level of the cervical spine as explained above in the angle of pull. The hold and rest periods and treatment are selected. The traction force is increased gradually to its peak point. Most of the mechanical traction units have safety switch which is given to the patient during the treatment. Instruct the patient to press the button if there is any alarming situation or discomfort.

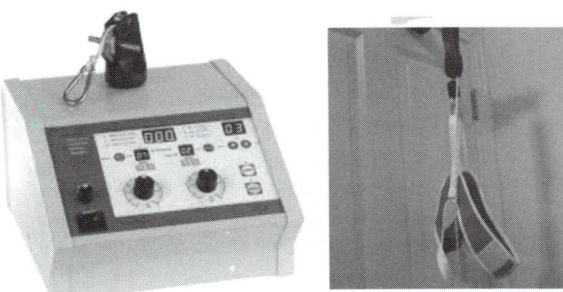

Figure 14.1 Cervical traction unit with the halter

B.   **Lumbar Traction**

a.   **Position of the Patient** –The most important position for treating the lumbar disorder is the patient comfort. The position which centralizes the symptoms must be preferred over the position that peripheralizes the symptoms. Lumbar traction can be given in supine, prone and side lying depending upon the symptoms of the patient. The lumbar spine may be kept neutral, flexed or extended. To achieve flexion the patient lies supine with both the hips and knees flexed to 45 degrees to 90 degrees. Flexion of the hip joints from

45 degrees to 60 degrees of flexion increase the laxity in the L5-S1, 60- 75 degrees in the L4-L5 segment, and 75 to 90 degrees in the L3-L4 segment[17]. Flexing the hips 90 degrees increases the posterior intervertebral space. The flexion is advised for the apophyseal joint dysfunctions or hypomobility as it opens them. To achieve neutral and minimal flexion the patient lies in the prone with minimal pillow under the pelvis. Traction in neutral and extension of the lumbar spine can be given in supine position with the hip and knees extended or in prone position without the pillows. The pain in the lumbar spine with radiation to the legs or sciatica due to soft disc herniation can be treated in the neutral or extension position of the spine. The ideal position of the patient for neutral is prone without the pillows. The traction in extension opens the anterior intervertebral joint space and allows the postero lateral protruded disc into the intervertebral joint space.

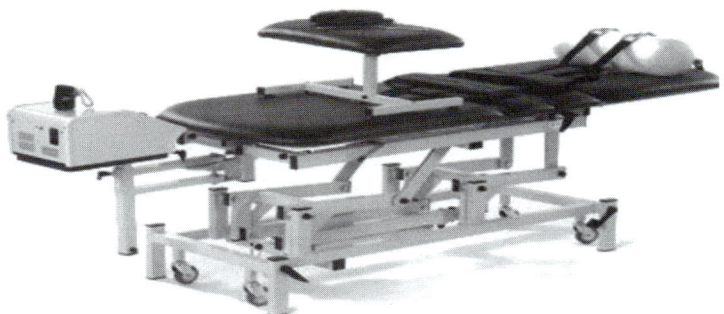

Fig: 14.2 Traction Unit with pelvic and dorsal belts

b. **Angle of Pull** – The angle of pull of the traction for the lumbar is changed by the increasing and decreasing the height of the bar attached to the end of the traction bed. If the aim of traction is to apply to the spine in a neutral or in extension, the angle of pull is adjusted by lowering the bar to the level or in the line of the spine. To apply traction in flexion, the hip and knees are flexed and the bar is raised appropriately.

c. **Tension** – The traction force to achieve significant separation of the vertebral joints should be of an appropriate weight. The traction force between 3o% to 50% of body weight is considered be an effective to overcome muscle contraction, ligamentous resistance and friction of the body on the couch surface. The general rule is that the treatment should be started with the traction force between 25 and 50 pounds to avoid any exaggeration in the symptoms. However, the traction force may be increased if the symptoms improve and the patient tolerates it. The traction force increases gradually and reaches to the peak which is held for few seconds. It is known as hold period. The traction force is gradually falls to the rest period which is usually kept half of the traction force. For an example if the traction force is 3opounds, the traction force at rest period would be 15pounds. However, the traction force at rest period may vary from the 5o% of the total traction force. Total release of the traction force to the zero is not recommended as the large difference in force application may irritate sensitive or painful tissues and aggravate the symptoms.

d. **Procedure** – The patient should lie in a comfortable position with minimal cloths as the application of the belts over the clothes may cause slipping, however the privacy should be the priority with an appropriate treatment. There are two belts thoracic and pelvic. The thoracic belt is attached around the thorax just below the xiphoid process and over the inferior rim of rib 8 through 10. The pressure of the belt on the thoracic cavity should not cause difficulty in breathing. The top of web of the pelvic belt should cross approximately at the umbilical line. Pelvic belt is applied first over the pelvis followed by the thoracic belt over the thorax. The lumbar traction couch has three sections. The middle section is a mobile section and fixed with the wedge during the application of belts. The lumbar spine should be over the mobile section of the couch which moves with the traction force. The most of mechanical traction units have preset hold and relax periods and also the preset treatment time which may be selected as per the conditions of the patients. After selecting the parameter of the traction the traction force is increased to its peak value. Immediately after that the wedge is remove from the mobile section that allows the mobile section to move with the increase and release traction force.

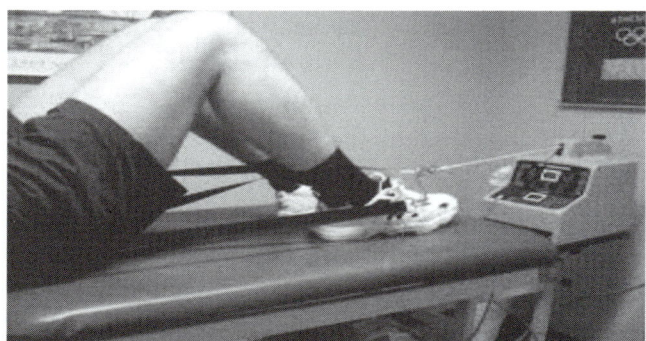

Fig: 14.3 Lumbar traction

Cervical Radiculopathy

Cervical radiculopathy is characterized by pain in the neck with radiation to the shoulder, arm, forearm and hand. It can either be acute radiculopathy or chronic radiculopathy. Acute radiculopathy is due to soft disc herniation into the posteriorly or posterolaterally which compresses the nerve roots. The pain is more intense in the arm and forearm and hand than the neck, that is often relieved with the hand on the head, however, symptoms aggravates with the arm hanging position. The symptoms usually start with the twist, jerk or injury to the cervical spine. The chronic radiculopathy is due to the degenerative changes in the disc and the vertebral bodies where the degenerated disc prolapses into the posteriorly and posterolaterally which put pressure on the nerve roots. The pain is more intense in the neck and less in the arm and forearm. The onset is usually gradual without the history of injury or trauma. Chronic radiculopathy usually occurs in the elderly patients whereas the acute radiculopathy may occur at any age but commonly occur before the fourth decade of life. If both the acute radiculopathy and chronic radiculopathy remains untreated for more than four weeks, the patient may present with weakness, parasthesia, sensory deficit and diminished or absent of triceps or biceps jerks.

Acute Radiculopathy – To treat the patients with acute radiculopathy the patient is placed in a supine position with the hip and knees flexed. A lucid history is taken for any contraindication to traction. A proper head halter is used that position the head slightly in flexion, enabling the traction pull to be exerted from the occiput, not the chin. Such halters concentrate the traction force posteriorly, where it is most beneficial. The angle of pull for the acute cervical radiculopathy should be neutral or slightly be in the extended position as this position would open the anterior intervertebral joint space and closes the posterior intervertebral joint space that forces the protruded soft disc back into the intervertebral joint space.

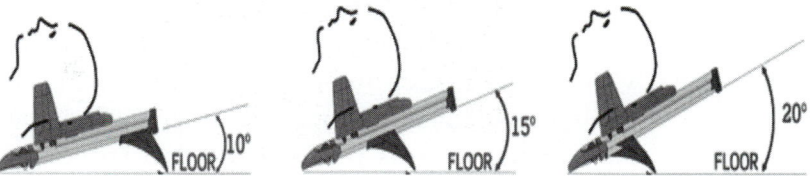

Figure 14.4 cervical traction in 10°, 15° and 20°.

Chronic Radiculopathy – To treat the patients with chronic radiculopathy the patient is placed in a supine position with both the hips and knees flexed to 45 degrees. The chronic radiculopathy is because of the degenerated disc herniation and osteophytes projected posteriorly or posterolaterally. Therefore, the angle of pull should be flexed as the flexion opens the posterior intervertebral joint foramen space. The increase posterior intervertebral joint space relieves the pressure on the nerve roots exerted by the osteophytes and degenerated disc.

Cervical Manual Traction

The localized pain caused by degenerative changes and hypomoblity of the facet joints can be treated with the manual traction. The manual traction can be given in neutral, flexion, extension, side flexion and rotation or in combination of movements. The lucid history is taken to rule out any contraindication to the traction, especially vertebro basillary insufficiency (VBI). To test VBI the patient is placed in a supine position with the head out of the couch. The examiner holds the head and extends, rotates, flexes to the opposite side of the vertebral artery which is being tested. The combinations of movements are held for twenty seconds for the delayed response. Any feeling of giddiness, vomiting, blurred vision and diplopia are the signs of VBI.

The Patient is placed in a supine position with hip and knees flexed to 45 degrees, the therapist stands at the top of the patient head and holds the occiput with one hand and chin with other hand. The patient slightly slides up to take the head out of the couch. The therapist flexes his right hip and knees slightly and places it on the foot on approximately six inches as this would reduce the load on the lumbar spine. Both the hands of the therapist should be close to the abdomen to avoid excessive stress. The therapist holds the head of the patient comfortably and firmly with both the hands and tucks in slightly to bring the neck into the flexion. A distraction force is applied with the hands through the body by taking body backward. The traction is held for an appropriate time at least six seconds and then the traction force is released. Several repetitions are performed to place significant amount of traction. The traction may be given in flexion, extension, rotation and sideflexion with care. To place a significant traction in posterior pillars of the cervical spine an appropriate flexion is required. Minimal flexion of 5-10 degrees is required for the upper cervical spine, 10-20 degrees for the mid cervical and 25-35 for the lower cervical spine.

References

1. Bernadette Hecox, Tsega Andemicael Mehreteab, Joseph Weisbeerg, Physical Agents A comprehensive Text for Physical Therapist, Appleton & Lange Norwalk, Connecticut, pp397

2. Basanta Kmar Nanda, Electrotherapy Simplified, second edition, Jaypee Brothers Medical Publishers (P) Ltd, pp464.

3. cyriax J, Russell G. Textbook of orthopaedic Medicine, vol. 2: Treatment oby manipulation, Massage and Injection, tenth ed. London: Bailliere Tindall, 1980 from Susan L. Michlovitz, Thomas P. Nolan, Jr., Modalities for Therapeutic Intervention, fourth edition, Contemporary Perspectives in Rehabilitaiton.

4. Nadine Graham, Anita R Gross, Charlie Goldsmith. Mechanical traction for mechanical neck disorders: A Systemic Review, J Rehabil Med 2006; 38:145-152

5. Mathews JA: Dynamic discography: Astudy of lumbar traction, Ann Phys Med 9:275-279, 1968

6. Cheatle R: Low Back Pain Syndrome, Philadelphia: FA Devis Company, 1988.

7. Pellecchia GL. Lumbar traction: A review of the literature. J Orthop Sports Phys Ther 20:262-267, 1994 from Susan L. Michlovitz, Thomas P. Nolan, Jr., Modalities for Therapeutic Intervention, fourth edition, Contemporary Perspectives in Rehabilitaiton.

8. Susan L. Michlovitz, Thomas P. Nolan, Jr., Modalities for Therapeutic Intervention, fourth edition, Contemporary Perspectives in Rehabilitaiton pp166.

9. cyriax J: Textbook of orthopedic Medicine, Volume I: Diagnosis of soft tissue Lesions, London: Bailliere Tindall, 1982

10. Coldish GD: Lumbar traction. In: Tollison CD, Kriegel ML eds, Interdisciplinary rehabilitation of Low Back Pain, pp 305-321. Baltimore: Williams and Wilkins, 1989.

11. Saunders HD, Saunders R, Evaluation, Treatment and prevention of Musculoskeletal Disordrs: Spine, vol 1, third edition Bloomington MN: Educational Opportunities 1995.

12. Colachis SC, Strohm BR. Effects of intermittent traction on separation of lumbar vertebra. Arch Physs Med Rehabil 50:251-253, 1969,

13. Pellecchia GL.. Lumbar traction: a review of the literature. J Orthop Sports Phys Ther 20:262-267, 1994.

14. Onel D, Tuzlaci M, Sari H, D emir K. Computed tomographic investigation of the effect of traction on lumbar disc herniations. Spine 14:82-90, 1989.

15. Deets, D, et al: Cervical traction: A comparison of sitting and supine positions. Phys Ther 57:225,1979.

16. cyriax J, Russell G. Textbook of orthopaedic Medicine, vol. 2: Treatment oby manipulation, Massage and Injection, tenth ed. London: Bailliere Tindall, 1980 from Susan L. Michlovitz, Thomas P. Nolan, Jr., Modalities for Therapeutic Intervention, fourth edition, Contemporary Perspectives in Rehabilitaiton.

17. Reily JP, et al: Effect of pelvic femoral position on vertebral separation produced by lumbar traction. Phys Ther 59:282, 1979.

Chapter 15

Extracorporeal Shockwave Therapy

Extracorporeal shockwave therapy is a mechanical therapeutic approach consists abrupt, low to high amplitude acoustic energy similar to the ultrasound waves. Extracorporeal refers to the pressure waves outside of the body that violently impact biological tissues for therapeutic purposes.[1] Shockwave patterns differ from ultrasound wave that is typically biphasic and has a peak pressure of .5 bar. Shockwave pattern is uniphasic with the peak pressure as high as 500bar.[2] The peak pressure of shockwave is approximately 1000 times that of ultrasound waves.

The shockwaves enter into the body and creates 'controlled explosions' in the tissues. Shockwaves travel nearly unchanged through fluids, and hence soft tissues of the body, exerting their effects only where there is a change in acoustic impedence along their path. The waves similar to the ultrasound may reflect, refract and absorbs in the tissues. The reflection and refraction depends upon the impedance between the interfaces. The shockwave energy will be reflected and creates compression and shear loads on the surface of the material with the greater impedance. This rapid interaction between compression and shear forces results in what is commonly referred to as cavitation. Cavitation is considered a central mechanism of action of shockwaves on the musculoskeletal tissues. The shockwave has capability to produce cavitation of 15Hz are more stronger than at 1Hz. Some equipments generate persistent cavitation at 15Hz. The microscopic gas bubbles are built up on the surface of the material (the one with the greater impedance) and the collapse of these bubbles creates a small jet of liquid (fast flowing) that causes high local stress. Some authors believe cavitation is responsible for the effects of ESW.

The depth a concusive shockwave can reach depends upon the force at which shockwaves are generated. The shockwave generated at high force has capability of producing energy into the more deeper structures. The radial shockwave energy declines rapidly in proportion to the distance from the site of the generation (the end of the gun). Therefore, the shockwaves loose energy the deeper they go into the body. The area of most energy is referred to as the energy flux area.

Production

The shockwaves are divided into two categories based on the propagation patterns. Focused and Unfocussed. The focused waves are sometimes also referred to as hard shockwaves, whereas, the unfocused radial (dispersive) wave sometimes called a 'soft' shockwaves. The focused shock waves are produced using electro-hydraulic, electromagnetic, and piezoelectric systems. The unfocussed shockwaves are referred to in the literature as radial shock waves. These waves are produced pneumatically using compressed air to accelerate a projectile onto a solid applicator that is in contact with the skin surface overlying the affected tissue.

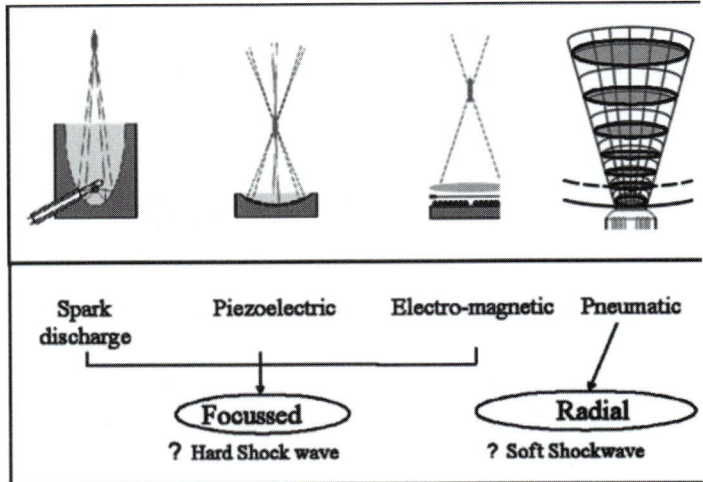

FIG. 15.1 Various types of shockwave generators

Electro hydraulic shockwaves are generated under water expansion with high voltage electrode spark discharge and the acoustic waves are then focused with an elliptical and transmitted to the tissues. Electromagnetic technique consists production of strong electric field. A lens is used to focus the waves with focal therapeutic point being defined by the lens of focus lens. Piezoelectric shockwave technique consists of a large number less than 1000 of piezocristals mounted in a sphere and receives a rapid electrical discharge that induces a pressure pulse in the surrounding water steepening to a shockwave. The pneumatic shockwaves are generated by a generator consists of compressed air rapidly accelerating a projectile, which hits the impact surface of the applicator and causes a shock wave. This wave immediately propagates in the tissues in a radial fashion, resulting in unfocussed shock waves. The pneumatic shockwaves are also known as radial or ballistic shockwaves.

Radial or soft shock waves are characterized by lower wave energies, slower rise time and a negative component that is of the same magnitude as the preceding positive component or an even larger negative component.

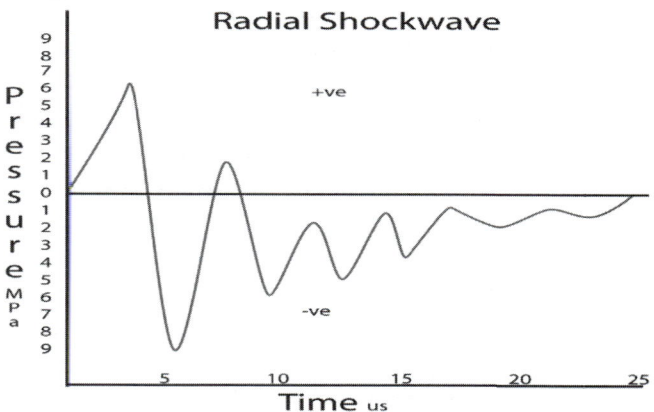

Fig. 15.2 Character of the shockwave.

High speed cavitation bubbles consequent to the negative phase of the propagation of radial shockwave are generated in the tissues. Cavitation is considered a central mechanism of action of shockwaves on the musculoskeletal tissues. The shockwave has capability to produce cavitation of 15Hz are more stronger than at 1Hz. Some equipments generate persistent cavitation at 15Hz.

The equipment is designed to produce either high energy focused or low energy focused shockwaves. Some equipments are designed to produce both the focused and unfocused shockwaves these are known as duel or combined type units. The focused type unit is mounted with an integrated image guiding system that can be adjusted along its axis to allow precise localization for therapy. The multi joint articulated arm allows individual adjustment for all treatment position with the patient lying or sitting. The radial shockwave therapy device is made of a pneumatic system to which a handheld pistol like applicator is attached with the radial or divergent projection of the waves.

Therapeutically the most commonly employed generation method is based on the pneumatic system or radial (nonfocused) shockwave, and the key reason for this is that a radial wave results. The focused shockwaves are essentially used for the surgical interventions, given their destructive nature, they are less appropriate for therapeutic uses.

Physiological Effects

The exact physiological mechanism at this stage is poorly understood, but it appears that the cells undergo microtrauma which promotes the inflammatory and catabolic processes that are associated with removing damaged matrix constituents.[3] The body responds by increasing metabolic activity around the source of pain. The series of high energy percussions break down the scar tissues and possible calcification as well. The shockwaves stimulate the body's natural self healing process.

One of the most important physiological effects of shockwave on the tissues is that it effectively takes a tissue from a more chronic state to acute state, by breaking down the scar tissues and possible calcification as well and in doing so, provide a stimulus to a stalled repair sequence. Hyperemia is one of the basic effects of the shockwave therapy in the tissues. The process of repairing of the tissue begins as soon as it reaches to the acute state from the chronic. Hence, the shockwave energy promotes regenerating and reparative process of the bones, tendons and other tissues. The other soft tissue manipulation techniques such as deep transverse friction massage also has similar physiological effects on the chronic or calcified tissues.

The following are the established physiological effects of the shockwave –

    i.   Mechanical stimulation,
    ii.   Increased local blood flow,
    iii. Increase in cellular activity – release of substance P, prostaglandin and other inflammatory cytokines,
    iv. Transient analgesic effect on afferent nerves and
    v. Break down of calcific deposits (primarily, but not exclusively in tendon)

Indications

Extracorporeal shockwave therapy began with an incidental observation of osteoblastic response pattern during animal studies in the mid 1980 that generated an interest in the application of ESWT to in musculoskeletal disorders,[4] including planter fasciitis,[5] lateral epicondyle of the elbow, calcific thendinitis of the shoulder and non union of long bone fracture. The rationale behind the use of shockwave is to provide a safe, non invasive alternative intervention to surgical for chronic and recalcitrant tendinopathies and delayed or nonunion fractures.

Shock waves, as applied in urology and gastroenterology, were introduced in the middle of the last decade in Germany to treat different pathologies of the musculoskeletal system, including epicondylitis of the elbow, plantar fascitis, and calcifying and noncalcifying tendinitis of the rotator cuff. With the noninvasive nature of these waves and their seemingly low complication rate, extracorporeal shock wave therapy (ESWT) seemed a promising alternative to the established conservative and surgical options in the treatment of patients with chronically painful conditions.[6]

Contraindications and Risks

i. Over uterus – The shockwaves may disrupt fetal development
ii. Over electronic implant
iii. Blood Coagulation therapy – The application of shockwaves may cause severe bleeding.
iv. Acute injuries – The shockwaves may aggravate the symptoms of inflammation and delay the process of healing
v. Over large vessels and nerves – Shockwave may rupture the blood vessels and nerves if apply directly over them. This may cause loss of blood supply and sensation of the area.
vi. Over epiphysis – Shockwaves may alter the normal growth of the bone if applied directly over the epiphysis.
vii. Risks – The application of the surges of shockwaves may cause local tissue damage that may lead to pain, swelling, ecchymosis, and bruising.

Application

The therapist should evaluate the patient thoroughly for the contraindications of the shockwave therapy. The energy, doses, medium, number of shocks and treatment sessions are the parameters to be determined before administering the shockwave therapy for optimal results.

Coupling Medium – Similar to ultrasound therapy a medium is required to propagate energy. An aquasonic gel between the applicator and the treatment area is required to maximize the acoustic transmission.

Energy and Flux Density – Expression of the shockwave energy produced in the tissues depends on the focused and non focused modes. The focused extracorporeal shockwave therapy energy is measured in milli joules per square millimeter. The concentration of shockwave energy per area is thus an important dosimetery. The energy is obtained by calculating the energy density(EFD) which is defined as the amount of mechanical acoustic energy per unit area (A) per shock. Therefore EFD is represented as EFD = E/A or millijoules per square millimeter. EFD may be low, medium, or high. FED of focused shockwaves is much larger than the unfocussed shockwaves. Radial shockwaves have significantly lower pressure waves and longer pulse duration than focused shockwaves therefore FED may not be suitable for the unfocused shockwaves. The alternative way to represent unfocussed shockwaves is pressure level in bar.

Applicator – The shockwaves are delivered to the tissues through the applicators. The applicator of unfocused or radial shockwaves is comparatively smaller that the applicator of focused shockwaves. The kinetic energy of the projectile, created by compressed air is transferred to the transmitter at the end of the applicator and further into the issue. There are various sizes and shape of applicators to deliver the shockwaves. The most commonly used heads are 15mm across and are described as convex, the grater energy at the centre than the edges. The head with smaller in the size (diameter) would produce more energy at the same power setting than a head with a bigger diameter. The convex shape helps in focusing the shockwaves. The radial head may also be concave shaped. The shape of the head is designed by the manufacture as per the requirement of the penetration.

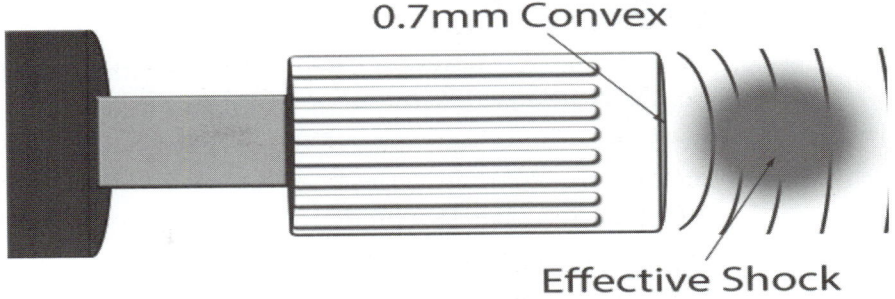

A.

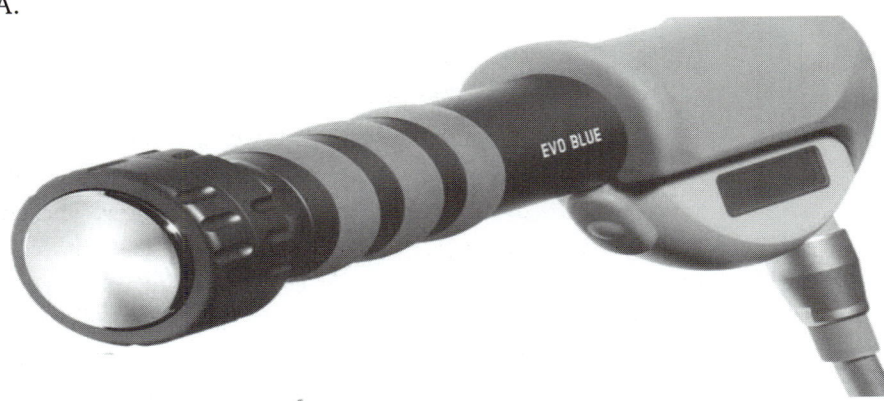

B.

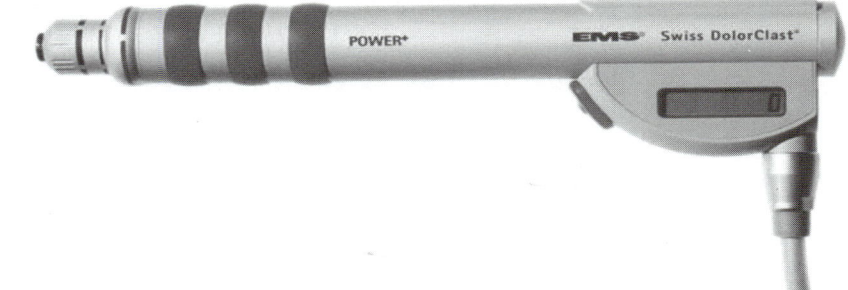

C.

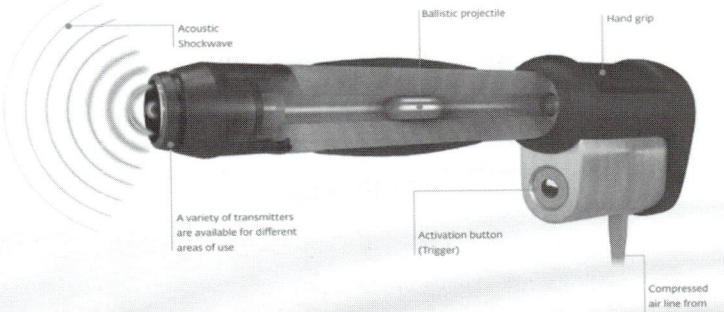

D.   Fig:15.3 A-D Various size of applicators of shockwave

Extracorporeal Shockwave Therapy

Frequencies – The shockwaves are generated with the range of frequencies from 1Hz to 22Hz. The patients experience pain and discomfort at the lower frequencies. The authors believe that the initial treatment should be given with the higher frequencies to familiarize the patient to the sensation of the shockwaves. The low frequencies from .5Hz to 5Hz produce less cavitations in the tissues whereas high frequencies above 5Hz produce larger number of cavitations in the tissues. The increase in the frequency produces more cavitations but does not change the size of the cavitations. The shockwaves produced at the high frequencies travel less deeper than the shockwaves produced at the lower frequencies. To produce shockwaves at the deeper tissues the shockwaves should be produced at the lower frequencies.

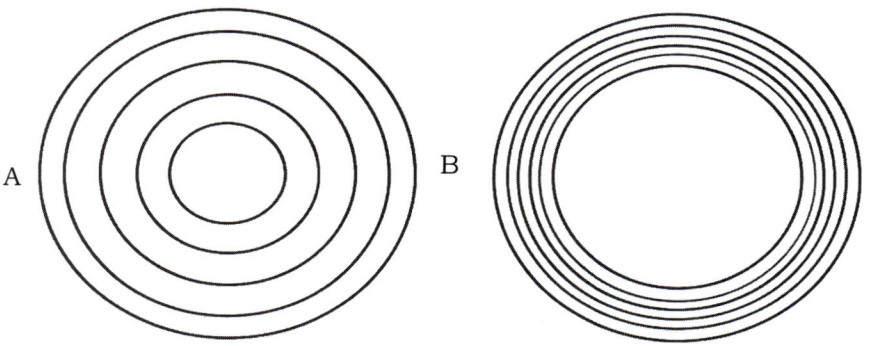

FIG: 15.4. A Low frequency shockwaves with deeper penetration, B high frequency shockwaves with less penetration

Below is a table showing approximations of the energy delivered:

Compressed Air Bar	Magnetic mJ	Energy per mm using 15mm head mJ/mm2
1	60	
2	90	
3	120	0.12
4	150	
5	180	0.38

Table15.1. approximation of energy delivered

Procedure- The patient is placed in a comfortable position. The part which is being treated should be exposed adequately. The therapist should ensure that the treatment area should be stable throughout the treatment session. Select the appropriate type of shockwave. Electrohydraulic, electromegnatic, and piezoelectric are chosen if the objective of the treatment is focused high energy (higher than $0.29Mj/MM^2$). The focused energy is preferred if the shockwaves are required to be produced into the deeper area (more than 5cm). Application of focused shockwaves is required to the use of in or off image guiding system, mounted on the applicator head, to direct the small focused beam area over the targeted tissue area.

The radial shockwaves mode is selected when the area to be treated is superficial (less than 5cm) and require less energy (less than $0.29Mj/MM^2$). The radial shockwaves do not require image guiding system. All the applicators of radial shockwaves have pistol – like shape. The applicator is selected according to the size of the area.

The area which is being treated is localized and marked with the marker. Aquasonic gel is spread over the marked area. The applicator is placed over the marked area and appropriate shocks area applied. Remove the applicator from the treatment area at the end of the treatment and place it on the holder. Clean the skin and inspect it for any side effects such as redness, light bruising and swelling. These may be considered normal if subside within few hours to two days.

Extracorporeal Shockwave Therapy in Tennis Elbow

Yasser A. Radwan conducted study on the tennis elbow to see the efficacy of shockwave versus percutaneous tenotomy. Fifty-six patients of chronic persistent tennis elbow of more than six months duration were randomly assigned to both the groups. Group 1 included 29 patients received high-energy extracorporeal shock wave treatment (1,500 shocks) at 18 kV (0.22 mJ/mm^2) without local anesthesia; group 2 which included 27 subjects underwent percutaneous tenotomy of the common extensor origin. Both groups achieved improvement from the base line at three weeks, six weeks, 12 weeks and 12 months post-intervention. The success rate at three months in the ESWT group was 65.5% and in the tenotomy group was 74.1%. ESWT appeared to be a useful noninvasive treatment method that reduced the necessity for surgical procedures.[7]

Extracorporeal Shockwave Therapy in subacromial Bursitis

Shockwave therapy should be considered for chronic pain due to calcific tendinitis which is resistant to conservative treatment. M. Loew conducted the study and found that the results of shockwaves on the subacromial bursitis are dose dependant. In their prospective study 195 patients were included which were divided into the control and subgroups of shockwave therapy. The subgroups of shockwaves were treated with low-energy and high-energy shock waves.The results showed energy-dependent success, with relief of pain ranging from 5% in the control group and up to 58% after two high-energy sessions.[8]

Rompe and et al conducted a prospective quasi randomized study to compare the effects of surgical extirpation with the outcome after high energy extracorporeal shock wave therapy (3000 impulses of an energy flux density of .6mj/mm^2 in patients with a chronic calcifying supraspinatus tendinitis. The symptoms and demographic data of the two groups were comparable. They found surgery superior compared with high energy shockwave therapy for patients with homogenous deposits. For patients with homogenous deposits, high-energy extracorporeal shockwave therapy was equivalent to surgery and should be given priority because of its noninvasiveness.[9]

Shockwave in Chronic Planter Fasciitis

Planter fasciitis is a common cause of heel and foot pain. More than 90% patients find relief in symptoms with the conservative treatment, however; it takes several days to months. John A. and at al. utilized metanalysis study on shockwave therapy for chronic proximal planter fasciitis. They hypothesized that extracorporeal shockwave therapy provided a reasonable nonoperative therapeutic alternative to surgical intervention in the treatment of chronic proximal plantar fasciitis. Statistically significant improvement in pain and functional capacity was found after completion of treatment in comparison with baseline.

The patient is placed in comfortable position with adequate exposure of the heel and foot. A coupling medium is poured on the treatment area this helps in transmitting the waves. The probe of the shockwave of an appropriate size is placed over the treatment area. The shocks of 2500 per session at a pressure of 2.5 bars are ideal for the chronic planter fasciitis.

References

i.   Rompe J, Schoellner C, Nafe B, Heine J. Evaluation of low energy extracorporeal shock wave application for treatment of chronic plantar fasciitis. J Bone Joint Surg (A), 84:335-3341

ii.   Ogden JA, Totch – Kischkat A, Schultthesis R: Priniciples of shockwave therapy Clin Orthop. 2001, 387:8-17

iii.   Waugh CM, Morrissey D, Jones E, Riley GP, Langberg H, Screen HR (2015). IN Vivo biological response to extracorporeal shockwave therapy in human tendinopathy. European cells and materials, 29:268-80.

iv.   Chin –Jen Wang, Extracorporeal shockwave therapy in musculoskeletal disorders, journal of orthopaedi Surgery and Research 2012, 7:11

v.   Buch M, Knorr U, Fleming L, Theodore G, Amendola A, Bachmann C, Zingas C, Siebert WE; Extracorporeal shockwave therapy in symptomatic heel spur. An overview orthopede 2002, 31 (7) 637-44)

vi.   Seil R, Wilmes P, Nührenbörger C. Extracorporeal shock wave therapy for tendinopathies. Expert Rev Med Devices. 2006 Jul;3(4):463-70.

vii.   Yasser A. Radwan, Gamal ElSobhi, Walid S. Badawy, Ali Reda, and Sherif Khalid Resistant tennis elbow: shock-wave therapy versus percutaneous tenotomyInt Orthop. 2008 Oct; 32(5): 671–677.

viii.   M. Loew, W. Daecke, D. Kusnierczak, M. Rahmanzadeh, V. Ewerbeck Shock-wave therapy is effective for chronic calcifying tendinitis of the shoulder. Bones and Joint Journal Formerly known as JBJS, published on 01. 1999.

ix.   Rompe, Jan D. MD; Zoellner, Jan MD; Nafe, Bernhard MD. Shock Wave Therapy Versus Conventional Surgery in the Treatment of Calcifying Tendinitis of the Shoulder. Clinical Orthopaedics & Related Research, June 2001, volume 387 –issue pp72-82.

Chapter 16

Electrodiagnosis

Electromyography

Electromyography involves recording of action potentials from muscle fibers during voluntary contraction as well as spontaneous action potentials, if any, from muscle fibers at rest. Electromyography may either by recorded from surface electrode placement or needle insertion into the muscle fibers. The patient is asked to contract the particular muscle voluntarily when the said muscle is at rest and during minimal to maximal contraction. The voluntary potentials in the form of motor units are displayed and recorded on the oscilloscope. The following features should be evaluated on oscilloscope:

    i.   Electrode insertion
    ii. Oscilloscope observation during rest
    iii. Oscilloscope observation of voluntary motor unit action potentials during a minimal contraction and
    iv. oscilloscope observation during a level of muscle contraction graded from weak to strong

A series of skeletal muscles are chosen for testing on the basis of nerve root distribution and peripheral nerve innervations. The skin overlying that particular muscle is cleaned with sterile pads. All efforts are made to prevent blood borne infection especially when needle insertion technique of EMG is chosen.

The evaluator must observe the insertional activity on oscilloscope during needle insertion into the muscle fibers and at rest. The insertional activity on the oscilloscope occurs due to injury potential which remains for less than few milliseconds in the form of burst.

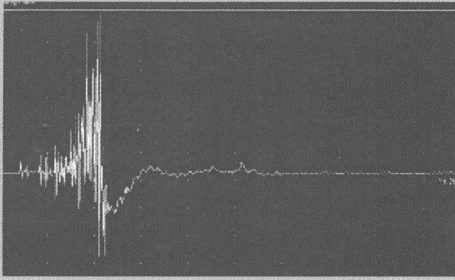

Fig. 16.1 Insertional Activity on Oscilloscope

However, insertional activity increases in duration in muscles with disruption of nerve supply (irritable muscles) as the needle is moved into the muscle. The fibrotic muscles do not show insertional activity on the oscilloscope, whereas, inflammatory and degenerative muscles show insertional activity after inserting the electrode and when the muscle is at rest. After insertion of the needle into the muscle, the patient is asked to contract that particular muscle isometrically from weak to strong contraction. The contraction should be isometric which does not allow movement at the joint. The action potentials generated following contraction of muscle are evaluated for the shapes, sizes, durations and firing rate. These parameters may vary from muscle to muscle as morphometric and histochemical composition of all the muscles is not same. The shape of the voluntary motor on the oscilloscope should be of two or three phases. At least 10-15 voluntary motor units should be examined for their duration, amplitude and phases in at least eight different anatomic areas of the skeletal muscles.

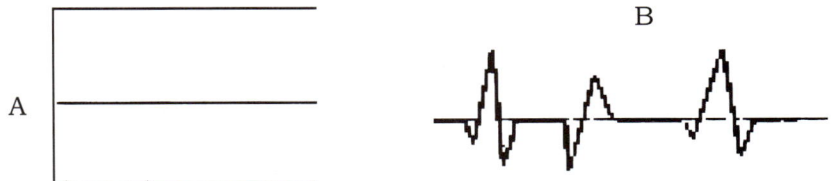

Fig. 16.2 Normal EMG readings. A- Muscle at rest, B- Muscle at minimal contraction with biphasic wave.

During regeneration, the nerves become healthier and better insulated through regrowth of their sheaths. The muscle fibers become stronger and gain mass. However, not all nerve fibers regenerate. Fibers that do regenerate usually branch more extensively than they did before the injury, and they spread to innervate as many denervated muscle fibers as possible.The motor unit potentials that are produced as a result of this ongoing regeneration have greater amplitudes than normal. These motor unit potentials have a prolonged duration and are often described as giant polyphasic potentials. Previous nerve injury can be inferred from their presence.

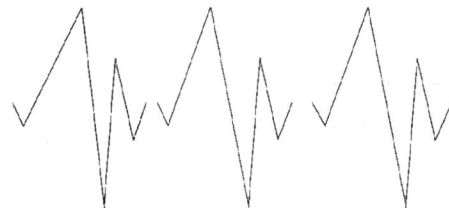

Fig. 16.3 EMG Polyphasic waves

As the muscle tension increase, the motor units discharge progressively which results in higher and higher amplitude. In addition to increasing the amplitude of motor unit discharge, the active units should also increase in their firing rate. Therefore, during strong muscle contraction motor unit potentials get superimposed on each other to obliterate the oscilloscope grid. This condition is known as interference or recruitment pattern which is the characteristic feature of the normal electromyography. The EMG interference pattern, built up of single motor unit action potentials, may be analyzed subjectively, or objectively by computer aided, quantitative methods, like counting of zero-crossings, counting of spikes, amplitude measurements, integration of the area under the curve, decomposition techniques, power spectrum analysis and turn/amplitude analysis. The shape of the interference pattern of healthy muscles is dependent on age, sex, force, muscle, temperature, fatigue, fitness level. The most well-evaluated methods are those using turn/amplitude analysis, like the cloud methods and the peak-ratio analysis. Peak-ratio analysis has the advantage that reference limits are easy to obtain and that its utility is well established and confirmed by several investigations.

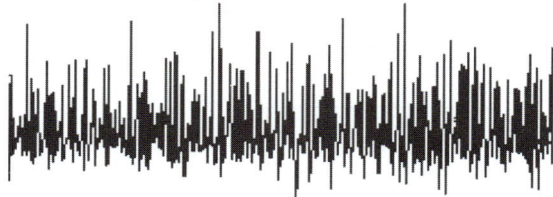

Fig. 16.4 Interference Pattern a normal feature of EMG during strong contraction of muscle.

Endplate potentials - If the electrode is placed in the endplate area of any muscle, it can irritate terminal axons and generate spontaneous electrical activity consisting of rapidly firing, biphasic, small amplitude (100 to 200 µV), short duration (3 to 4 ms) spikes with negative (upward) onset. Electrode placement in the endplate area is usually more painful than elsewhere in the muscle.

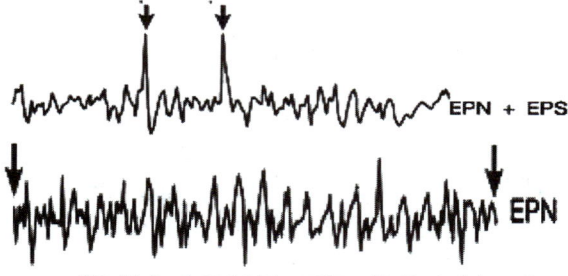

Fig. 16.5. A end plate spikes, B- End plate noises

Electrodiagnosis

Fibrillations - Fibrillation potentials occur when an individual muscle fiber is denervated. Fibrillation potentials are small (<500 µV), short (<5 ms in duration), biphasic or triphasic, and fire regularly or sometimes irregularly. The sound accompanying them has been likened to "rain on a tin roof." Fibrillations have an initial positive (downward) deflection (not to be confused with the initial upward/negative deflection of the endplate potential). Fibrillation potentials, if observed, are scored according to a semiquantitative grading system of 1+ when spontaneous activity is rare, to 4+ when spontaneous potentials fill the oscilloscope screen.

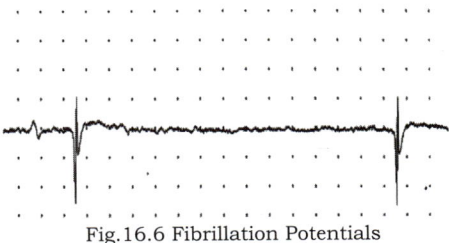

Fig.16.6 Fibrillation Potentials

Positive sharp Wave - Positive sharp waves also emanate from denervated muscle fibers and have the same clinical significance as fibrillations. They have a sharp initial positive deflection followed by a longer, lower amplitude negative phase than fibrillation potentials. The positive sharp wave can be considered a 'blocked' fibrillation potential.

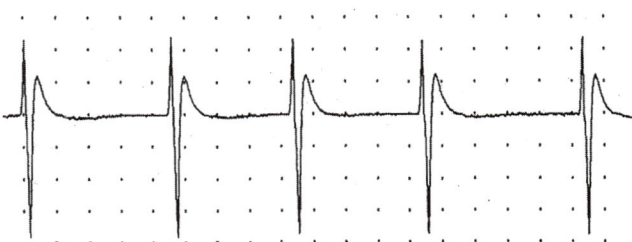

Fig.16.7 Positive Sharp Wave Potentials

Complex repetitive discharges (CRD)- Complex repetitive discharges (CRDs) are bursts of potentials, each having the appearance of grouped fibrillations or positive sharp waves that begin and end suddenly. Each burst is multiphasic and composed of up to 10 spike components representing the firing of individual muscle fibers, and can last for up to 100 ms. The bursts end when muscle fibers become fatigued, but can start up again when a new pacemaker starts firing again. The bursts sound like a "machine gun." Most often present in myopathies (e.g. muscular dystrophies and the Schwartz-Jampel syndrome). The abrupt onset and offset of the CRD helps to discriminate it from the myotonic discharge (which tends to fade away to nothing).

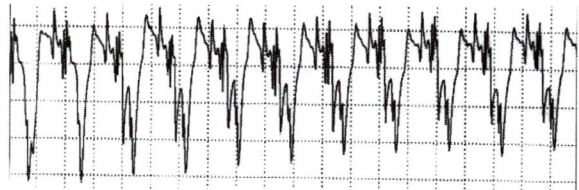

Fig.16.8 Complex Repetitive Discharges

Fasciculations

Single motor unit potentials, activated spontaneously. They look like normal or polyphasic voluntarily activated MUAPs, but fire irregularly. In general, benign fasciculations have faster firing rates and occur in muscles below the knees. Common in amyotrophic lateral sclerosis (ALS), but also in many other conditions.

Nerve Conduction Velocity

Nerve conduction study, also known as nerve conduction velocity test is a measurement of the speed of conduction of an electrical impulses to determine the level of nerve injury. Conduction of electrical impulses through the nerve are affected by various factors such as age, sex and pathological conditions. Cutaneous sensory receptors such as proprioceptors type (Ia, Ib and II), mechanoreceptors (type II &III sensory fibers), nociceptors, and thermoreceptors (type III and type IV) receive the information regarding position of joints, limbs, movments, nechanical pressure or distortion, pain and temperature, which travels through the peripheral nerves to the central nervous system. Normal impulses in peripheral nerves of the lower legs travel at the speed of 40-45 m/s, and in the upper extremity at the speed of 50-65 m/s. Largely generalized, normal conduction velocities for any given nerve will be in the range of 50-60m/s.[1]

Conduction of electrical impulses through peripheral nerve depends upon various factors such as age, sex, local temperature and other anthropometric factors such as hand sex and height.[2-3] Stetson, PhD, Diana S, James W, Albers; Barbara A. Silvertein; Robert. The normal impulse conduction value in the newborns and toddlers tend to be about half the adult values, however, it reaches to the adult value at the age of four years. The nerve conduction velocities in the upper extremities decrease by about 1m/s for every 10 years of age. The conduction velocities of most motor and sensory nerves are positively and linearly associated with body temperature. Nerve at the low temperature show slow nerve conduction whereas, higher temperature increase the nerve conduction velocity. The conduction velocities of impulses in the median sensory and ulnar sensory nerves are negatively related to an individuals height.

Measurement of Nerve conduction Velocity

The conduction of electrical impulses along the peripheral nerve is measure to determine the sites of lesion. Therefore, nerve conduction velocity of a peripheral nerve is measured at different segments of the course of nerve; from distal to the proximal. Each segment is studied by comparing different segments to each other to determine if there is relative slowing in one portion versus the other or if there is drop in amplitude in one segment versus another. The clinical nerve conduction velocities and nerve amplitude should be compared with normal values of the same age group individuals.

To measure the nerve conduction velocities the clinician should have a electrograph instrument with frequency response from 10Hz to 10000Hz, sweep speed from 2to 5 msec/div. and sensitivity or gain from 1000 to 5000 MV/div. three electrode namely active also known as recording electrode, reference electrode and ground electrode.

Median Motor Nerve Conduction Velocity Measurement

The below mentioned procedure should be followed to measure the median motor nerve conduction

i. Place the patient in a comfortable supine position with arm abducted to 45°, forearm fully supinated and wrist in neutral position

ii. Clean the skin with alcohol to remove dirt, and to reduce the skin resistance.

iii. Use sensitivity setting of 2.5 mV.

iv. Use a sweep speed of 5 ms/division

v. Use a stimulus rate of 1/s and a duration of .1 ms

vi. Active or Recording Electrode – place the cathode (negative) recording electrode directly over the anatomy center of the abductor pollicis brevis muscle. The electrode is placed one half the distance between the metacarpophalangeal joint of the thumb and midpoint of the distal wrist crease.

vii. Reference Electrode - Place anode reference electrode (stimulating electrode) all over the tendon of the same muscle.

viii. Ground Electrode- Place the ground electrode between stimulating and recording electrodes.

ix.   Secure all the electrodes firmly.

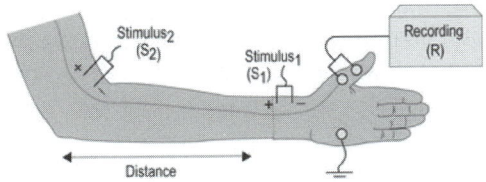

FIG. 16.9 Median motor nerve conduction velocity measurement procedure

x.   Ensure the temperature of the room should not be below 35°C. Low temperature can reduce the nerve conduction velocity. Record the skin temperature.

xi.   Measure the distance between the distal cathode stimulating electrode and proximal cathode recording electrode. The measurement of distance should approximate the anatomic course of the nerve being tested. All distance measurement should be taken with a metal tape measure.

xii.   Apply the stimulating electrodes with the cathode (negative) directed distally towards the muscle.

xiii.   Increase the intensity of the stimulus gradually until a muscle twitch contraction is seen and a response appears on the oscilloscope screen.

xiv.   A supramaximal stimulus 10% more intensity of twitch contraction is applied to ensure that all axons got stimulated. The different nerve fibers have different thresholds of excitation, therefore, a supramaximal stimulus is necessary to be certain that all of the fasted conducting nerve fibers are being monitored which are stored on the oscilloscope screen.

xv.   Record three response from the proximal point.

xvi.   Record proximal and distal latencies and measure distance from the proximal to the distal point.

xvii.   The nerve conduction velocity is calculated as under-

NCV = <u>Distance in Millimelier</u>

      Time difference between latencies from two stimulus sites.

Distance – it is the distance between two stimulating sites

Latencies – latency is a time interval between the stimulations and response, or, from a more general point of view, a time delay between the cause and the effect of some electrical change in the nerve being stimulated. To determine nerve conduction time in motor nerve fibers exclusively, two sites are stimulated and the latency from the more distal site is subtracted from the more proximal latency, leaving a difference that is the time of conduction between the two sites of

stimulation. A proximal latency is measured from a site of stimulation as far as possible from the recording electrode (terminal end of the electrode). It is usually recorded from the stimulus artifact to the beginning of the evoked muscle action potential (upward deflection of negative of the muscle response), the latency is expressed in milliseconds.

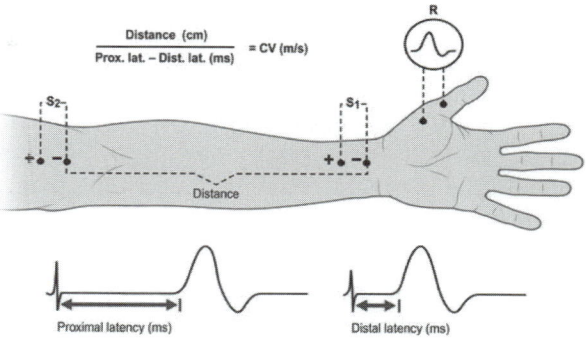

Fig. 16.10 Nerve Conduction Velocity Study.

More than one segment of the nerve can be stimulated to determine the level of nerve lesion. Next segment may be stimulated above the elbow proximal and medial to the antecubital space and proximal to the elbow crease between the belly of the biceps muscle and the medial head of the biceps muscle. The third segment which is more proximal is stimulated in the axila at least 10cm proximal to the above elbow site and immediately lateral and anterior to the brachial artery.

Sensory Nerve Conduction Velocity Measurement

There are two methods of measuring the sensory nerve conduction velocity – antidromic and orthodromic. In the antidromic method both the sensory and motor nerves are stimulated. To study median sensory nerve conduction active recording electrode is attached to the index finger at the midpoint of the distance between the phalangeal flexion crease and the web space of the index finger so that a distance of at least 10 cm, but not more than 14 cm is maintained between the stimulating electrode and active electrode. The reference electrode is positioned at or about the distal interphalangeal flexions crease of the index finger so that a distance of at least 3 cm is maintained between the active and reference electrode. The ground electrode is positioned on the dorsum of the hand between the active and stimulating electrodes. The stimulation is applied at the wrist between the Palmaris langus and flexor carpi radialis muscle tendons proximal to the tranverse carpal ligament. A low amplitude stimulus is enough to elicit the antidromic sensory response. Latency is usually measured to the peak amplitude of the response because the exact initial deflection of the response is often difficult to determine. The procedure of study of median sensory nerve conduction velocity by using orthodromic remain same like of antidromic method, but the nerve is stimulated at a distal. Latency is usually measured to the peak amplitude of the response latencies recorded using antidromic and orthodromic are not significantly different. The sensory nerve conduction irrespective of either methods is calculated by using a below mentioned formula-

$$\text{SNCV} = \frac{\text{distance 10 (mm)}}{\text{time (ms)}}$$

Distance is measured with metal tape from recording electrode to the reference electrode. Latency (time in millisecond) is the peak amplitude of the response.

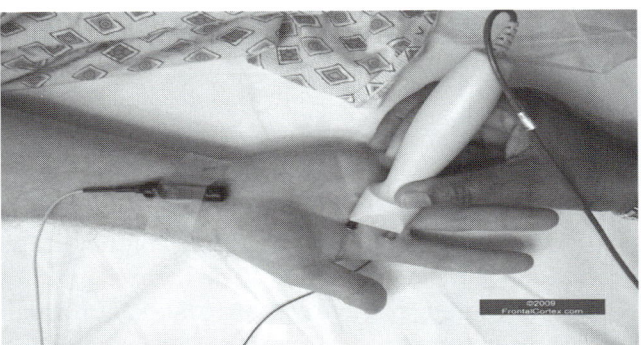

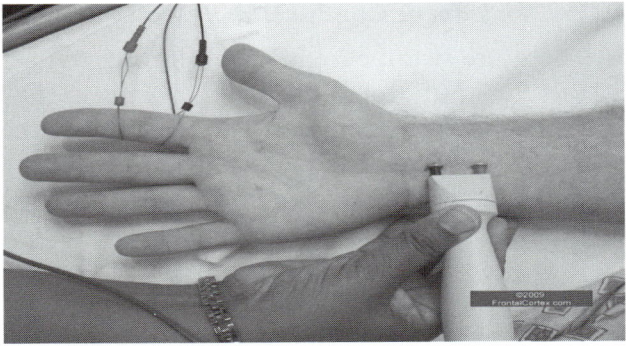

Fig. 16.11 Median Nerve Sensory Nerve Conduction Study. a - Orthodromic, b – Antidromic.

Motor Unit Duration- The normal motor unit potential duration is seven milliseconds with the standard deviation of 3.5 milliseconds. The motor unit duration depends upon the area of the end plate zone in the concerned muscle. The end plate zone in the smaller muscles is spreaded in the large area whereas, in the larger muscles the end plate

Electrodiagnosis

zone is spreaded in the smaller portion. The end plate zone in the abductor pollicis bravis covers 50% length of the muscle; on the other hand, the end plate zone in the biceps brachii covers the 10% length of the muscle. Therefore the motor unit duration of abductor pollicis bravis is higher (8-9 milliseconds) than the biceps brachii muscle (5-6 milliseconds).

Motor Unit Amplitude – The normal motor unit potential varies from 300 microvolt to 5000 microvolt. Amplitudes represent the size of an active membrane area of the total size of the muscle. The small muscle which has larger number of muscle fibers will have high amplitudes than the larger muscle with the same muscle fibers, the amplitude of motor unit is measured from base line to the negative (upward) phase.

References

i   Parry, Gareth J. 2007. Guillain –Barre Syndrome. New York. NY: Demos medial publishing pp1-9

ii   A. WALFE (October 1992), Effects of age, sex, and anthropometric factors on nerve conduction measure". Muscle and Nerve. 15:1095-1104).

iii   Thankiatpinyo, MD, Thanitta, Gulapar Srisawasdi (2013). Effects of hand size on the stimulation intensities required for median and ulnar sensory nerve conduction studies". Archives of Pysical Medicine and Rehabilitation on 94:925-929.

Index